STRENGTH ZONE TRAINING

The Most Effective Method for Maximizing Muscle Development

CONTENTS

STRENGTH ZONE TRAINING

The Most Effective Method for Maximizing Muscle Development

Nick Tumminello

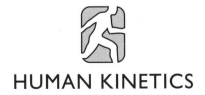

HUMAN KINETICS

Library of Congress Cataloging-in-Publication Data

Names: Tumminello, Nick, author.
Title: Strength zone training / Nick Tumminello.
Description: Champaign, IL : Human Kinetics, [2023] | Includes
  bibliographical references.
Identifiers: LCCN 2021051508 (print) | LCCN 2021051509 (ebook) | ISBN
  9781718211476 (paperback) | ISBN 9781718211483 (epub) | ISBN
  9781718211490 (pdf)
Subjects: LCSH: Weight training. | Muscle strength. | Physical
  fitness--Physiological aspects.
Classification: LCC GV546 .T86 2023 (print) | LCC GV546 (ebook) | DDC
  613.7/13--dc23
LC record available at https://lccn.loc.gov/2021051508
LC ebook record available at https://lccn.loc.gov/2021051509

ISBN: 978-1-7182-1147-6 (print)

Senior Acquisitions Editor: Roger W. Earle; **Developmental Editor:** Amy Stahl; **Managing Editor:** Miranda K. Baur; **Copyeditor:** Annette Pierce; **Permissions Manager:** Martha Gullo; **Graphic Designer:** Denise Lowry; **Cover Designer:** Keri Evans; **Cover Design Specialist:** Susan Rothermel Allen; **Photograph (cover):** cosmonaut/iStock/Getty Images; **Photographs (interior):** © Human Kinetics; **Photo Production Specialist:** Amy M. Rose; **Photo Production Manager:** Jason Allen; **Senior Art Manager:** Kelly Hendren; **Illustrations:** © Human Kinetics; **Printer:** Versa Press

We thank The ZOO Health Club in Oakland Park, Florida, for assistance in providing the location for the photo shoot for this book.

Human Kinetics books are available at special discounts for bulk purchase. Special editions or book excerpts can also be created to specification. For details, contact the Special Sales Manager at Human Kinetics.

Printed in the United States of America   10 9 8 7 6 5 4 3 2 1

The paper in this book is certified under a sustainable forestry program.

Human Kinetics
1607 N. Market Street
Champaign, IL 61820
USA

United States and International
Website: **US.HumanKinetics.com**
Email: info@hkusa.com
Phone: 1-800-747-4457

Canada
Website: **Canada.HumanKinetics.com**
Email: info@hkcanada.com

E8518

Tell us what you think!
Human Kinetics would love to hear what we
can do to improve the customer experience.
Use this QR code to take our brief survey.

EXERCISE FINDER

Chapter 10 The Best Quadriceps Exercises

Chapter 11 The Best Glute and Hip Exercises

ACKNOWLEDGMENTS

This book would not be possible if it weren't for several people. My thanks to my good friend and business associate David Crump, Chris and Dani Shugart (editors at T-Nation.com), and Nick Collias (former editor at Bodybuilding.com) for their help in the creation of this book. Thank you to Eileen Escarda, who took all of the exercise pictures, along with my exercise models: Juli Lopez, Joe Drake, Lexi Northway, Chris Bozeman, and Patrick Miller. My thanks to Gil Krohn and the staff at Zoo Health Club in Oakland Park, Florida, for allowing us to do the photo shoot at this facility. And many thanks to the Human Kinetics family—with special thanks to Roger Earle, Amy Stahl, Annette Pierce, Jenny Lokshin, and Alexis Koontz for their involvement and hard work on this book. It's truly a privilege to work with these professionals in bringing this project to life, and I'm honored that they'll forever be a part of this book.

I owe a big debt of gratitude to Romina Marinaro, Jay Bileau, and Steve Tripp for their help with filming videos during my time in Rhode Island. I also want to thank all my clients—past, present, and future—for allowing me to continue to do what I love.

I'm so lucky that I get so much love and support from my mother, Faith Bevan; her husband, John Cavaliere; my father, Dominic Tumminello; and my close friends Marc and Brenda Spataro, Kate and Daniel Blankenship, Ryan and Tina Huether, Rob Simonelli, Joe Drake, Deanna Avery, and Paul Christopher from Gravity + Oxygen in Boca Raton, Florida.

I like to say that training is the art of applying the science. Like other artists, I have built my work upon the ideas of others who have come before me. I therefore owe those who came before me my gratitude and recognition for paving the way in categorizing strength exercises based on the muscle range of motion they target. To my knowledge, Steve Holman was the first to write a book on this type of training, with his 1994 work titled *Critical Mass: The Positions-of-Flexion Approach to Explosive Muscle Growth*. He would likely credit others who came before him for their influences, but I wanted to recognize his work for popularizing a similar concept in consumer book format.

INTRODUCTION

Strength training in its purest form isn't about moving loads by getting better at exercising—that's powerlifting and Olympic weightlifting. Strength training is about loading movements to develop a better-looking and better-functioning body that is stronger, more fit, and more resistant to injury. That's what *Strength Zone Training* is all about!

Unlike most books on strength training that focus on simply doing exercises, this book focuses on what those exercises are and aren't doing for you so you know how to save time by avoiding the mistakes that cause workout redundancy and inefficiency. You'll use the strength zone training exercise lists to choose the exercises your program needs to build strength through the true full range of motion. This will make you stronger in more ways and therefore capable of functioning at a higher level in any environment, not just inside the gym.

Put simply, strength zone training isn't just about helping you to build muscle; it's your workout blueprint to building muscle with a purpose.

You want to be strong through the full range of motion that each of your joints can move through in order to be more functional and less susceptible to injury. However, as you'll discover in chapter 1, You Don't Know What True Full Range of Motion Means, it's a myth that getting stronger through the true full range of motion is accomplished by moving through the full range of motion involved in any given exercise. Instead, it's accomplished by training each muscle group in each of the strength zones based on which aspects of the range of motion each exercise does and doesn't strengthen your body in.

Also, Chapter 1 covers the redundant exercises you don't need, the missing exercises you need for building full-range strength, and the four advantages strength zone training provides you over traditional strength training methods.

Training to develop strength through the true full range of motion is essential for building complete strength and preventing injury. Chapter 2, The New Rules of Full Range of Motion, listed the principles that'll help you to avoid wasting your time on workouts that are leaving large gaps in your strength or loading you up with unnecessary, redundant movements. These are the basic principles that everyone who enters the gym should follow for building muscle with a purpose!

For complete strength and injury prevention, doing only the big basic exercises leaves gaps in your strength. That's why chapters 3 through 13 provide you a list of exercises in each strength zone. By completing exercises from each strength zone each week, you'll build strength through the true full range of motion in every muscle group and ensure you don't skip key exercises that will leave strength on the table.

These chapters also provide detailed descriptions of the best exercises for the chest (chapter 3), lats (chapter 4), shoulders (chapter 5), traps (chapter 6), biceps (chapter 7), triceps (chapter 8), hamstrings (chapter 9), quadriceps (chapter 10), glutes and hips (chapter 11), calves (chapter 12), and core (chapter 13) in each strength zone for building strength through the true full range of motion.

Chapter 14, Beginner Workout Program, provides a workout plan for those who are just starting out or who haven't done regular strength training in a while. This ensures your body is ready to safely perform the more intense workouts.

Chapters 15, 16, and 17 provide a multitude of workout programs for you to choose from depending on how many days per week you prefer to exercise. Chapter 15 provides workout programs for training two or three times per week, chapter 16 provides workout programs for training four times per week, and chapter 17 provides workout programs for training five or six times per week.

All of the workout programs in chapters 15, 16, and 17 include the exercises in each strength zone you need to do each week for every muscle group to ensure your workouts are complete. The workouts are designed to maximize your valuable training time while helping you to build a better-looking body that's all-around stronger and more adaptable.

Additionally, the workout programs have been designed with the big-box gym member in mind. For instance, the programs can be done during the busiest times in a gym because they combine exercises in a strategic way without you having to walk all over the gym and lose the equipment to another member before you're finished.

To ensure that you continue to achieve the best full-range of motion strength training results, the final chapter, The Most Effective Muscle-Building Strategies, provides you with best splits, sets, reps, tempos, and more that are science-backed and gym-proven for gaining muscle.

Chapter 18 also takes a look at some of the biggest training and diet trends. Did you follow any of them? You'll see what lessons we've learned so far and what you need to keep in mind in order to forget the fitness and nutrition fads and stick to proven principles that always work and will never go out of date.

What You Need and Don't Need to Get Stronger

Cut out looking for the magic bullet. Add in proven exercise programming. A magic bullet is that mystical training secret that will change everything and give you everything you want. The problem is it doesn't exist. Strength program design continues to confuse people. Too many of us don't search for the key elements of successful programming and instead look for the shortcut. This demand has brought on an explosion of exercise programming information that instead of producing simplicity and clearer understanding has produced more complexity and confusion.

Strength Zone Training isn't about trying to reinvent the wheel. It's about making a better tire by simplifying the strength programming process and ensuring you do the basics better. We're in this together! I'm going to give you the tools, but you're the one who needs to use them. Be patient, be realistic, and be consistent. Smart training, hard work, and consistency cannot be beat.

GUIDE TO MUSCLES

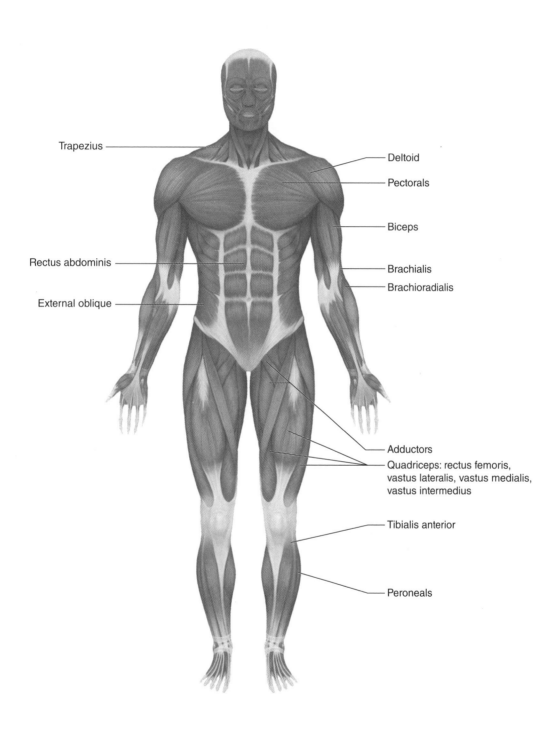

Trapezius

Rectus abdominis

External oblique

Deltoid

Pectorals

Biceps

Brachialis

Brachioradialis

Adductors

Quadriceps: rectus femoris, vastus lateralis, vastus medialis, vastus intermedius

Tibialis anterior

Peroneals

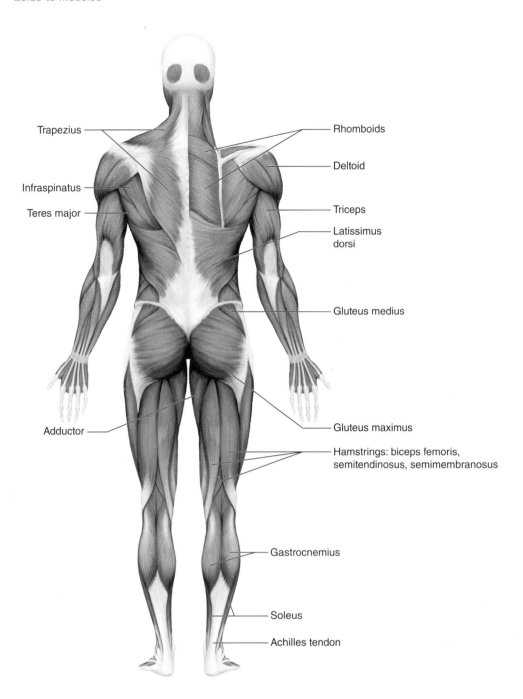

Trapezius

Rhomboids

Deltoid

Infraspinatus

Teres major

Triceps

Latissimus dorsi

Gluteus medius

Adductor

Gluteus maximus

Hamstrings: biceps femoris, semitendinosus, semimembranosus

Gastrocnemius

Soleus

Achilles tendon

CHAPTER 1

You Don't Know What True Full Range of Motion Means

The first things we're told about how to properly strength train is to maintain good exercise form and use a full range of motion. Yet many people, even experienced lifters and trainers, don't understand what strength through the true full range of motion is and how to successfully build it.

It's common to think of full range of motion as exercise range of motion, which is certainly needed to gain muscle. However, what matters most is possessing strength throughout your full anatomical range of motion at each joint. Otherwise you end up doing redundant exercises you don't need while missing the exercises you do need to fill gaps in your strength.

For most of us, the goal is to build a more fit, stronger body that's more functional and less prone to injury. To accomplish this goal, you need to build strength throughout your full anatomical range of motion at each joint. That way, you're stronger and more resistant to injury in all positions.

Strength zone training is strength training through the true full range of motion because it ensures you're strong through your full anatomical range of motion at each joint. This is what makes it so effective for developing complete strength and preventing injury.

The Missing Exercises for Complete Strength and Injury Prevention

Strength training through the true full range of motion is based on your anatomical range of motion, not on exercise range of motion. The workout programs in this book are about getting you strong through your full anatomical range of motion at each joint. This isn't accomplished by focusing on performing mainly compound (multi-joint) lifts along with random isolation (single-joint) exercises and moving through the full range of motion in all of your reps. It's accomplished by understanding which portion of your anatomical range of motion each exercise does and doesn't strengthen. Otherwise, you're sure to have gaps in your strength, which means your body is less functional and more susceptible to injury in the ranges of motion you've neglected.

Compound exercises provide a great foundation for strength training programs. These are squats, presses, deadlifts, rows, and other big movements. However, doing just the big basic exercises leaves gaps in your strength.

For example, having strong and functional glutes can help you perform better in sports, better stabilize your knees, and help keep your back healthy. That said, because of the mechanics involved, squats, Romanian deadlifts, and lunges create plenty of mechanical tension on your glutes when your hips are flexed at the bottom of the movement (see figure 1.1). However, there is very little mechanical tension on your glutes at the top when you're standing upright and the weight is nearly in line with the hips (see figure 1.2).

To build strength through the true full range of motion of hip extension so your glutes are stronger in all positions, you need to use isolation exercises such as a dumbbell one-leg hip thrust, weight plate one-leg hip lift, and NT Loop glute walk to train your glutes in the short-ened-to-midrange strength zone of hip extension that is neglected by most squat, deadlift, and lunge varia-tions (see figure 1.3).

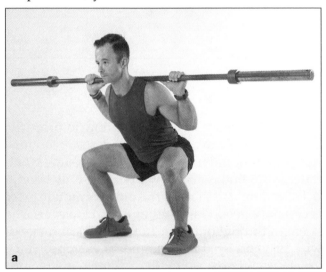

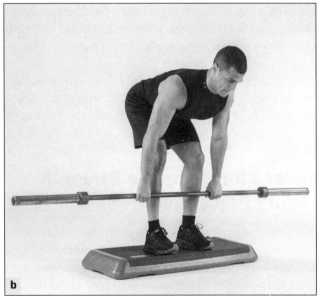

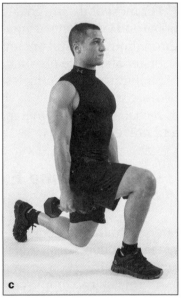

FIGURE 1.1.

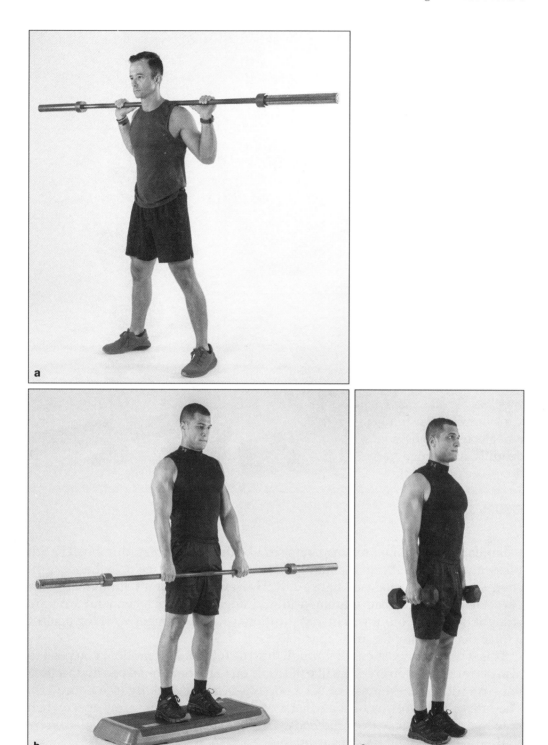

FIGURE 1.2.

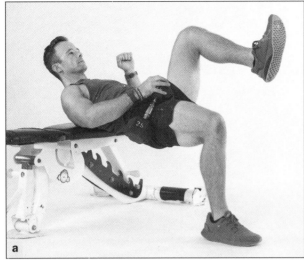

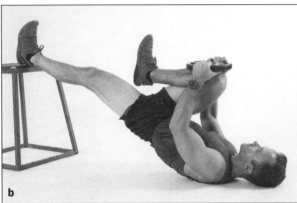

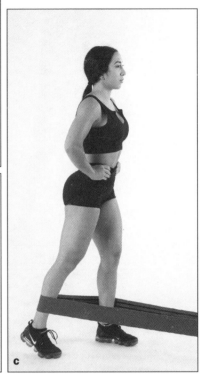

FIGURE 1.3.

Similarly, horizontal pressing exercises like the bench press, dumbbell bench press, and push-up effectively strengthen your pecs when they're in their length-ened-to-midrange zone (see figure 1.4). However, they don't strengthen your pecs when they're in their shortened-to-midrange zone, like when your arms are straight out from your torso. In that position, you're no longer working against a force that's pulling the arms apart.

This is why, for pec strength through the true full range of motion, you need to also perform isolation exercises like the cable one-arm horizontal pec fly, machine one-arm rotated chest press, or NT Loop one-arm pec deck fly (see figure 1.5). They make you work against a resistance that's pulling your arms apart when they're extended away from the body. This is a range that's often neglected by traditional compound pressing exercises.

"So what?" you might be asking. "I'm not a powerlifter struggling with locking out my deadlift or bench press. Why does this matter to me?" Here's why: Life and sports don't always happen in the ranges of motion used in compound exercises.

If you do only compound exercises like squats, Romanian deadlifts, and lunges for your lower body, you might find that you lack optimal strength when your hips are in the shortened range of hip extension—which, in any sport, they often will be. This means you're leaving muscle gains on the table. It might also mean you're building unbalanced strength and you're leaving yourself open to pain or injury.

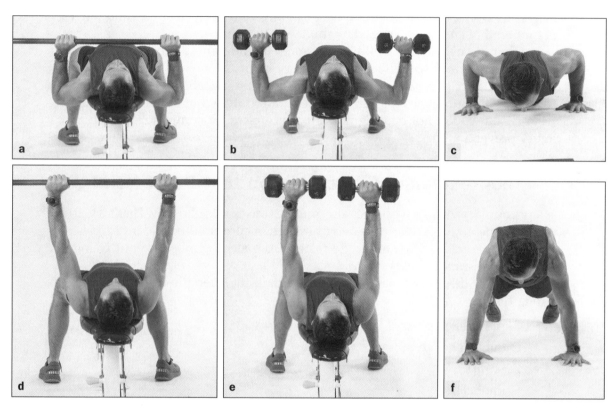

FIGURE 1.4.

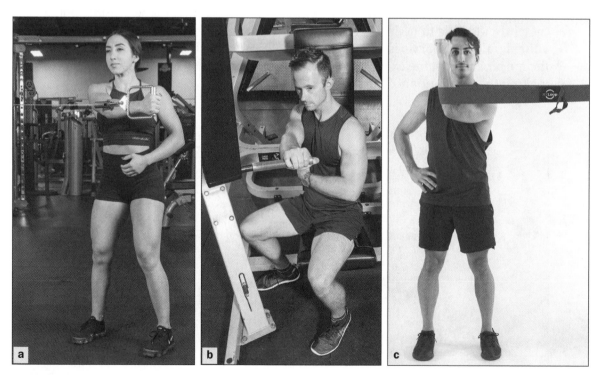

FIGURE 1.5.

The same can be said if you do only compound exercises for your upper body. This is where isolation, or single-joint, exercises can be truly helpful. They can help you achieve full-range strength by training your body in angles and ranges of motion that are not optimized by multi-joint exercises.

In other words, you can build bigger, nicer-looking muscles by doing mainly compound lifts and sprinkling in random isolation. However, if you also want to have better-performing muscles and have a more durable body, you need to cover the strength zones for each muscle group outlined in chapters 3 through 13 to ensure you're not missing important exercises for complete strength and injury prevention.

The Redundant Exercises You Just Don't Need

Many popular exercises work the same muscles the exact same way. That's a waste of your time. In this section are two examples of common redundant exercises, along with exercises you should do instead to make the most of your training time and get stronger.

All four of these exercises work your pecs in their lengthened-to-midrange strength zone:

- Barbell bench press
- Dumbbell bench press
- Push-up
- Dumbbell fly

In other words, they're basically the same exercise when it comes to how they load your pecs because they all create the most mechanical tension on the pecs when your humerus (the bone in your upper arm) is parallel to the ground, and they provide little to no load on your pecs when your wrists are directly above your shoulders. That doesn't mean they're not valuable, but it means they're for the most part the same exercise when it comes to how they load your pecs, thus making them redundant (see figures 1.4 and 1.6).

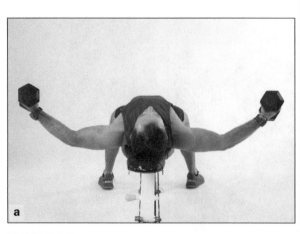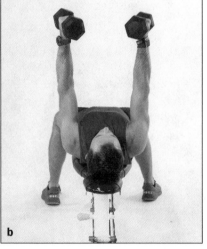

FIGURE 1.6.

Here's a better way: Once you've done one or two of these presses in your workout, perform an isolation exercise like the cable one-arm horizontal pec fly, machine one-arm rotated chest press, or one-arm NT Loop peck dec fly because they don't duplicate the way compound horizontal pressing exercises load your pecs. Why? They create the most mechanical tension on your pecs in their shortened-to-midrange strength zone, when your hands are more in front of your shoulders and torso (see figure 1.5).

The many popular biceps curl exercises are also redundant variations of the same theme. For example, let's compare the cable lying biceps curl (see figure 1.7) to any standing curl variation using free weights (dumbbell curls, EZ-bar curls, or barbell curls).

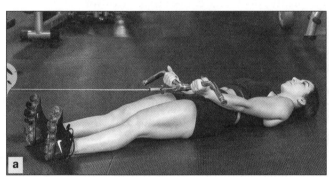 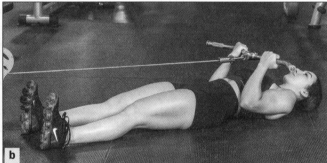

FIGURE 1.7.

Sure, the cable lying biceps curl is performed with a cable instead of a free weight, and it's also performed while lying supine on the floor instead of standing upright. However, when you look at how the cable lying biceps curl places mechanical tension across the biceps during elbow flexion, it becomes obvious that it's not much different from the standing variations.

During any biceps curls, the most mechanical tension is on the biceps when your forearm is at 90-degree angle to the line of force because this is where you have the least mechanical advantage on the load. Therefore, during all standing free weight biceps curls, the most mechanical tension is on the biceps—provided you don't cheat by allowing your elbows to drift forward—when your elbow is bent at 90 degrees (see figure 1.8). The trouble is, we see the same thing happening when you do cable lying curls.

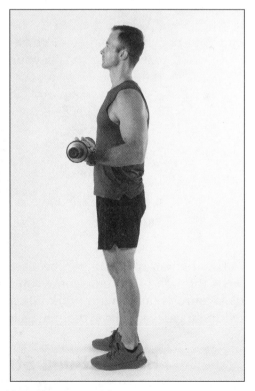

FIGURE 1.8.

What this means is that not only are cable lying biceps curls and standing free weight curls redundant, but the standing free weight curl variations duplicate one another. Although these exercises may appear different, they basically work the biceps in the same way.

Don't get me wrong! This isn't saying that cable lying biceps curls are a waste of time. This simply means that you don't need to go through the extra trouble of getting on the floor to do this exercise thinking it provides unique strength benefits to your biceps, different from doing dumbbell standing biceps curls with free weights. If you like doing lying cable biceps curls because it helps you keep your elbows back against the floor, there's no reason to stop doing them. Just know that you can accomplish the same thing more easily by standing with your back and elbows against a wall while doing free weight biceps curls.

The main point is, if you've already gotten everything you can from an EZ-bar curl or dumbbell biceps curl, there's no reason to add lying cable curls or other standing biceps curl variations. You aren't stimulating the muscles differently; you're training your biceps in the same strength zone, which is shortened to midrange.

If you're trying to maximize your training time and build true full range of motion biceps strength, you'd be far better off using less redundant biceps exercises in the lengthened-to-midrange strength zone, such as preacher biceps curls or cable face-away biceps curls. During preacher curls and cable face-away biceps curls, your forearm is perpendicular to the line of force (i.e., the load) when your elbow is straighter, thus working your biceps in a different manner and strengthening your biceps in their lengthened to midrange strength zone (see figure 1.9).

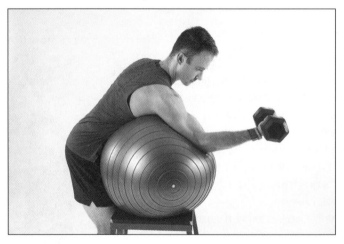

FIGURE 1.9.

The strength zone training checklists for each muscle group provided in chapters 4 through 14 not only show you the exercises you need to do each week to make sure your strength workouts are more complete, but they also remove redundancies so you can build muscle faster.

How to Build Strength Through the True Full Range of Motion

On any given training day, there are hundreds of exercises you could perform. With all the choices, it's no wonder that a lot of workouts end up looking—to put it generously—confusing or overwhelming. Minimalist workouts often rely on just a couple of big lifts to accomplish the athlete's goals, whether or not those lifts are up to the task. Higher-volume bodybuilding-style workouts use a lot of different movements and are often packed with redundant exercises, which is inefficient.

A better way to build your workout or audit a program that you're thinking of following is to determine how an exercise or group of exercises targets a muscle either when it is lengthened or when it is shortened. I call these two categories of muscle targeting the *strength zones*.

What Is a Strength Zone?

Every type of strength training exercise we do is most difficult at a certain portion in the range of motion. Or to think of it in more anatomical terms, it makes the target muscles work the hardest at a certain joint angle.

It can be different for every movement, but I've found that there are two general categories of strength training exercises, based on what range of motion for any given muscle they target. The two strength categories—what I call "strength zones"—are:

1. **The Lengthened to Midrange Strength Zone:** These are exercises that make certain muscles work hardest during the stretched, or lengthened, position through the middle of the range of motion

2. **The Shortened to Midrange Strength Zone:** These are exercises that make certain muscles work hardest during the contracted, or shortened, position through the middle of the range of motion

This might seem like a minor distinction, but plenty of research indicates that when we strength train, the gains we make are specific to the joint positions trained (1, 2, 3). This has been one of the criticisms of isometric training: It makes you strong, but only in a specific range of motion. This is also a reality with non-isometric exercises.

To illustrate, let's compare two common shoulder exercises: the dumbbell rear-deltoid fly and the dumbbell side-lying rear-deltoid fly. When performing the traditional dumbbell rear-delt fly, the point where it's most difficult is when the arm is farthest from the side of your torso; when your arm is roughly parallel to the floor (see figure 1.10a). How can you tell? Try to hold that position and you'll see how difficult it is. This is where you have the least mechanical advantage over the load because the lever arm is the longest and where the most mechanical tension is created on the involved musculature. In this position, your rear deltoid is in a contracted or shortened position.

By contrast, the point within the range of motion where the movement is easiest is when your arm is in front of your shoulders and your rear deltoids are closer to being in a stretched position (see figure 1.10b). Pausing at this point is easy. You could probably hang out there until your grip gives out. At this point, the least mechanical tension is being created on the involved muscles. Therefore, no strength is being gained in this portion of the range of motion. For this reason, a dumbbell rear-delt fly exercise strengthens your rear-deltoids in their shortened-to-midrange strength zone.

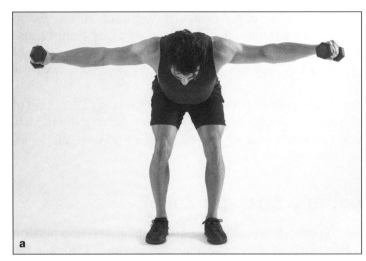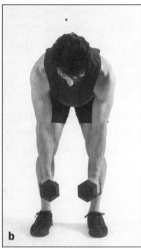

FIGURE 1.10.

On the other hand, when performing a dumbbell side-lying rear-deltoid fly, the situation is reversed. The movement is easiest when your arm is away from the side of the torso, or above you, and the muscle is shortened (see figure 1.11*a*). It's hardest on the involved muscles when your arm is directly in front of the torso, and the muscle is more lengthened (see figure 1.11*b*).

Thus, the dumbbell side-lying rear-delt fly trains the lengthened-to-midrange strength zone of your rear deltoids.

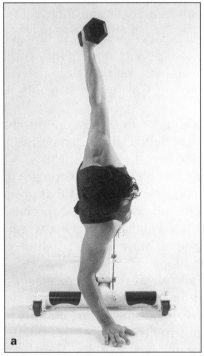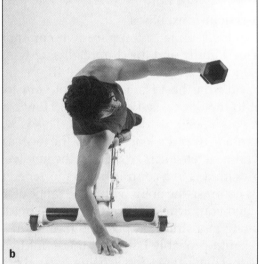

FIGURE 1.11.

Without the strength zone frame of reference, it could be easy to think that the two exercises I just discussed are interchangeable. After all, they're both rear-delt isolation movements, right?

But it's more accurate to say that they're complementary and that a complete approach to training the rear delts should include both. That way, you strengthen different aspects of the range of motion and ensure you possess true full anatomical range of motion strength through horizontal shoulder abduction (moving your arms from in to out; see figure 1.12).

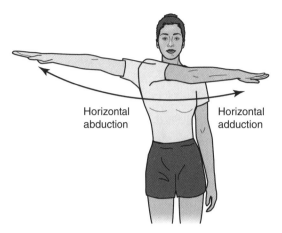

FIGURE 1.12 Anatomical action of shoulder horizontal abduction and adduction.

Keep It Simple and Efficient!

Over the years, other coaches have talked about similar concepts to what's presented in this book. However, they've historically been geared towards advanced bodybuilders. My unique contribution is coining the term *strength zones* and trying to improve these ideas by simplifying them and applying them in a way that is practical for everyone, regardless of knowledge, lifting experience, or fitness level. And I've made these concepts apply to wanting to gain muscle, but also wanting to have a more functional body.

That said, it's important to understand that the strength zones are just that: zones. These zones are areas within the range of motion of an exercise, not specific points within the range of motion of an exercise. You're not only getting stronger at one specific joint angle, but you're also getting stronger within a specific range of motion where the most mechanical tension on the involved muscles occurs. The farther an exercise gets away from creating the most mechanical tension at a joint angle, the less strength it builds at that joint angle.

This explains why just two strength zones are needed to build strength through the true full range of motion and also explains why there is no need to separate strength exercises into three strength zones:

1. Shortened range
2. Midrange
3. Lengthened range

Although this approach isn't wrong, it adds unnecessary length and complexity to your workouts because the exercises listed for the two strength zones for each muscle group in chapters 3 through 13 also develop strength in the midrange position. This is why the two strength zones are not simply shortened-range exercises and lengthened-range exercises. Instead, the zones include movements through the range of motion for each muscle from the lengthened end to the middle of the range and from the shortened end to middle of the range.

Four Advantages of Strength Zone Training

Perks you can expect from building true full range of motion strength using strength zone training include functional performance, improved physique, improved flexibility, and reduced injury risk.

Functional Performance

Strength zone training helps create a body that can get things done. You now know that some lifts train only the shortened end to the middle of the range of motion, while others mainly train the lengthened end to the middle. Strength zone training ensures you develop strength throughout your full anatomical range of motion at each joint so you're stronger in more ways and therefore capable of functioning at a higher level in any environment, not just inside the gym.

Improved Physique

There's a reason why seasoned bodybuilders try to hit all angles of a muscle. Doing so brings up the appearance of less-developed areas. To maximize the aesthetics of a muscle group, you wouldn't train it with exercises that emphasize only one range of motion, would you? That's not the best way to get a complete look. Plus, when you fill in the strength gaps, you get stronger overall, and it's simply easier to make strong muscles bigger.

Improved Flexibility: Better Than Stretching

Training at longer (stretched) muscle lengths not only causes muscles to be stronger at long lengths, it also can improve flexibility as well as, if not better than, typical static stretching (4,5). This is why one of the strength zones involves performing exercises that emphasize the target muscles in the lengthened end to the middle of the range of motion. These are exercises that create the most tension on the working muscles while they're being stretched. A great example is the Romanian deadlift (RDL), which can be considered a standing hamstring stretch while holding weight.

In short, the best way to prevent tight muscles is to regularly do exercises that create a stretch without overstretching by forcing the range of motion. So unless you simply enjoy stretching because it feels good, you won't need to spend extra time trying to work on flexibility limitations because you won't have any if you're training each muscle group in its lengthened range.

Reduced Injury Risk

Of course, you can't prevent all injuries, but strength training is proven to help reduce injury risk by a significant margin. Injury risk is a modifiable risk factor that can be improved with proper strength training. (That's what I mean when I use terms like *injury prevention* throughout this book.)

Strength gaps in your range of motion are injury liabilities. They're making you more prone to injury in the ranges of motion you've not trained in. So, training in both strength zones will help you build a more resilient, adaptable body and prepare it for whatever life and sport throws at it. It's no mystery that you're more susceptible to injury when your tissues and joints are asked to deal with force in positions they're not prepared for. Therefore, you'll be more physically prepared when you use strength zone training because it builds a stronger body through the true full range of motion.

This will not only help you build true full range of motion strength, but it will also successfully improve both flexibility and joint stability. You won't have to spend extra time with boring, corrective exercises and stretching because strength zone training prevents common movement deficiencies that can lead to injury while helping you to build muscle.

For complete strength and injury prevention, muscles need to be worked in the lengthened-to-midrange and shortened-to-midrange positions. Because most exercises don't require you to produce a constant force at all points throughout the range of motion, to fully strengthen a muscle usually requires at least two exercises. Therefore, you need to train it in both strength zones. You don't have to do exercises for both strength zones within one workout. If you train a muscle several times a week, you can distribute these exercises across multiple sessions, as is done in the workout programs in chapters 14 through 17.

With strength zone training there are no redundant exercises. The exercises in each strength zone for each muscle group in chapters 3 through 13 target a specific portion of the joint's range of motion, and they work synergistically to develop strength through your true full anatomical range of motion.

Strength zone training isn't just about helping you to build muscle, it's about building muscle with a purpose!

CHAPTER 2

The New Rules of Full Range of Motion

The strength zone training approach plays very well with pretty much every type of lifting schedule: body-part splits, full body, upper and lower body, and all points in between. It can help you determine whether an exercise belongs in your workout based on how it complements—or just repeats—the stimulus of other exercises. It'll help you direct more energy to the exercises that will offer the best payoff and less to those that make you feel more fatigued without much payoff. But most important, it will help you build balanced strength and muscularity, while making your training carry over to sports and life.

This book includes what you need to know to create an effective strength training plan. Chapters 3 through 13 provide a comprehensive list of the best exercises in each strength zone for each muscle group. Chapters 14 through 17 offer a multitude of workout programs that get you stronger through the true full range of motion. You'll be able to put one together that fits your weekly schedule.

Training to develop strength through the true full range of motion is essential for building complete strength and preventing injury. Next are the new rules of full range of motion for building muscle with a purpose.

Rule 1: Avoid Redundant Exercises

A positive consequence of thinking of exercises in terms of which strength zone they do and don't build strength in is that you quickly realize that plenty of popular movements don't necessarily send a dramatically different stimulus to their target muscles. In effect, many exercise variations are redundant.

To be clear, some redundancy is OK when you're trying to emphasize an aspect of your training for whatever reason. However, don't let redundancy get in the way of building strength through the true full range of motion at each joint. Dialing back redundant exercises will increase the productivity, efficiency, and effectiveness of your workouts.

Rule 2: Build Strength Through the Full Anatomical Range of Motion

Based on what you learned in chapter 1, you know that some strength exercises train only the range of motion from the shortened end to the middle, while others mainly train the range from the lengthened end to the middle. Because strength adaptions are specific to a joint position, the flipside to minimizing exercise redundancy is to train both ends of the range of motion by using strength zone training to ensure you strengthen your full anatomical range of motion at each joint. See figure 1.12 in chapter 1 and figure 2.1 for examples of full anatomical range of motion at specific joints.

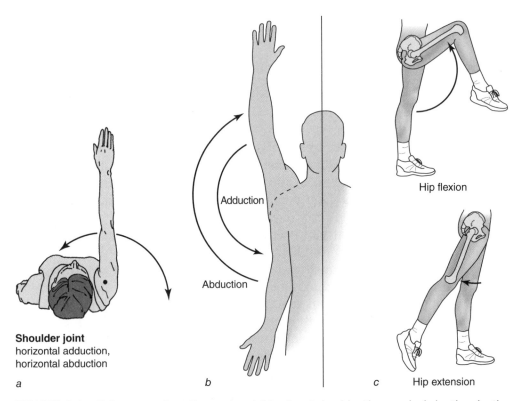

Shoulder joint
horizontal adduction,
horizontal abduction

a

Adduction

Abduction

b

Hip flexion

Hip extension

c

FIGURE 2.1 Full range of motion using *(a)* horizontal adduction and abduction in the shoulder joint, (b) vertical adduction and abduction in the shoulder joint, *(c)* flexion and extension in the hip joint.

Think about it this way: Olympic weightlifting and powerlifting require mastering a limited number of movements and positions in order to gain strength in them. But the principles I'm recommending expose you to a wider variety of movements and positions so you're stronger in more ways and therefore capable of functioning at a higher level in any environment, not merely in the gym. This is what complete strength training and injury prevention is all about. This book will show you how to build an all-around stronger, more adaptable body that's not limited to the competition lifts, although they have their value as well.

Strength Training Versus Powerlifting

Although this book talks about lifting weights, we're not talking about powerlifting. We're talking about strength training.

Many people, including trainers, commonly mistake the fundamentals of competitive powerlifting for the fundamentals of strength training. The differences between powerlifting and strength training are illustrated in table 2.1.

Table 2.1   Differences Between Powerlifting and Strength Training

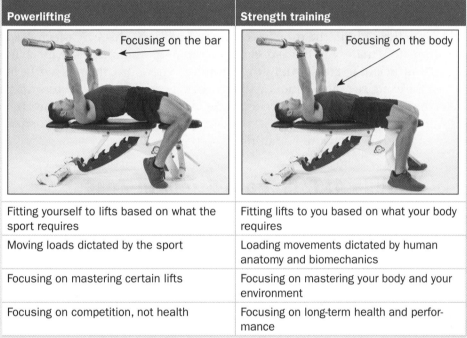

Powerlifting	Strength training
Focusing on the bar	Focusing on the body
Fitting yourself to lifts based on what the sport requires	Fitting lifts to you based on what your body requires
Moving loads dictated by the sport	Loading movements dictated by human anatomy and biomechanics
Focusing on mastering certain lifts	Focusing on mastering your body and your environment
Focusing on competition, not health	Focusing on long-term health and performance

Photos adapted from the 1996 book, *Biomechanically Correct* by Everett Aaberg. Published by Realistic Individualized Professional Training Service.

With this reality in mind, it's clear that the main thing that separates a powerlifting program from a strength, or lifting, program is the desired outcome of the program. While the purpose of a powerlifting program is to master specific exercises, the purpose of a strength program is to achieve an all-around stronger, healthier, and more adaptable body.

For athletes and everyone else, the conventional deadlift, squat, and bench press are simply exercises—optional tools that train the hip-hinging, knee-bending, and pushing actions of the human body. But their toolbox contains many other exercise options to train those same main functional movement patterns.

Sure, the big barbell lifts are a great way to create progressive overload because they provide a lot of value, but they're not the only way. Resistance exercises are just a way to put force across joints and tissues to help them to grow stronger. That's it! Barbells, dumbbells, cables, machines, and bands are all just tools that allow us to apply force across joints and tissues.

So for athletes and anyone else who lifts, sticking to the basics isn't about honoring a list of specific exercises. It's about honoring the principles of anatomy and biomechanics to build strength throughout your full anatomical range of motion at each joint because that's foundational to improving your long-term health and performance in any physical endeavor. And no system does that better than strength zone training.

Rule 3: Exercise Range of Motion Doesn't Equal Effective Range of Motion

The body gets stronger by creating mechanical tension across tissues and joints. This can be accomplished by loading them through movement against resistance, which we call strength training exercises. All strength training exercises that involve free weights and cables have areas within the range of motion where the exercise is hardest on the working muscles, and where the exercise is the easiest, based on the mechanical tension involved.

As demonstrated in chapter 1, the majority of strength training exercises involving free weights and cables do not provide the same level of mechanical tension at all points throughout the exercise's range of motion. This can affect strength adaptations too, mainly in the aspect of the range of motion where mechanical tension is sufficient to create strength adaptions. Therefore, there is a difference between the exercise range of motion of a given exercise and the effective range of motion that offers strengthening benefits. So in order to get stronger throughout your full anatomical range of motion at each joint, you need to do exercises in each strength zone to ensure you don't have weak points.

Rule 4: Train Both Strength Zones

To get strong, and to avoid wasting your time on workouts that are leaving large gaps in your strength, use at least one exercise from each strength zone for each muscle group. This will strengthen different portions of the range of motion in each main joint movement.

When you're choosing exercises, this strategic approach guarantees that you'll build strength through the true full range of motion. In each exercise chapter, you'll find a multitude of examples of how this approach works for each muscle group.

Rule 5: Use Isolation Exercises to Fill Gaps Left by Compound Exercises

In the strength zone training system, every exercise has a purpose. This is why I say this book is about how to build muscle with a purpose.

When it comes to the goal of building strength through your full anatomical range at each joint, the smarter way to use isolation (i.e., single joint) exercises is to train in ranges of motion and movements missed by the compound (i.e., multijoint) exercises. A strength training program that focuses exclusively on either compound or isolation exercises will leave potential strength gains untapped because each type of exercise trains a strength zone the other misses. In contrast, a lifting program that combines both compound and isolation exercises in a strategic manner that minimizes redundancy will help you to achieve superior results in your overall strength and muscle gains.

It's important to note that many trainers and serious lifters bring up the fact there's really no such thing as an isolation exercise. This is because other muscles may be working to stabilize you or resist unwanted movement somewhere else on your body while you perform a certain exercise that's targeted at a certain

Free Weights Versus Machines: The Final Word

A false dichotomy is a logical fallacy in which only two choices are presented when, in fact, other possible choices exist. These dilemmas reflect oversimplified thinking and are usually characterized by a black and white approach and *this versus that* language. A common false dichotomy in fitness is the debate pitting free weights against machines.

The idea of pitting free weights against machines is like pitting fruits against vegetables. Both training modalities offer a unique benefit the other misses, so it makes sense to do them both in order to make your workouts more comprehensive, just like eating both fruits and vegetables will make your diet more nourishing.

Free weights excel by forcing you to use your stabilizer muscles, allowing you to move naturally and requiring you to control not just the load being moved, but also the path of the movement. Free weights fall short when it comes to keeping consistent tension on the working muscles throughout the range of motion. And that's the area that selectorized machines (with the weight-stack and pin) excel in better than free weight exercises. Selectorized machines use a cam system, in which a bean-shaped mechanism on the machine rotates as you do each rep. The cam offers much more consistent resistance throughout a larger range of motion than when using free weights.

While you can build plenty of muscle using free weights exclusively, there's no reason to avoid machines. To build strength and muscle, machines can and should be used in conjunction with free weights, which is why machines are used in the strength zone training system.

muscle group. For example, during a standing biceps curl with dumbbells, an EZ-bar, or barbell, the muscles that move your shoulder blade are working to keep your shoulder posture from rounding forward as you perform the lift, and your back extensor muscles are also working to keep your torso from being pulled forward by the weight that's in front of you. Therefore, it's more accurate to use the term *targeted exercise* when referring to exercises that are commonly called isolation exercises because they're targeted at a specific muscle group while not necessarily involving only that muscle group. That said, I'm using the term *isolation exercise* in this book because it's such a commonly used term that nearly everyone is familiar with.

Rule 6: Train Movements *and* Muscles!

The world of strength and conditioning has gone from viewing muscles purely in isolation to recognizing more integrated movement patterns that show how these muscles create coordinated movement. As a result, some trainers now say to "train movements, not muscles" to direct people away from isolation exercises.

But as you know now, exercise redundancy and gaps in your strength are the result of following the "train movements, not muscles" mantra because it leads to repeatedly loading the same areas and ranges of motion while failing to load others. This is not good. Isolation exercises are needed to train the movements and ranges of motion missed by the compound exercises. So saying "train movements, not muscles" is like saying eat vegetables, not fruits. Avoiding one or the other will leave your diet deficient.

Here we train movements and muscles because muscles create movements. And using isolation exercises to train the muscles in important ranges of motion neglected by the compound movement exercises is needed for complete strength and injury prevention.

Strength Zone Training Exercise Checklist

Next is a strength zone training checklist of exercises you need to do each week to make sure your strength workouts are more complete.

Exercise chapters 3 through 13 provide you with a strength zone checklist for building true full-range of motion strength in each muscle group. They also describe how to perform the best exercises in each strength zone for every muscle group. These checklists ensure you avoid redundant exercises and train each muscle group in the most effective manner possible for creating strength throughout the true full range of motion.

Each exercise outlines the setup and provides action and coaching tips. The exercises are categorized to match table 2.2.

The strength zone workout programming in chapters 14 through 17 put the exercise checklists into practice by providing you workout plans that make the most of your training time and ensure your workouts will be effective at building strength through the true full range of motion.

Let's get started!

TABLE 2.2   Strength Zone Training Exercise Checklist

UPPER-BODY STRENGTH ZONES

Muscle group	Movement or range of motion		
Pecs	Lengthened to mid-range: horizontal or decline pressing exercise	Lengthened to mid-range: diagonal pressing exercise	Shortened to mid-range: horizontal or diagonal shoulder adduction exercise
Lats	Lengthened to mid-range: vertical or diagonal pulling exercise with arms outside	Lengthened to mid-range: vertical or diagonal pulling exercise with arms inside	Shortened to mid-range: horizontal pulling exercise
Middle delts	Lengthened to mid-range exercise	Shortened to mid-range exercise	
Rear delts	Lengthened to mid-range exercise	Shortened to mid-range exercise	
Traps	Scapular elevation exercise	Scapular retraction exercise	
Biceps	Lengthened to mid-range exercise	Shortened to mid-range exercise	
Triceps	Lengthened to mid-range exercise	Shortened to mid-range exercise	

LOWER-BODY AND CORE STRENGTH ZONES

Muscle group	Movement or range of motion		
Hamstrings	Lengthened to mid-range: hip-hinging exercise	Shortened to mid-range: knee flexion exercise	
Quads	Lengthened to mid-range: knee-bending exercise	Shortened to mid-range: knee extension exercise	
Hips	Abduction exercise	Adduction exercise	
Glutes	Lengthened to mid-range: hip-hinging exercise	Shortened to mid-range: hip extension exercise	
Calves	Straight-knee exercise	Bent-knee exercise	
Core	Linear exercise	Lateral exercise	Rotational exercise

How to Use the Strength Zone Training Exercise Chapters

Chapters 3 to 13 start with some composite photos showing the starting position and ending position of an exercise blended into one image. These photos include a gradient bar showing what strength zone the exercise creates the most mechanical tension in and where in the range of motion the tension drops off.

Although there is some level of tension of the involved muscles throughout each exercise's range of motion, the darkest area of the gradient bar in each photo represents the strength zone where your involved musculature gets the most mechanical tension during the exercise. The lighter portion of the gradient bar represents where your involved musculature gets the least mechanical tension during the exercise.

As you'll see in the composite photos at the beginning of each exercise chapter, one exercise will have the gradient bar darkest on one end, while the other exercise for the other strength zone with be darkest on the opposite end.

It is important to note that the gradient bars are a representation of how the tension changes through the exercise and are not an exact science. They are there to provide you with a simple and clear visual of strength zone training.

It is also important to understand that the arrows included in these photos are pointing to the starting position and ending position of the exercise and not at a particular joint or muscle in the body.

I chose to limit the number of exercises in order to make this book easier to use. The exercises included are by no means an exhaustive list, and this book could be much longer with all the exercises I could include. You may have other exercises you enjoy for each included muscle group. Use the sample exercises I included in this book as a guide, and then apply them to the exercises and muscle groups in your daily workouts.

CHAPTER 3

The Best Chest Exercises

Your chest contains your pectoral muscles (pecs). Training to develop chest strength through the true full range of motion involves performing at least one exercise for each of the following strength zones:

- Lengthened-to-midrange strength zone: horizontal or decline pressing exercise
- Lengthened-to-midrange strength zone: incline pressing exercise
- Shortened-to-midrange strength zone: horizontal or diagonal shoulder adduction exercise

Picking at least one exercise from each category on this list maximizes your workout efficiency and helps you develop full-range chest strength.

Chest Exercise Mechanics

Both the incline pressing exercise and the horizontal or decline pressing exercise train your chest in the lengthened-to-midrange strength zone. Even though these exercises hit the same general strength zone for your chest, it's important to do both because varying the bench angle during pressing exercises has been shown to bias activation in either the sternal or clavicular portion of the pectoralis musculature.

Muscle activation of the sternocostal head of the pectoralis major is significantly greater during the decline hip bridge press (see figure 3.1), whereas activation of the clavicular

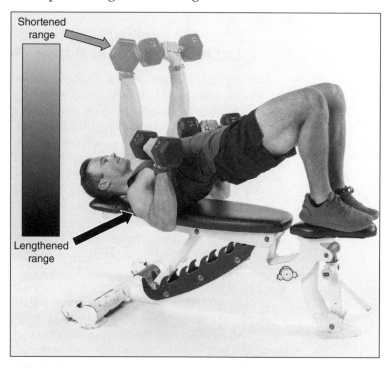

FIGURE 3.1 Dumbbell decline hip bridge press in the lengthened-to-midrange strength zone: horizontal or decline pressing exercise.

head of the pectoralis major was significantly greater on an inclined bench (1,2,3).

Because pressing from a flat or declined position offers different chest-training benefits than pressing from an incline, it's important to do chest exercises from a horizontal or declined angled and exercises from an inclined angled each week (see figure 3.2).

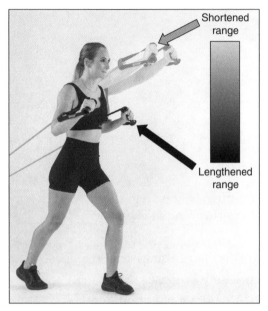

FIGURE 3.2 Band incline press in the lengthened-to-midrange strength zone: incline pressing exercise.

That said, as established in chapter 1, presses in the flat, decline, and incline position all create the most tension on the pecs when the humerus (upper-arm bone) is parallel to the ground, which is in the lengthened-to-midrange strength zone. However, these exercises provide little mechanical tension on your pecs when your wrists are directly above your shoulders, which is in the shortened-to-midrange strength zone of your pecs. It is important to include an exercise in the shortened-to-midrange strength zone that forces your pecs to deal with a large load (relative to your current strength level) when your hands are directly in front of your shoulders and torso. This trains your body in the strength zone missed by the compound pressing exercises, and you get stronger pecs in all positions of horizontal and diagonal arm adduction (moving your arm from out to in). See the following sidebar on why cable pec flys are better than dumbbell pec flys in the shortened-to-midrange strength zone for a horizontal or diagonal shoulder adduction exercise.

Cable Pec Flys Are Better Than Dumbbell Pec Flys

Not only do dumbbell flys and dumbbell or barbell bench presses involve horizontal shoulder adduction, they also create the most mechanical tension on the pecs when the humerus (upper-arm bone) is parallel to the ground (see figure 3.3). So both exercises load your pecs in the same way, which makes doing both of them redundant.

The reason you can use much more weight when doing a dumbbell bench press is because it allows the triceps to contribute. The weight is also much closer to your shoulder joints, which gives your pecs and front delts a bigger mechanical advantage.

That said, cable flys and dumbbell bench presses aren't redundant because they load the pecs differently (see figure 3.4).

Dumbbell flys provide little or no force on your pecs when your wrists are directly above your shoulders. However, because cable flys work against a 45-degree line of force (the cables themselves), your pecs handle a great deal of load when your hands are directly in front of your shoulders.

So it's not that dumbbell pec flys are a waste of time. It's simply that, if you're already doing horizontal compound pressing exercises like push-ups, bench press, or dumbbell press, you don't need to do dumbbell flys because you've already trained in that strength zone. This is why cable pec flys with the cable at an angle to your body, along with the other exercises listed in the section on horizontal or diagonal shoulder adduction in the shortened to midrange strength zone, are better at building pec strength through the true full range of motion.

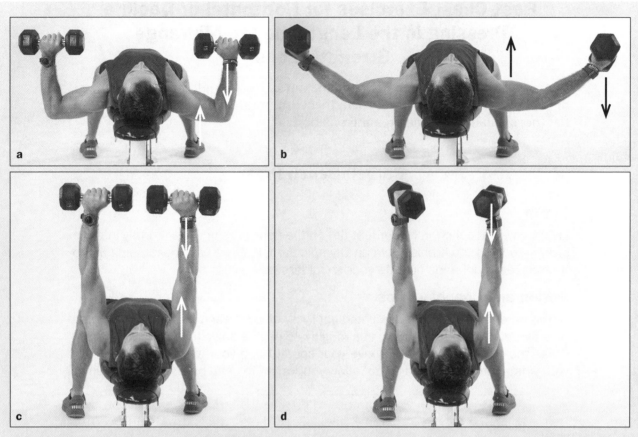

FIGURE 3.3.

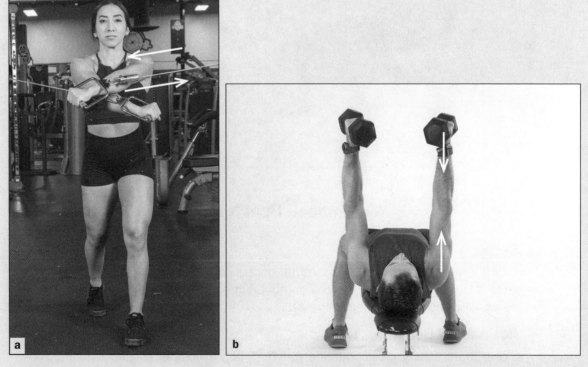

FIGURE 3.4.

Best Chest Exercises for Horizontal or Decline Pressing in the Lengthened-to-Midrange Strength Zone

The exercises in this section help you maximize the strength and development of your chest musculature in the lengthened-to-midrange strength zone from a flat (horizontal) or decline pressing position.

Barbell Bench Press

Setup

Lie on a weight bench with your feet flat on the floor, pressing them firmly into the ground to keep you stable. Hold an Olympic barbell above your head using a grip that places your hands outside your shoulders (see figure *a*).

Action and Coaching Tips

Slowly lower the bar toward your chest until your elbows reach just below your torso (see figure *b*). Keep your elbows at a roughly 45-degree angle relative to your torso. Press the bar toward the sky above your chest. Keep your elbows directly under your wrists throughout, and do not allow your wrists to bend backward at any time.

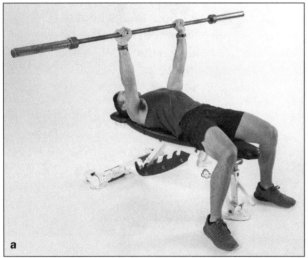
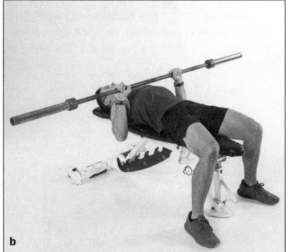

Dumbbell Bench Press

Setup

Lie on a weight bench with your feet flat on the floor, pressing them firmly into the ground to keep you stable. Hold a dumbbell in each hand above your shoulders, with your arms straight (see figure *a*).

Action and Coaching Tips

Slowly lower the dumbbells outside your body at a 45-degree angle relative to your torso, stopping when your elbows go just below torso level (see figure *b*). Press the dumbbells back toward the sky, above your shoulders.

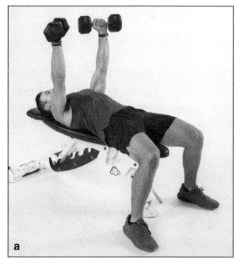

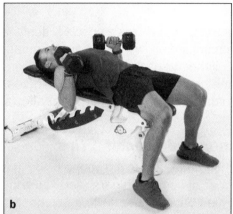

Dumbbell Decline Hip Bridge Press

You can use a decline bench to perform this exercise, but I'm highlighting this variation because many facilities don't have a special decline bench, nor do you need one to perform this exercise.

Setup

Lie on your back (supine) on a weight bench or the floor with your knees bent and heels on the bench or floor. Lift your hips as high as you can without overextending your lower back. Maintain this lifted hip position while holding a dumbbell in each hand above your shoulders, with your arms straight (see figure *a*).

Action and Coaching Tips

Without allowing your hips to drop, slowly lower the dumbbells outside your body at a 45-degree angle to your torso, stopping when your elbows lightly touch the sides of the bench or the floor (see figure *b*). Press the dumbbells back toward the sky, above your shoulders.

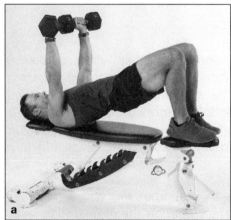

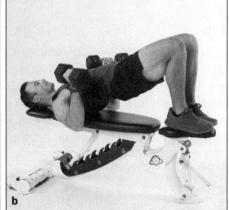

Machine Chest Press

Setup

This exercise requires a specially designed machine that is available in most gyms. The machine allows you to push its handles horizontally away from your body. Sit tall, with your back in front of the pad. Hold the handles at midchest level, with your elbows directly behind the handles and your arms bent (see figure *a*). Find a comfortable foot placement that allows you to perform the exercise with proper technique.

Action and Coaching Tips

Without fully locking out your elbows, press the handles so your arms are straight in front of your shoulders (see figure *b*). Slowly reverse the motion, bringing the handles back to the starting position.

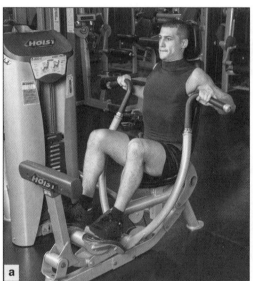 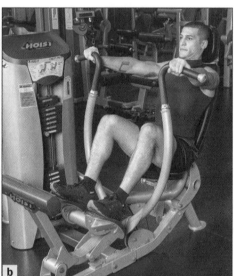

Band Step and Chest Press

Setup

Face away from a heavy-duty resistance band attached at mid-torso to shoulder height to a stable structure or inside a doorjamb (many resistance bands come with a doorjamb attachment). With your knees slightly bent and your feet roughly hip-width apart, hold a handle in each hand. Your arms are at a 45-degree angle to your sides, and your forearms are slightly parallel to the floor (see figure *a*). The band should create enough tension that it forces you to lean slightly forward.

Action and Coaching Tips

Step forward with one leg while performing a chest press with both arms; maintain your slightly forward torso lean with your rear heel off the ground (see figure *b*). Step your lead leg back to the starting position while allowing your arms to come back as well. Alternate legs on each repetition. Explode into each repetition as if you were shoving someone. The resistance band should create enough tension to make you work to hold your position from the start of each repetition—not just at the end when your arms are extended.

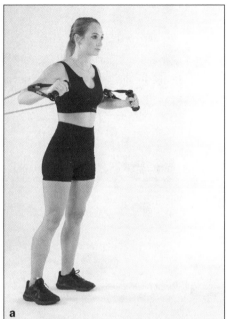 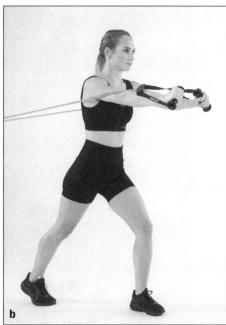

NT Loop Resisted Push-Up

Setup

You can do this exercise using a superband, but I prefer using the NT Loop, an exercise band I designed to be more comfortable and stable when it is around the body.

Place an NT Loop around your upper back and place your fingers (but not your thumbs) inside the band from the bottom up (see figures *a* and *b*). Position your hands on the floor shoulder-width apart, with your elbows straight (see figure *c*). Turn your hands slightly outward so that your fingers point at roughly 45 degrees.

Action and Coaching Tips

Perform a push-up by lowering your body to the floor while keeping your elbows directly above your wrists (see figure *d*). At the bottom of each push-up, position your arms at a 45-degree angle so your torso forms the shape of an arrow. Once your elbows are at an almost 90-degree angle, reverse the motion by pushing your body up so that your elbows are straight again. At the top of each push-up, instead of finishing with your shoulder blades pinched together, protract (push apart) your shoulder blades while keeping your body in a straight line from your head through your hips to your ankles. Do not allow your head or hips to sag toward the floor at any point.

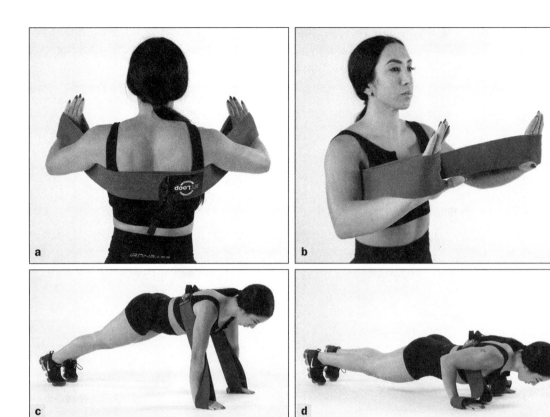

Push-Up

Setup

Place your hands on the floor just wider than shoulder-width apart, with your elbows straight. Turn your hands slightly outward so that your fingers point at roughly 45 degrees (see figure *a*).

Action and Coaching Tips

Lower your body to the floor while keeping your elbows directly above your wrists (see figure *b*). Once your elbows are at an almost 90-degree angle, reverse the motion by pushing your body up so that your elbows are straight again. At the top of each push-up, instead of finishing with your shoulder blades pinched together, protract (push apart) your shoulder blades while keeping your body in a straight line.

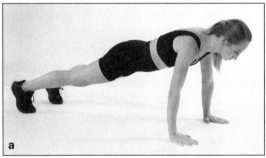
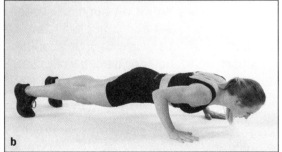

Box Crossover Push-Up

Setup

Begin in a push-up position, with both hands on top of a platform or ball and your feet just wider than shoulder-width apart (see figure a).

Action and Coaching Tips

Without moving your feet, step one hand off the platform or ball to the floor while performing a push-up (see figure b). As you come out of the push-up, bring your hand back to the platform or ball. Repeat the same action on the other side (see figure c). Do not allow your head or hips to sag toward the floor at any point.

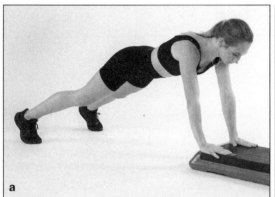
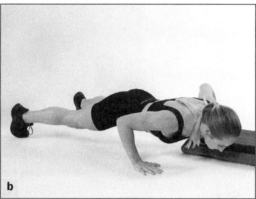

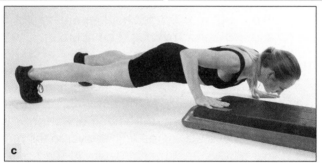

Lock-Off Push-Up

Setup

Begin in a low push-up position, with your feet shoulder-width apart, one hand on top of a medicine ball or platform, and your other hand on the floor (see figure a).

Action and Coaching Tips

Press up with one hand on top of the platform or medicine ball. At the top of the push-up, lock off by fully straightening the elbow of the arm resting on the platform or ball (see figure b). Place the other arm at your opposite shoulder and pause for 1 or 2 seconds at the top of each repetition (see figure c), then slowly lower yourself. Perform half of the repetitions with your right arm elevated and the other half with your left arm elevated. Do not allow your shoulders or hips to rotate at any time; keep your torso parallel to the ground throughout.

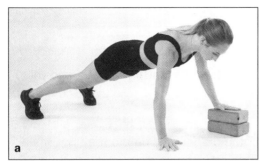

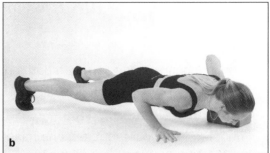

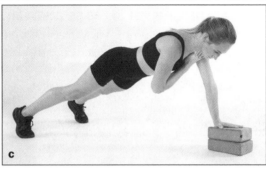

Feet-Elevated Push-Up

Setup

Begin in a push-up position, with your hands shoulder-width apart on the floor and your feet elevated on a weight bench or chair (see figure *a*).

Action and Coaching Tips

Perform a push-up by lowering your body to the floor while keeping your elbows directly above your wrists (see figure *b*). At the bottom of each push-up, position your arms at a 45-degree angle to form the shape of an arrow with your torso. Once your elbows are almost at a 90-degree angle, reverse the motion by pushing your body up so that your elbows are straight again. At the top of each push-up, instead of finishing with your shoulder blades pinched together, protract (push apart) your shoulder blades while keeping your body in a straight line from your head through your hips to your ankles. Do not allow your head or hips to sag toward the floor at any point.

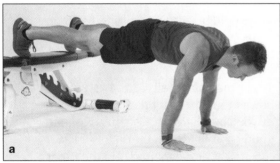

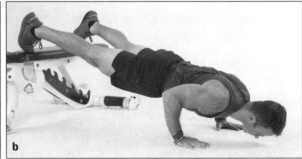

Hands-Elevated Push-Up

Setup

Assume a plank position, with your hands on top of a weight bench and outside of your shoulders (see figure *a*).

Action and Coaching Tips

Perform a push-up by lowering your body to the bench while keeping your elbows directly above your wrist (see figure *b*). Once your elbows reach an angle just below 90 degrees or your chest touches the bench, reverse the motion by pushing your body up so that your elbows are straight again. At the top of each push-up, do not finish with your shoulder blades pinched together; instead, protract (push apart) your shoulder blades while keeping your body in a straight line. Do not allow your head or hips to sag at any point.

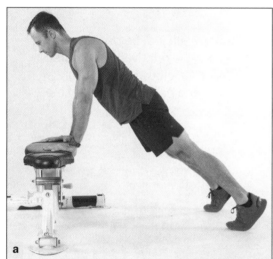
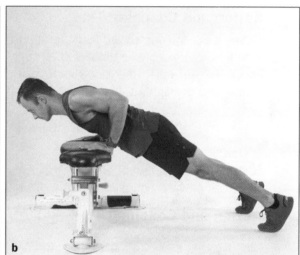

Best Chest Exercises for Incline Pressing in the Lengthened-to-Midrange Strength Zone

The exercises in this section help you maximize the strength and development of your chest musculature in the lengthened-to-midrange strength zone from the incline (diagonal) pressing position.

Barbell Incline Bench Press

Setup

Lie on a weight bench angled at about 45 degrees, with your feet flat on the floor, pressing them firmly into the ground to keep you stable. Hold an Olympic barbell overhead using a grip that places your hands outside your shoulders (see figure *a*).

Action and Coaching Tips

Slowly lower the bar toward your chest until your elbows reach just below your torso (see figure *b*); keep your elbows at a roughly 45-degree angle relative to your torso. Press the bar up to the sky above your chest. Keep your elbows directly under your wrists throughout, and do not allow your wrists to bend backward at any time.

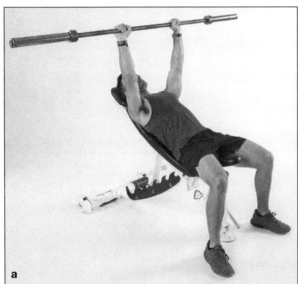
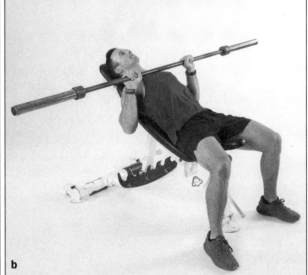

Dumbbell Incline Bench Press

Setup

Lie on a weight bench angled at about 45 degrees, with your feet flat on the floor, pressing them firmly into the ground to keep you stable. Hold a pair of dumbbells above your head, slightly outside your shoulders (see figure *a*).

Action and Coaching Tips

Slowly lower the dumbbells outside your body at a 45-degree angle to your torso, stopping when your elbows are below your torso level (see figure *b*). Press the dumbbells back up toward the sky, above your shoulders. Keep your elbows directly under your wrists throughout, and do not allow your wrists to bend backward at any time.

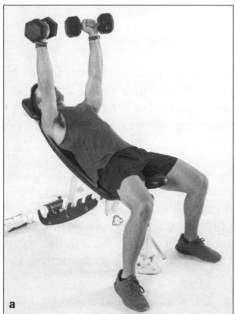

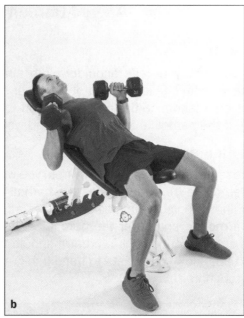

Angled-Barbell Shoulder-to-Shoulder Press

Setup

Stand tall, with your feet parallel to one another and a little wider than shoulder-width apart. Hold on to the end of the barbell with both hands stacked one over the other and with the end of the barbell in front of your left shoulder (see figure *a*).

Action and Coaching Tips

Press the barbell out and away from you so that when your arms reach full extension, the barbell is directly in line with the center of your body (see figure *b*). Slowly reverse the motion and lower the barbell to your right shoulder (see figure *c*). Press it out and away again so that it ends up in the middle of your body. Do not allow your shoulders or hips to rotate during this exercise.

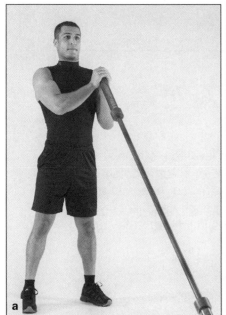

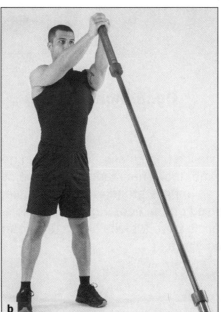

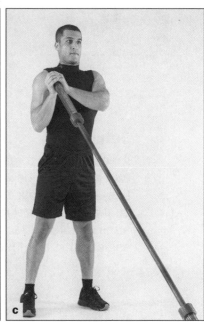

Angled-Barbell One-Arm Press

Setup

Stand with your legs shoulder-width apart in either parallel (as shown) or split stance with one leg in front of the other. Place one end of a barbell in a corner or inside a landmine device and hold on to the other end of the barbell (see figure a). If the barbell is in your right hand, your right leg is your back leg.

Action and Coaching Tips

Press the barbell up and away from you while keeping your torso upright and stable (see figure b). Do not press the barbell toward the midline of your body; keep it in line with your same-side shoulder as you press it up and out. Slowly reverse the motion and lower the barbell back in front of your shoulder. At the bottom of each repetition, your forearm should form a 90-degree angle with the barbell. Do not allow your wrists to bend backward at any time; keep your wrists straight throughout this exercise.

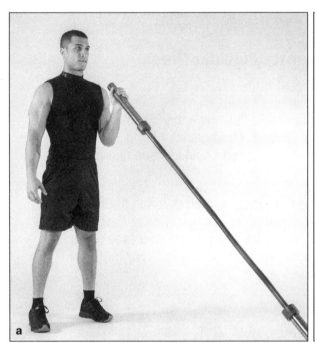
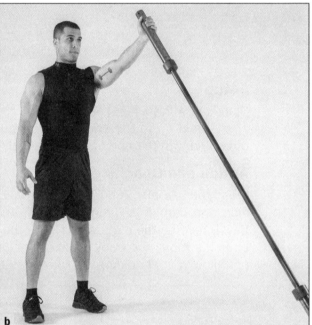

Band Incline Press

Setup

Face away from a resistance band that's attached at knee level to a stable structure or inside a doorjamb (many resistance bands come with an attachment for this). Keeping your torso upright, stand in a split stance, with your knees slightly bent and back heel raised off the floor. Holding a handle in each hand, keep your arms at a 45-degree angle to your sides and your forearms in line with the same angle as the band (see figure a).

Action and Coaching Tips

Without overextending at your low back, press your arms straight out at a 45-degree angle (see figure *b*). Keep your arms at the same angle as the band. Slowly bring your arms back to your sides to complete the rep. Stand far enough away from the band to keep tension from the start of each rep. Stand farther away from the band if you need more tension.

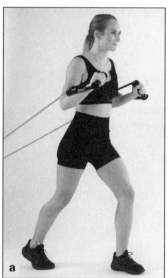
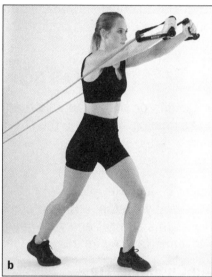

Machine Incline Chest Press

Setup

This exercise requires a specially designed machine that is available in most gyms. The machine allows you to push its handles diagonally upward away your body. Sit tall, with your back in front of the pad. Hold the handles at midchest level, with your arms bent and elbows directly behind the handles. Your forearms point in the direction you will press (see figure *a*). Find a comfortable foot placement that allows you to perform the exercise with proper technique.

Action and Coaching Tips

Press the handles so your arms are straight and above your shoulders (see figure *b*). Slowly reverse the motion, bringing the handles back to the starting position.

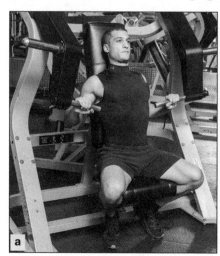
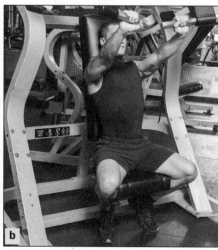

Best Chest Exercises for Horizontal or Diagonal Shoulder Adduction in the Shortened-to-Midrange Strength Zone

The exercises in this section help you strengthen and develop the chest musculature that was missed by the previous two exercise categories by focusing on horizontal and diagonal shoulder adduction in the shortened-to-midrange strength zone.

Dumbbell Squeeze Press

The squeeze action on the dumbbells that occurs as your arms are above your torso creates a training stimulus in the shortened-to-midrange of horizontal shoulder adduction.

Setup

Lie on a weight bench, with your feet flat on the floor, pressing them firmly into the ground to keep you stable. Hold a dumbbell in each hand above your shoulders, with your arms straight and your palms facing each other and squeeze the dumbbells together (see figure *a*).

Action and Coaching Tips

While continuing to squeeze the dumbbells together as hard as you can, bend your elbows and lower the dumbbells to your chest as your elbows go out to the sides (see figure *b*). Reverse the motion by pressing the dumbbells back up while squeezing them together.

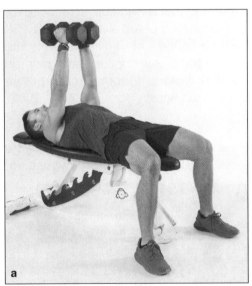
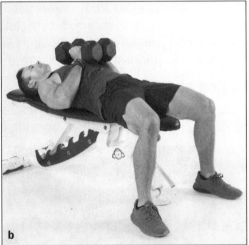

Cable One-Arm Horizontal Pec Fly

Setup

Stand tall, in either a split stance or a parallel stance, just in front of the middle of a cable crossover machine or next to a resistance band. With one hand, hold a handle attached at shoulder level. Extend your arm out to your side, with a slight bend in the elbow (see figure a).

Action and Coaching Tips

Bring your arm across your torso while keeping a soft bend in your elbow (see figure b). Slowly reverse the motion until your arm is back out to your side and your elbow is just behind your shoulder. Perform all reps on the same side before switching sides.

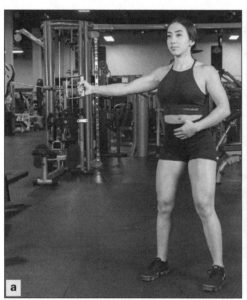 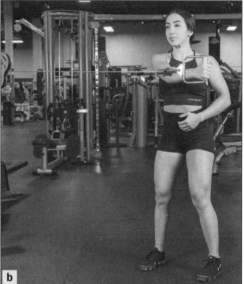

Cable One-Arm Diagonal Pec Fly

Whereas the cable one-arm horizontal fly uses the shoulder motion involved in a flat chest press, these cable one-arm diagonal pec flies use the shoulder motion involved in a decline chest press. So although they're not technically a horizontal shoulder action, the motion is similar enough to be in this category because of the similar chest activation involved in flat and decline pressing actions.

Setup

Stand tall, in either a split stance or a parallel stance, just in front of the middle of a cable crossover machine. With one hand, hold a handle attached just above your head. Your arm should be extended to your side and slightly above your shoulder, with a slight bend in the elbow (see figure a).

Action and Coaching Tips

Bring your arm across your torso at a slight downward angle while keeping a soft bend in your elbow (see figure b). Slowly reverse the motion until your arm is back out to your side and your elbow is just behind your shoulder. Perform all reps on the same side before switching sides.

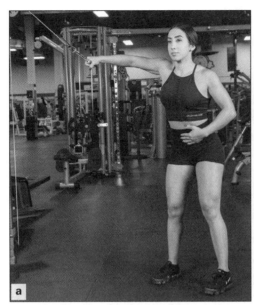
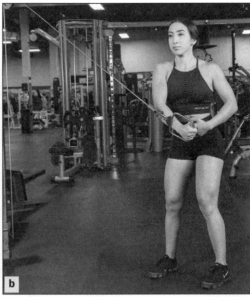

Machine One-Arm Rotated Chest Press

Setup

This exercise requires a specially designed machine that is available in most gyms. The machine allows you to push its handles horizontally away from your body. Sit tall at a 45-degree angle to the machine, with your right side resting against the pad. Hold the handle with your right hand at midchest level, with your elbow directly behind the handle and your arms bent (see figure a). Find a comfortable foot placement that allows you to perform the exercise with proper technique.

Action and Coaching Tips

Without fully locking out your elbow, press the handle so your arm is straight and across your body (see figure b). Slowly reverse the motion, bringing the handle back to the starting position.

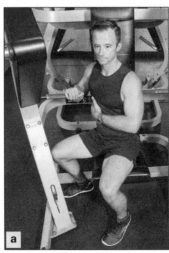
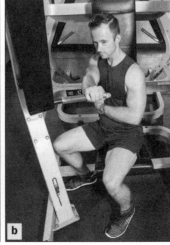

NT Loop One-Arm Pec Deck Fly

You can do this exercise using a superband, but I prefer using an NT Loop, an exercise band I have designed to be more comfortable and stable when it is around the body.

Setup

Stand tall, in either a split stance or a parallel stance, just in front of the middle of a cable crossover machine or next to a resistance band. With one hand, insert your upper forearm into an NT Loop attached to a stable structure or inside a doorjamb (many resistance bands come with an attachment for this) at shoulder level. Extend your arm out to your side, with a 90-degree bend in the elbow (see figure a).

Action and Coaching Tips

Bring your arm across your torso while keeping a soft bend in your elbow (see figure b). Slowly reverse the motion until your arm is back out to your side and your elbow is just behind your shoulder. Perform all reps on the same side before switching sides.

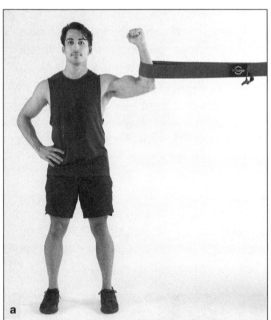
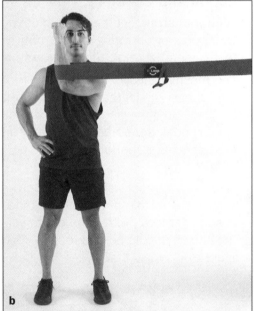

Cable Crossover Pec Fly

Setup

Stand tall, in either a split stance or a parallel stance, just in front of the middle of a cable crossover machine. In each hand, hold the handles attached at shoulder level. Your arms extend out to your sides with a slight bend in the elbows. The cables should be at roughly a 45-degree angle behind you on each side (see figure a).

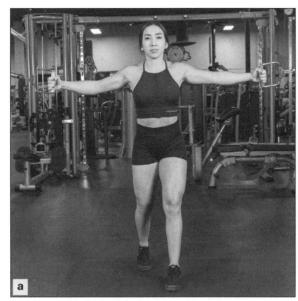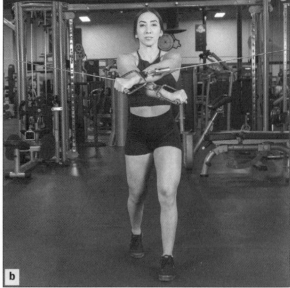

Action and Coaching Tips

Bring your arms together in front of you while keeping a soft bend in your elbows, as if you were hugging a tree, until your hands cross over one another in the center (see figure *b*). Slowly reverse the motion until your arms are back out to your sides and your elbows are just behind your shoulders.

Wide-Cable Crossover Chest Press

Setup

Stand tall in a split stance with your rear heel elevated off the floor and just in front of the middle of a cable crossover machine. Grip the handles in each hand at shoulder level, with arms out to your sides and your elbows bent 90 degrees. The cables should be at a roughly 45-degree angle behind you on each side (see figure *a*).

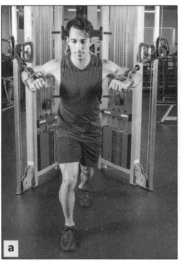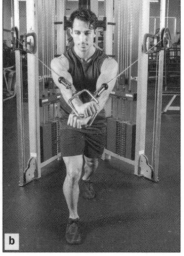

Action and Coaching Tips

Press into the handles by extending your arms toward the midline of your body and crossing your arms over one another at the top of each rep (see figure *b*). Slowly reverse the motion until your arms are back out to your sides and your elbows are bent. Be sure to keep your torso upright and your forearms in line with the angle of the cables throughout.

Machine Pec Fly

The machine pec fly trains your pecs in both strength zones. It is included in this category because it provides a great deal of mechanical tension on your pecs in their shortened-to-midrange strength zone when your arms are more in front of your body. This is the strength zone missed by the majority of the exercises in the Best Chest Exercises in the Lengthened-to-Midrange Strength Zone section.

Setup

This exercise requires a specially designed machine that is available in most gyms. It allows you to push its handles horizontally to the midline of your body. Sit tall, with your back in front of the pad. Hold the handles at shoulder height with a neutral grip, your palms facing forward (see figure *a*). Find a comfortable foot placement that allows you to perform the exercise with proper technique.

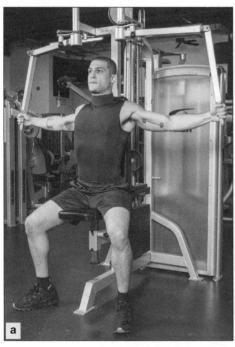 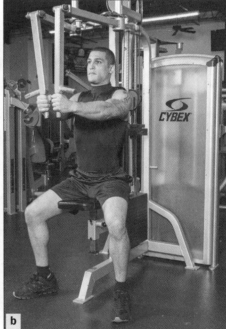

Action and Coaching Tips

Keeping your elbows slightly bent, close your arms in front of your body until the handles touch. Slowly reverse the movement, allowing your hands to go out to the sides of your body (see figure *b*). Be sure to keep a stable spine and minimize overarching in your lower back when performing this exercise.

The best way to complement the development of a chest that is strong through the full range of motion is to do the same for your back. The next chapter provides you with a comprehensive list of the best exercises for lats in each strength zone.

CHAPTER 4

The Best Lats Exercises

Training to develop lat strength through the true full range of motion involves performing at least one exercise for each of the following strength zones:

- Lengthened-to-midrange strength zone: vertical or diagonal pulling with arms outside
- Lengthened-to-midrange strength zone: vertical or diagonal pulling with arms inside
- Shortened-to-midrange strength zone: horizontal pulling

Picking at least one exercise from each category in this list maximizes your workout efficiency and helps you develop full-range back strength.

Lat Exercise Mechanics

Anatomically, the latissimus dorsi is divided into three regions—thoracic, lumbar, and pelvic—based on the anatomical location. Each of these regions produces slightly different contributions during common back exercises.

Vertical or diagonal pulling with your arms outside and with your arms inside train your lats in the lengthened-to-midrange strength zone. Even though both of these arm positions hit the same general strength zone for your lats, it's important to use both because the lumbar and pelvic regions of the lats contribute more to shoulder adduction, which occurs during exercises with the arms outside the torso, such as pull-ups (see figure 4.1a) and lat pull-downs. On the other hand, the thoracic region of the lats contributes more to shoulder extension, which occurs during exercises with the arms inside (i.e., in front) of the torso, such as chin-ups (see figure 4.1b) and neutral-grip lat pull-downs (1, 2).

That said, because different regions of the lats respond differently to vertical pulling from different shoulder positions, it doesn't make sense to look at all vertical pulling exercises as interchangeable. Instead, it makes sense to look at vertical pulling movements as either shoulder adduction (with the arms outside the torso) or shoulder extension (with the arms inside or in front of the torso) and to choose at least one exercise from each category.

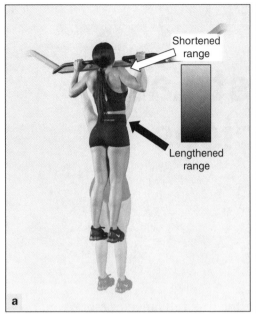
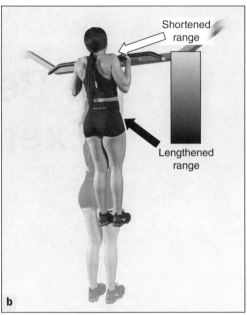

FIGURE 4.1 *(a)* Pull-up in the lengthened-to-midrange strength zone: vertical or diagonal pulling exercise with arms outside and *(b)* chin-up in the lengthened-to-midrange strength zone: vertical or diagonal pulling exercise with arms inside.

It's important to note that the teres major muscle is also involved in vertical pulling exercises. In fact, some coaches and lifters may argue the teres major muscle (a small muscle that also attaches to the scapula and upper-arm bone) is more heavily involved in vertical pulling exercises with the arms outside of the torso than with the arms in front of the torso. That might be the case, although research looking at various lat pulldown grips (both with the arms inside and outside of the torso) found no significant difference in teres major muscle activation among any of the hand positions (3).

Since research is limited, it's important we also use our common sense. For improved functional performance and injury prevention, you want to be stronger in both arm positions. So, it's important to perform vertical pulling exercises using both the arms outside the torso and inside the torso positions, regardless of the levels of contribution the lats and teres major muscles are involved in each movement.

Additionally, the thoracic region of the lats contributes more to horizontal pulling exercises, such as dumbbell rows (see figure 4.2) and seated rows. These train your lats in the shortened-to-midrange strength zone.

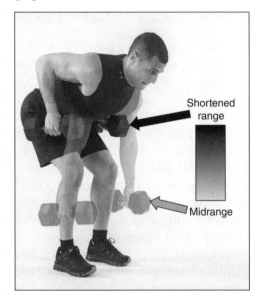

FIGURE 4.2 Dumbbell two-arm bent-over row in the shortened-to-midrange strength zone: horizontal pulling.

Medium or Wide Grip for Lat Pull-Downs?

Despite common belief among many lifters, all grip widths on the pull-down bar will hit your lats, and you can use a medium-width grip to target the biceps more. So find a width that feels most comfortable to you.

Here's why: It's generally believed that a wider grip on the pull-down bar activates the lats more than a narrow one does. This belief originates from bodybuilding dogma, but it also appears to be evidence based. One study found that the wide-grip pull-down produced greater muscle activity than pull-downs using a closer, underhand grip. The problem with this study is that it didn't compare different overhand grip widths (3).

However, another study compared a 6 repetition max (RM) load and muscle activity using three pronated grip widths. Lifters performed 6RM in the lat pull-down with narrow, medium, and wide grips: one, one and a half, and two times the biacromial distance, a measure of shoulder width (4). This study found that, aside from a bit more biceps involvement in the medium grip, all three grips produced similar levels of lat activation. This challenges the notion that a wide grip is best for targeting the lats when doing pull-downs.

You can mix up grip widths to add subtle variety to your lat pull-downs without feeling as if you're missing out on the lat-building benefit of a wide grip. If your objective is to add biceps work while doing lat pull-downs, a medium-width grip is just what the muscle doctor ordered.

Using Band Assistance for Chin-Ups and Pull-Ups

Regardless of whether you're doing chin-ups, pull-ups, or neutral grip pull-ups, you can use assistance to perform the movement with less than your body weight by placing one foot inside a resistance band loop that is anchored between your hand on the bar you are pulling yourself up to. See photos on page 49 for an example of using a resistance band loop for assisted pull-ups.

Best Vertical or Diagonal Pulling Exercises With Arms Outside in the Lengthened-to-Midrange Strength Zone

The vertical and diagonal pulling exercises in this section position your arms outside of your torso to produce shoulder adduction and maximize the strength and development of your lats in the lengthened-to-midrange strength zone.

Pull-Up

Setup
Hang from a pull-up bar using an overhand grip (see figure *a*).

Action and Coaching Tips
Bring yourself up so that your chin rises above the bar (see figure *b*). Don't swing your body. Slowly lower yourself with control.

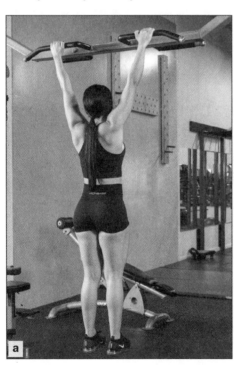 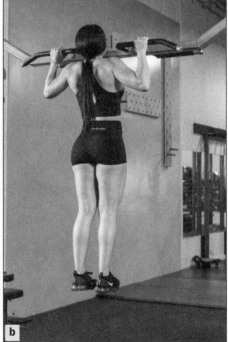

Assisted Pull-Up

Setup
Hang from a pull-up bar using an overhand grip. You can use assistance to perform the movement with less than your body weight by either placing your feet on the platform or by placing one foot inside a looped resistance band that's anchored on the bar you're pulling yourself up to (see figures *a* and *b* for an example using a resistance band).

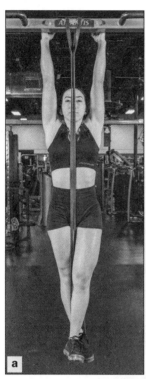
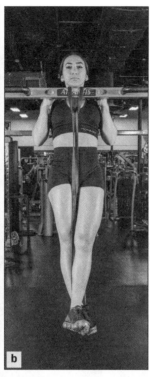

Action and Coaching Tips

Bring yourself up so that your chin rises above the bar (see figure b). Don't swing your body. Slowly lower yourself with control.

Overhand-Grip Lat Pull-Down

Setup

Position yourself just behind a traditional lat pull-down bar and hold it with an overhand grip over your head (see figure a).

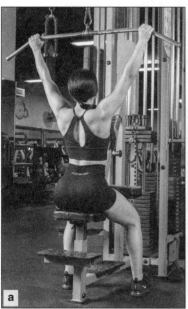
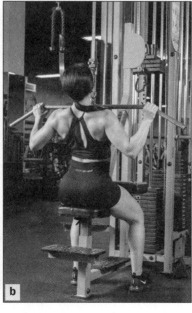

Action and Coaching Tips

Pull the bar down to the top of your chest while keeping your back straight and your elbows following a straight line (see figure b). Slowly reverse the motion, keeping control. You can also add variety to this exercise by performing it using an underhand grip, with your palms facing you and roughly shoulder-width apart.

One-Arm Lat Pull-Down

Setup

Position yourself on the seat, perpendicular to the lat pull-down machine. If the machine is on your left side, hold the handle with your right arm over your head in a neutral grip (see figure *a*).

Action and Coaching Tips

Pull the handle down to your right side while keeping your back straight and your elbow following a straight line (see figure *b*). Slowly reverse the motion, controlling the movement.

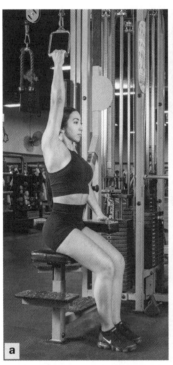
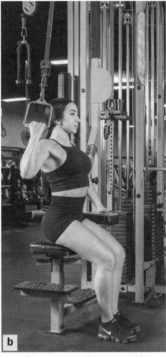

Cable One-Arm Half-Kneeling Lat Pull-Down

Setup

Position yourself in a half-kneeling position so you're perpendicular to a cable column, with the handle attached above your head. If the cable is on your right side, hold the handle with your right hand so your arm and the cable are at a roughly 45-degree angle over your head. You should be 1 to 2 feet (30-60 cm) away from the cable in order to get the proper arm angle (see figure *a*).

Action and Coaching Tips

Pull the handle down to your right side while keeping your back straight and your elbow outside of your torso (see figure *b*). Slowly reverse the motion, controlling the movement.

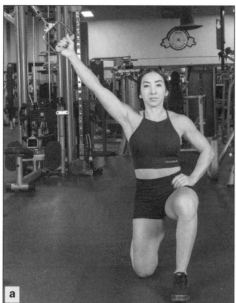
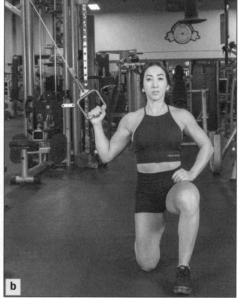

Cable Fighters Lat Pull-Down

I gave this exercise its name simply because the bottom position of the rep is similar to when boxers or kickboxers are blocking a body shot by slightly crunching their torso laterally while having their arm against their side.

Setup

You'll need a dual adjustable cable machine for this exercise. Sit between a set of cables that are above you. Hold a handle in each hand, with your arms straight at an angle roughly 45 degrees to your torso (see figure *a*).

Action and Coaching Tips

Pull one arm toward your body, bringing your elbow all the way down to your hip bone. Combine the pull-down motion with a small side crunch in a motion similar to that of a fighter blocking a body strike (see figure *b*). Reverse the motion in a controlled fashion. Once your arm becomes straight, repeat the action with the other arm (see figure *c*). Do not allow your torso to twist, and keep your forearms perpendicular to the floor throughout.

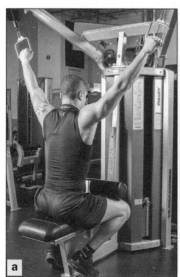
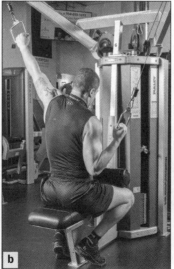
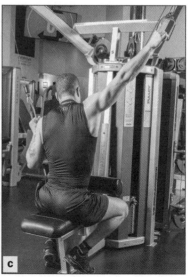

Band Lat Pull-Down

Setup

Stand with your feet shoulder-width apart and face a resistance band that is securely anchored at shoulder level. Hold one handle of the band in each hand and bend over at your hips with a slight bend at your knees, and arms extended above your head toward the anchor point of the band. Your arms should be stretched nearly above your head, forming a straight line between the band, your arms, and your torso (see figure *a*).

Action and Coaching Tips

Pull your arms into your sides the same as you would when using a lat pull-down machine so that your triceps come close to the sides of your body (see figure *b*). Reverse the motion by slowly straightening your arms again to complete one rep. Keep your spine straight and do not round your lower back at any point in this exercise. Maintain a 20-degree knee bend throughout.

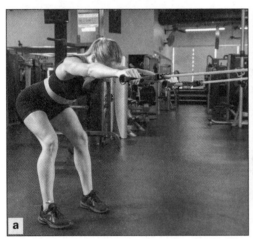 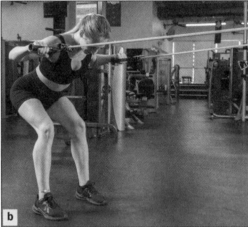

Band One-Arm Lat Pull-Down

Setup

Stand with your feet shoulder-width apart and face a resistance band that is securely anchored at shoulder level. Hold one or both handles of the band in one hand and bend over at your hips with a slight bend at your knees and arm extended above your head toward the anchor point of the band. Your arm should be stretched nearly above your head, forming a straight line between the band, your arm, and your torso (see figure *a*).

Action and Coaching Tips

Pull your arm close to your side the same as you would when using a lat pull-down machine so that your triceps come into contact with the same side of your body (see figure *b*). Reverse the motion by slowly straightening your arm again to complete the rep. Keep your spine straight, and do not round your lower back at any point in this exercise. Maintain a 20-degree knee bend throughout.

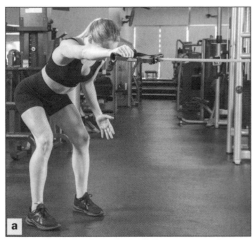
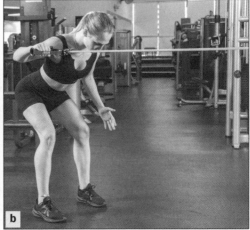

Best Vertical or Diagonal Pulling Exercises With Arms Inside in the Lengthened-to-Midrange Strength Zone

The vertical and diagonal pulling exercises in this section position your arms inside of your torso to produce shoulder extension and help you maximize the strength and development of your lats in the lengthened-to-midrange strength zone.

Chin-Up

Setup

Hang from a pull-up bar using an underhand grip (see figure a). Grip the bar at a width that feels comfortable for you. You can use assistance to perform the movement with less than your body weight by either placing your feet on the platform or by placing one foot inside a looped resistance band that's anchored on the bar you're pulling yourself up to.

Action and Coaching Tips

Bring yourself up so that your chin rises above the bar without swinging your body (see figure b). Pause for a second at the top of each rep before lowering yourself. Slowly lower yourself with control.

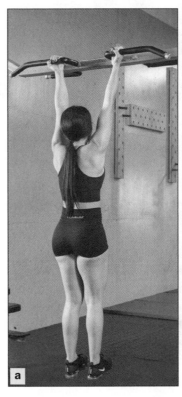
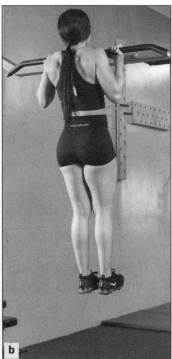

Neutral-Grip Pull-Up

Setup

Hang from a pull-up bar using a neutral grip that places your hands about shoulder-width apart (see figure *a*). You can use assistance to perform the movement with less than your body weight by either placing your feet on the platform or by placing one foot inside a looped resistance band that's anchored on the bar you're pulling yourself up to.

Action and Coaching Tips

Bring yourself up so that your chin rises above the handles without swinging your body (see figure *b*). Pause for a second at the top of each rep before lowering yourself. Slowly lower yourself with control.

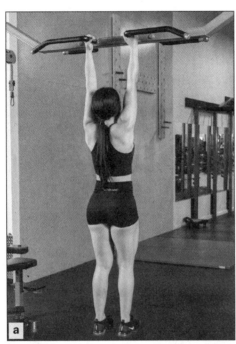 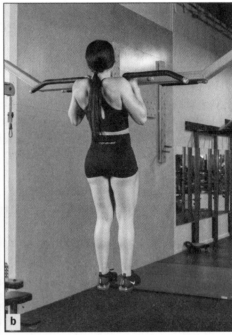

Neutral-Grip Lat Pull-Down

Setup

Position yourself just behind neutral-grip handles that are attached to the lat pull-down machine. Hold the handles so your arms are about shoulder-width apart over your head (see figure *a*).

Action and Coaching Tips

Pull the handles down to the top of your chest while keeping your back straight and your elbows following a straight line (see figure *b*). Slowly reverse the motion, controlling the movement.

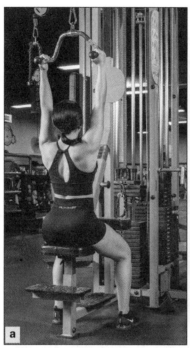
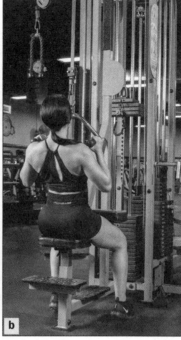

Underhand-Grip Lat Pull-Down

Setup

Position yourself just behind a traditional lat pull-down bar and hold it over your head with an underhand grip (see figure *a*).

Action and Coaching Tips

Pull the bar down to the top of your chest while keeping your back straight and your elbows following a straight line (see figure *b*). Slowly reverse the motion, keeping control.

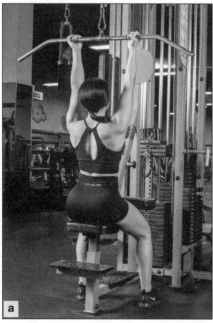
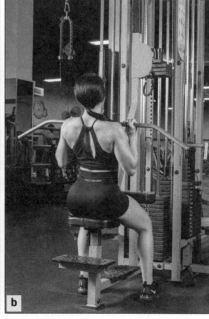

Neutral-Grip One-Arm Lat Pull-Down

Setup

Position yourself on the seat perpendicular to the lat pull-down machine. Position one of your shoulders directly under the handle. Grab the handle with the hand on the side that is directly above your shoulder, with the arm over your head in a neutral grip (see figure *a*).

Action and Coaching Tips

Pull the handle straight down in front of your same side while keeping your back straight and your elbow following a straight line with the cable (see figure *b*). Slowly reverse the motion, controlling the movement until your arm is straight above your head again to complete the rep.

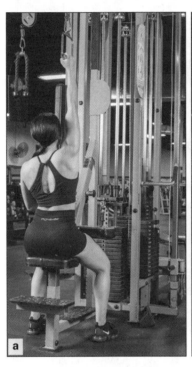 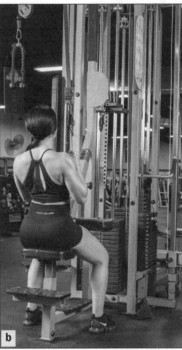

Cable One-Arm Half-Kneeling Neutral-Grip Lat Pull-Down

Setup

From a half-kneeling position, face a cable column with the handle attached above your head. Grip the handle so your same-side shoulder is directly in line with the origin of the cable. Lean your torso forward so your arm and torso form a straight line with the cable. You should be 1 to 2 feet (30-60 cm) away from the cable to get the proper arm angle (see figure *a*).

Action and Coaching Tips

Pull the handle down, keeping your arm in front of your same-side shoulder (see figure *b*). Slowly reverse the motion, controlling the movement.

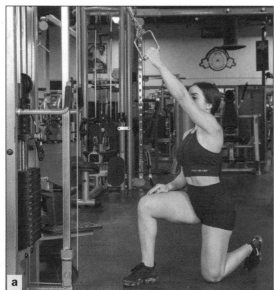
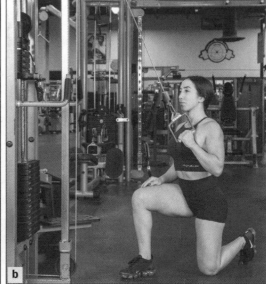

Cable Straight-Arm Compound Pull-Down

This is a hybrid exercise that could be listed in the shortened-to-midrange strength zone: horizontal pulling category because of the challenge it provides when your arms are at your sides at the bottom of each rep. It's listed here as a vertical pulling movement in the lengthened-to-midrange strength zone: vertical or diagonal pulling with arms inside category because it also provides a significant challenge when your arms are overhead.

Setup

Stand facing an adjustable cable column with your feet about hip-width apart and a rope attached to a cable column above your head at eye level. Hold one end of the rope in each hand with your palms facing one another. With a slight bend at your knees and your arms extended above your head, hinge at your hips (see figure a).

Action and Coaching Tips

At the same time you raise your torso to an upright position, pull the rope down, keeping a slight bend in your elbows, until the handles touch just outside of your hips (see figure b). Do not round your shoulders forward at the top of each repetition. Slowly reverse the motion, hinging at your hips and reaching your arms back above your head; use a controlled rhythm. Perform the exercise smoothly, with your arms lowering as your torso rises and vice versa.

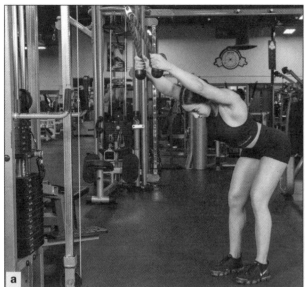 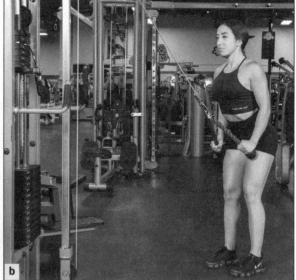

Band Neutral-Grip Lat Pull-Down

Setup

Stand with your feet shoulder-width apart and face a resistance band that is securely anchored at shoulder level. Hold one handle of the band in each hand and bend over at your hips with a slight bend at your knees. Your arms should be extended nearly above your head toward the anchor point of the band, forming a straight line between the band, your arms, and your torso (see figure a).

Action and Coaching Tips

Pull your arms in to your sides the same as you would when using a lat pull-down machine so that your triceps come into contact with the side of your ribs (see figure b). Reverse the motion by slowly straightening your arms again to complete the rep. Keep your spine straight, and do not round your lower back at any point in this exercise. Maintain a 20-degree knee bend throughout.

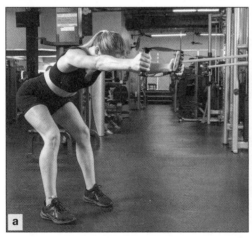 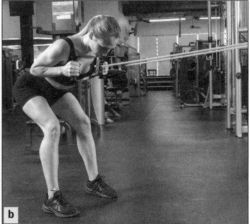

Band One-Arm Neutral-Grip Lat Pull-Down

Setup

Stand with your feet shoulder-width apart in a staggered stance and face a resistance band that is securely anchored at shoulder level. Hold one or both handles of the band in one hand and bend over at your hips with a slight bend at your knees and arm extended toward the anchor point of the band. Your arm should be stretched above your head, level with your shoulder, forming a line between the band, your arm, and your torso (see figure a).

Action and Coaching Tips

Pull your arm into your body the same as you would when using a lat pull-down machine so that your triceps come into contact with the side of your ribs (see figure b). Reverse the motion by slowly straightening your arm again to complete the rep. Keep your spine straight, and do not round your lower back at any point in this exercise. Maintain a 20-degree knee bend throughout.

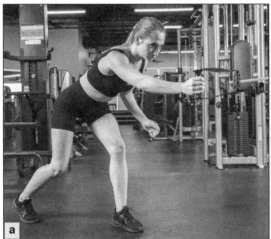 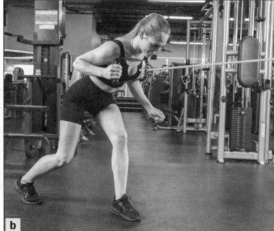

Best Horizontal Pulling Exercises in the Shortened-to-Midrange Strength Zone

The horizontal pulling exercises in this section help you maximize the strength and development of your lats in the shortened-to-midrange strength zone.

Barbell Bent-Over Row

Setup

Stand with your feet about hip-width apart. Hold a barbell with an underhand grip that is just wider than shoulder width. You can also perform bent-over rows with an overhand grip; however, many people find this to be a weaker gripping option. Bend over at your hips, keeping your back straight so that your torso is parallel to the floor (see figure a). Keep your knees bent 15 to 20 degrees.

Action and Coaching Tips

Row the bar into your body, just above your belly button (see figure *b*). Pause for a second and pinch your shoulder blades together at the top. Do not allow the fronts of your shoulders to round forward at the top of each repetition. Slowly lower the bar to complete the rep. Do not allow your back to round at any time.

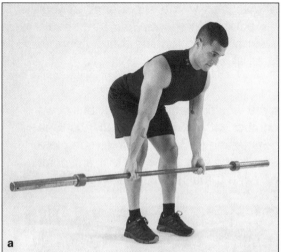
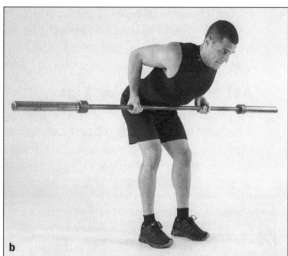

Dumbbell Two-Arm Bent-Over Row

Setup

Stand with your feet hip-width apart and hold a dumbbell in each hand. Bend over at your hips, keeping your back straight so that your torso is parallel to the floor (see figure *a*). Keep your knees bent 15 to 20 degrees.

Action and Coaching Tips

Row the dumbbells toward you while keeping your arms at a 45-degree angle to your torso; at the top, pinch your shoulder blades together (see figure *b*). Pause for a second at the top of each repetition. Slowly lower the dumbbells without allowing them to contact the floor until the set is completed. Do not allow your back to round at any time. At the top of each repetition, do not allow your wrists to bend or the fronts of your shoulders to round forward.

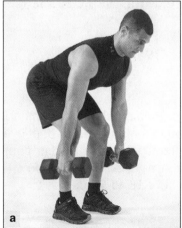
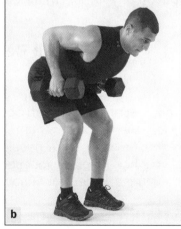

Dumbbell One-Arm Bench Row

Setup

Stand parallel to a traditional weight bench with your right hand and right knee on the bench and a dumbbell in your left hand using a neutral grip. Your left foot is on the floor, and the left knee is slightly bent. Keep a straight back that is roughly parallel to the floor. Rotate your torso slightly to the left so that your left shoulder—the same side you're holding the dumbbell on—is slightly below the level of your right shoulder (see figure a).

Action and Coaching Tips

While keeping your left shoulder slightly below the level of your right shoulder, perform the row by pulling the dumbbell toward your body so that your left elbow is at a roughly 90-degree angle (see figure b) while you drive your right shoulder blade toward your spine. Do not allow your rowing-side shoulder to move forward at the top of each rep. Slowly lower the dumbbell toward the floor until your arm straightens without allowing the dumbbell to touch the floor.

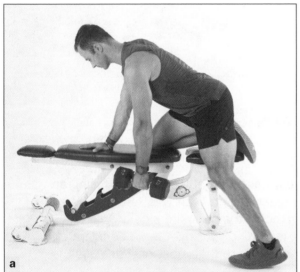 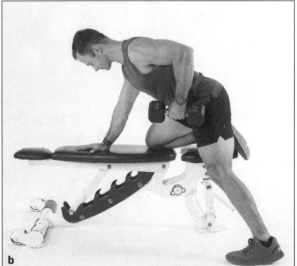

Dumbbell One-Arm Off-Bench Row

Setup

Stand perpendicular to a traditional weight bench, with your right hand on top of the bench and a dumbbell in your left hand using a neutral grip. Keep a straight back that is roughly parallel to the floor. Stand in a slightly staggered stance, with your left leg behind your right leg (see figure a). You can also stand in a parallel stance with your feet hip-width apart and your knees slightly bent.

Action and Coaching Tips

Perform the row by pulling the dumbbell toward your body so that your left elbow is at a roughly 90-degree angle while you drive your left shoulder blade toward your spine (see figure *b*). Do not allow your rowing-side shoulder to move forward at the end of each rep. Slowly lower the dumbbell toward the floor until your arm straightens, but don't allow the dumbbell to touch the floor. Repeat all reps on the same side before switching sides.

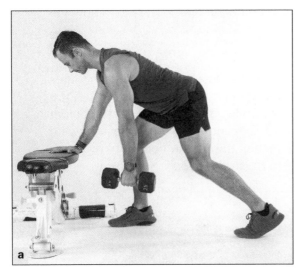 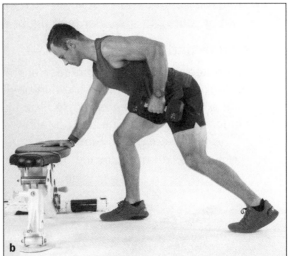

Cable One-Arm Row

Setup

Stand tall, with your spine straight and your knees slightly bent while facing an adjustable cable column set to about shoulder height. With your left hand, grab the handle in a neutral grip (i.e., your palm facing the opposite side of your body) and split your stance so that your left leg is behind your right leg (see figure *a*). Keep your back heel raised off the ground to ensure that most of your weight is on your front leg.

Action and Coaching Tips

Perform a row by pulling the cable toward your body, driving your shoulder blade back so that it's retracted at the end of the row (see figure *b*). Do not allow your rowing-side shoulder to move forward at the end of each rep. Maintain a stable spine, and keep your shoulders and hips from rotating more than a few degrees. Slowly reverse the motion by allowing your scapula to protract while your arm straightens. Perform all reps on one side before switching to the other side.

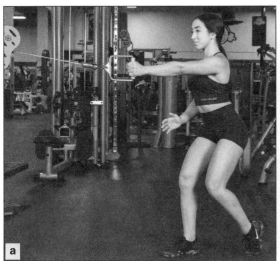

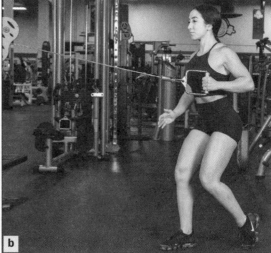

Cable One-Arm Compound Row

Although this hybrid exercise begins more like a vertical pulling movement with the arm inside, the majority of the exercise is more similar to a horizontal pulling movement, so it's listed in this category.

Setup

Stand facing an adjustable cable column that's set at midtorso level. Keep your feet about shoulder-width apart in a split stance, with your right leg in front and your knees slightly bent. Hold the handle in your left hand using a neutral grip (i.e., your palm facing the opposite side of your body). Keep your back heel raised off the ground to ensure that most of your weight is on your front leg (see figure *a*).

Action and Coaching Tips

Hinge at your hips, reaching your right arm in front of you toward the origin of the cable (see figure *b*). Do not allow your rowing-side shoulder to move forward at the end of each rep. Reverse this motion while performing a row. Finish the row as you return to the upright standing position. Slowly reverse the motion, hinging at your hips and reaching out; use a controlled rhythm. Perform all reps on one side before switching to the other side.

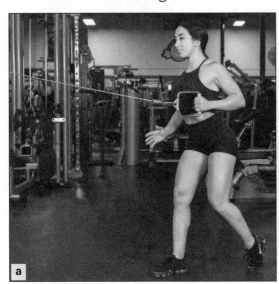

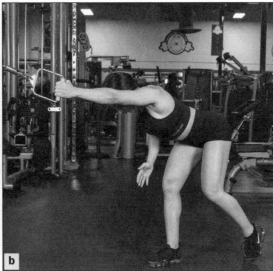

Seated Row

Setup

Sit on a cable row bench with your feet firmly planted on the foot plate. Grab the neutral-grip handle attached to the cable pulley, with your hands about shoulder-width apart. Keep your knees slightly bent and your back straight. Maintain a slight arch in your lower back and keep your chest out (see figure a).

Action and Coaching Tips

Pull the handle toward your midsection, focusing on driving your elbows back until the handle touches your lower abdomen (see figure b). Do not allow the front of your shoulders to round forward at the end of each repetition. After squeezing your shoulder blades together at the peak of the contraction, slowly return to the starting position.

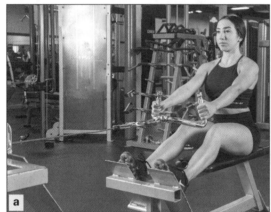
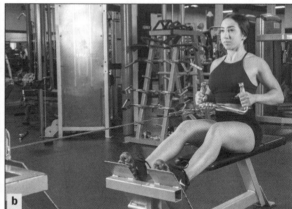

Machine Row

Setup

This exercise requires a specially designed machine that is available in most gyms. It allows you to pull its handles horizontally into your body. Sit tall, with your chest in front of the pad. Hold the handles at shoulder height using a neutral, overhand, or underhand grip, depending on the gripping options the machine allows (see figure a for an example using the neutral grip). Find a comfortable foot placement that allows you to perform the exercise with proper technique.

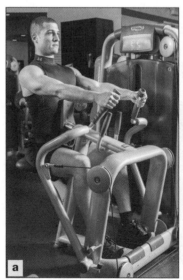
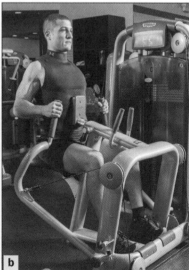

Action and Coaching Tips

Row the handles into your body, pinching your shoulder blades together at the top and without allowing the fronts of your shoulders to round forward (see figure b). Slowly reverse the motion until your elbows are straight to complete the rep.

Suspension Trainer Row

Setup

Using a suspension trainer, face the anchor point and hold on to the handles with your palms either facing each other or facing the sky and with your arms extended straight in front of your shoulders (see figure *a* for an example with the palms facing each other). Lean back with your body in a straight line from head to toe.

Action and Coaching Tips

Pull yourself up toward your hands by bending at your elbows. Keep your elbows tight to your sides and perform a rowing motion until the insides of your wrists are close to your bottom ribs, thus ensuring a full range of motion (see figure *b*). Pause at the top for a second, then slowly lower yourself until your elbows are straight. Keep your body in a straight line and do not lead with your hips when pulling yourself up. Do not allow your wrists to bend as you pull yourself up; keep your elbows directly behind your hands throughout. Do not allow the fronts of your shoulders to round forward at the end of each repetition.

To increase the difficulty, start the exercise from a more severe backward lean, bringing your body closer to the floor.

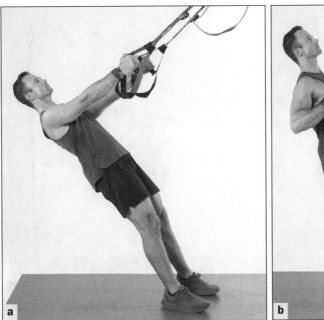
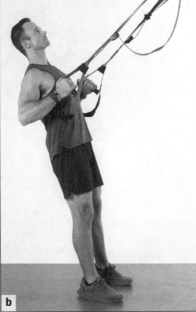

One-Arm Anti-Rotation Suspension Row

Setup

Face the anchor point of a suspension trainer and hold a handle in your right hand. Lean back, away from the anchor point, with your body forming a straight line and hold your left arm at a 90-degree angle by your side (see figure *a*).

Action and Coaching Tips

Without allowing your body to rotate at any point, perform rows by pulling your body toward the handle (see figure *b*) and going back down. Each time you pull yourself toward the handle, keep your elbow (on the rowing side) tight to your body. Keep your body in a straight line throughout; keep your shoulders and hips parallel to the floor, and do not allow your hips to sag toward the floor.

To increase the difficulty, walk your feet further in toward the anchor point to increase your body angle and bring you lower. To decrease the difficulty, decrease your body angle by walking your feet further away from the anchor point so that they're more under you.

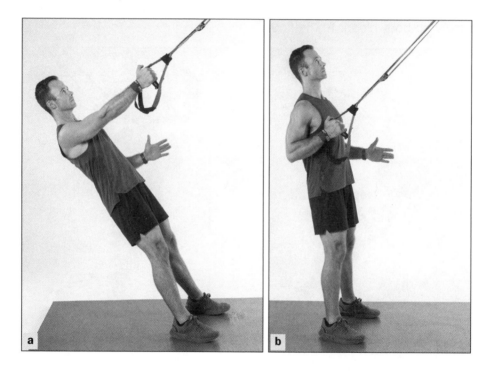

Now it's time to look at the best exercises for the shoulders. These will complement your chest and back exercises.

CHAPTER 5

The Best Shoulder Exercises

Training to develop shoulder strength through the true full range of motion involves performing at least one exercise for each of the following strength zones:

- Shortened-to-midrange strength zone: middle-delt exercise
- Lengthened-to-midrange strength zone: middle-delt exercise
- Shortened-to-midrange strength zone: rear-delt exercise
- Lengthened-to-midrange strength zone: rear-delt exercise

Picking at least one exercise from each category in this list maximizes your workout efficiency and helps you develop full-range shoulder strength.

Shoulder Exercise Mechanics

During any style of shoulder (overhead) press or side shoulder raise, the point that places the most mechanical tension on the muscles is when the lever arm is at its longest. This occurs when your humerus (bone in the upper arm) is at a 90-degree angle with the line of force (see figure 5.1).

If you're using free weights, gravity is your line of force. Therefore, the point of maximal mechanical tension on your shoulders during an overhead press or a side shoulder raise or rear-delt fly is when your humerus is parallel to the floor.

This is important to understand because not only do side-shoulder raises with a dumbbell and overhead presses with a dumbbell, barbell, or machine both involve shoulder

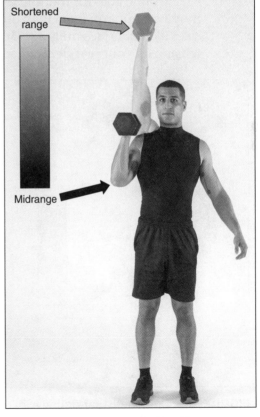

FIGURE 5.1 Dumbbell one-arm overhead press in the shortened-to-midrange strength zone: middle-delt exercise.

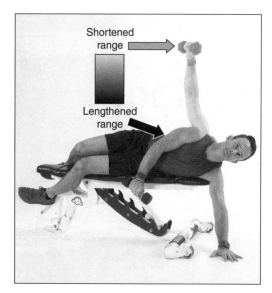

FIGURE 5.2 Dumbbell side-lying side shoulder raise in the lengthened-to-midrange strength zone: middle-delt exercise.

abduction (i.e., moving your arms upward while they are out to the side of your torso), but they also create the most mechanical tension on the shoulders when the humerus is parallel to the ground. For this reason, both exercises train in the same strength zone, which is in the shortened-to-midrange strength zone of shoulder abduction. So they load, and therefore strengthen, your shoulders in the same way, which makes doing both of them redundant.

The reason you can use much more weight when doing a dumbbell or barbell overhead press is because it allows the triceps to contribute. The weight is also much closer to your shoulder joints, which gives your shoulders a much better mechanical advantage.

That said, exercises like the cable side shoulder raise or dumbbell side-lying side shoulder raise (see figure 5.2) don't duplicate the action of the overhead presses because they load the shoulders in the lengthened-to-midrange strength zone of shoulder abduction, which the overhead press misses.

The same goes for training the motion of horizontal shoulder abduction (i.e., moving your arm from in to out while it is perpendicular to your torso). Exercises like cable face pulls and dumbbell rear-delt flys place the most mechanical tension on your rear delts when they're in the shortened-to-midrange strength

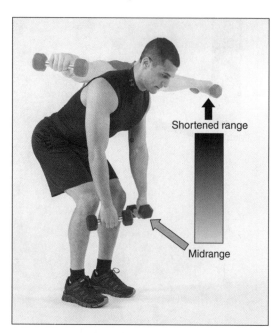

FIGURE 5.3 Dumbbell rear-delt fly in the shortened-to-midrange strength zone: rear-delt exercise.

zone when your arm is out to the side of your torso (see figure 5.3). On the flipside, when performing the dumbbell side-lying rear-delt fly, the situation is reversed. That exercise places the most mechanical tension on the involved muscles when your arm is extended in front of your torso, but it doesn't strengthen your rear delts and the rest of your posterior shoulder musculature when your arm is out to the side of your torso (see figure 5.4). So you need to do both exercises to achieve strength in your rear delts through the true full range of motion of horizontal shoulder adduction.

With that in mind, exercises like cable rope face pulls and dumbbell rear-delt flys do a great job of training your rear delts in their shortened-to-midrange strength zone of horizontal shoulder abduction, but they neglect to strengthen the aspect of horizontal shoulder abduction when your arm is in

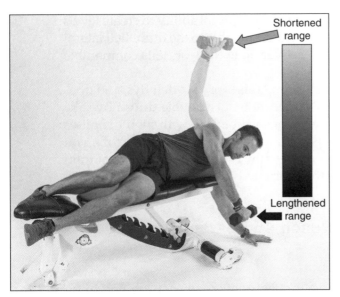

Shortened range

Lengthened range

FIGURE 5.4 Dumbbell side-lying rear delt fly in the length-ened-to-midrange strength zone: rear-delt exercise.

front of or across your torso, which is in the lengthened-to-midrange zone of your rear delts. This is where exercises such as cable rear-delt flys and dumbbell side-lying rear-delt flys are useful. They train you in the strength zone (the range of motion) neglected by the exercises in the shortened-to-midrange strength zone of horizontal shoulder adduction to create true full range of motion strength in your rear delts.

Redundant Exercises You Just Don't Need: Front-Delt Raises

Research on muscle activation shows that the front delts are stimulated during horizontal presses, stimulated to a higher degree during incline presses, and stimulated to an even higher degree during vertical (overhead) presses (1). In practical terms, you don't need to do exercises like dumbbell front raises if you're already doing compound pressing exercises at different angles by doing the horizontal or decline pressing exercises and incline pressing exercises described in chapter 3. Especially if you're also doing overhead pressing exercises, which are highlighted in this chapter for the middle delts in the shortened-to-midrange strength zone.

In other words, your front delts are being strengthened with overhead pressing, along with diagonal and horizontal pressing, even though these exercises are categorized in the book under different muscle groups. Your shoulder workout will be less redundant if you complement your compound pressing exercises from chapter 3 with shoulder exercises that target the middle and rear delts, which is what the exercises for each of the strength zones in this chapter accomplish.

Double-Duty Shoulder Exercises Your Upper Body Needs

A variety of exercises are needed to effectively train your shoulders. Presses, raises, reverse fly variations—they're all great and contribute in their own ways to building healthy, balanced shoulders that are full-range strong.

That said, a single move can build strength in both of these strength zones:

- Middle delts in the shortened-to-midrange strength zone
- Rear delts in the shortened-to-midrange strength zone

I'm talking about the 45-degree row.

Research has shown that the 45-degree row has a special ability to create levels of muscle activation in the middle delts that's comparable to the dumbbell lateral raise while also creating levels of muscle activation in the rear delts comparable to the dumbbell rear-delt fly (2).

Does this make it better than dumbbell lateral raises or rear-delt flys, and does it mean you should quit doing them? Absolutely not. But a double-duty move like the 45-degree row definitely can be rotated in or swapped out with shoulder raises and rear-delt flys. In addition to exercises for each strength zone category, you will find in this section the top three 45-degree row exercise variations that train both the middle delts and rear delts in the shortened-to-midrange strength zone.

Dumbbell Incline Bench 45-Degree Row

Setup

Position yourself facing the floor with your chest resting against the pad of an incline bench set to a roughly 45-degree angle. Hold a dumbbell in each hand with your arms straight below your shoulders and your palms facing your feet (see figure a). Most people perform these sitting on the seat, which forces them to bury their face in the bench pad. I don't recommend it. Instead, place your knees on the seat, which is far more comfortable and keeps your face above the bench.

Action and Coaching Tips

Pull your arms up and out to the sides of your torso so your elbows form a 90-degree angle to your torso at the top of each repetition (see figure b). Keep your elbows directly behind your hands throughout the rep. Put another way, don't allow your wrists to bend as you pull the weight up.

Pause for a second at the top of each rep without allowing the front of your shoulders to round forward. Slowly lower the weight until your arms are once again straight to complete the rep. Do not allow your back to round at any time.

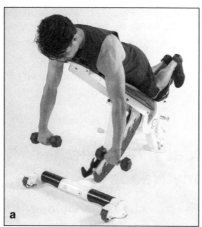 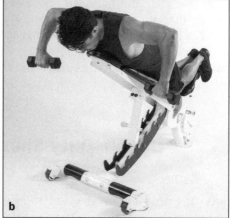

Dumbbell 45-Degree Row

Setup

With your feet roughly shoulder-width apart and your knees slightly bent, stand with your torso at a 45-degree angle to the floor. Hold a dumbbell in each hand with your arms straight below your shoulders and your palms facing your feet (see figure a).

Action and Coaching Tips

Pull your arms up and out to the sides of your torso, so your elbows form a 90-degree angle to your torso at the top of each repetition. Keep your elbows directly behind your hands throughout the rep (see figure b). Put another way, don't allow your wrists to bend as you pull the weight up.

Pause for a second at the top of each rep without allowing the front of your shoulders to round forward. Slowly lower the weight until your arms are once again straight to complete the rep. Do not allow your back to round at any time.

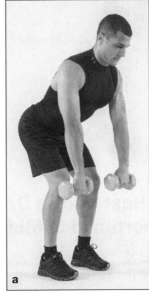 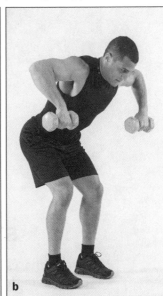

Barbell 45-Degree Row

Setup

With your feet roughly shoulder-width apart and your knees slightly bent, stand with your torso at a 45-degree angle to the floor. Hold a barbell using a wide grip with your hands placed about 5 inches (13 cm) outside of your shoulders (see figure a). Your arms should be straight and directly below your shoulders.

Action and Coaching Tips

Pull your arms up and out to the sides of your torso so your elbows form a 90-degree angle to your torso at the top of each repetition (see figure b). Keep your elbows directly behind your hands throughout the rep. Put another way, don't allow your wrists to bend as you pull the weight up.

Pause for a second at the top of each rep without allowing the front of your shoulders to round forward. Slowly lower the weight until your arms are once again straight to complete the rep. Do not allow your back to round at any time.

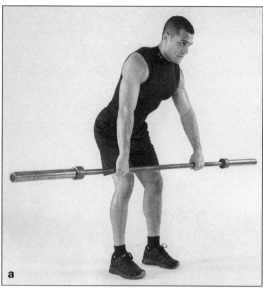

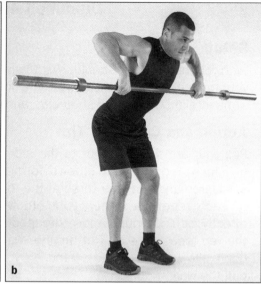

Best Middle-Delt Exercises in the Shortened-to-Midrange Strength Zone

The exercises in this section help you maximize the strength and development of your middle (lateral) deltoids in the shortened-to-midrange strength zone. The overhead pressing exercises in this section also are effective at strengthening your front (anterior) deltoids.

Dumbbell Side Shoulder Raise

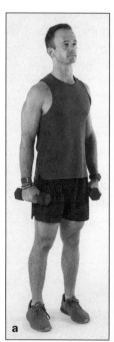 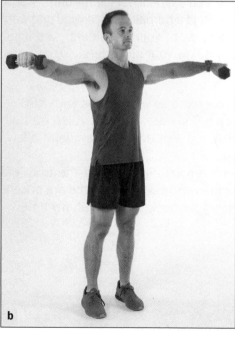

Setup

Stand tall, with your feet hip-width apart. Hold a pair of dumbbells at your sides (see figure a).

Action and Coaching Tips

With your elbows slightly bent, raise your arms out to the sides at a roughly 30-degree angle in front of your torso until your elbows rise just above your armpits (see figure b). Do not swing the weight up. Slowly lower the dumbbells to your sides. Use deliberate control on the lifting and lowering portion of each rep.

Kettlebell Shoulder-to-Shoulder Press

Setup

Stand tall with your feet parallel to one another and roughly shoulder-width apart. Hold on to the round part of a kettlebell with both hands and with your thumbs inside the handle above one shoulder (see figure a-b).

Action and Coaching Tips

Press the kettlebell overhead so that when your arms reach full extension, the kettlebell is directly in line with the center of your body (see figure c). Slowly reverse the motion and lower the kettlebell to your opposite shoulder (see figure d). Press it up again so that it ends up in the middle of your body, then lower it to the other shoulder to complete 1 rep. Do not allow your shoulders or hips to rotate. Do not allow your torso to bend to the side; maintain your upright torso position throughout.

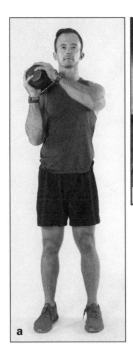
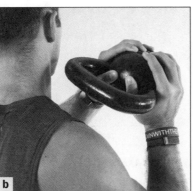
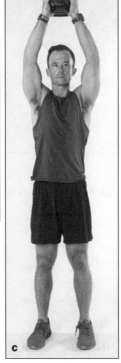
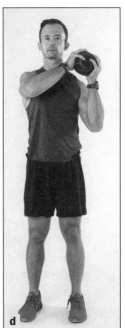

Dumbbell Rotational Overhead Press

Setup

Stand tall with your feet roughly shoulder-width apart. Hold a dumbbell in front of each shoulder (see figure a).

Action and Coaching Tips

Press one dumbbell into the air directly over your same-side shoulder as you rotate to the opposite side (see figure b). To better allow your hips to rotate, raise your heel off the ground as you turn. Lower the dumbbell in a smooth, controlled manner as you bring your torso back so it faces straight ahead. Then turn to the opposite side to perform the rep with the other arm to complete 1 rep (see figure *c*).

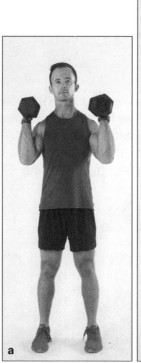
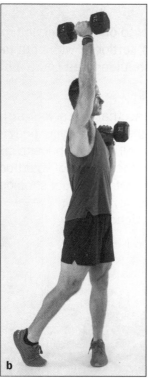
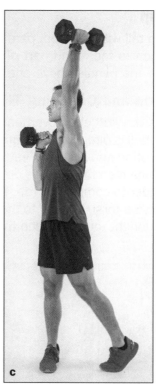

Dumbbell One-Arm Overhead Press

Setup

Stand tall with your feet shoulder-width apart. Hold a dumbbell at a roughly 45-degree angle in front of one shoulder (see figure *a*).

Action and Coaching Tips

Press the dumbbell into the air directly over your same-side shoulder, keeping your arm at a roughly 45-degree angle to your torso (see figure *b*). Lower the dumbbell smoothly and with control. Be sure to keep your wrist straight and your elbow directly under your wrist throughout each rep. Perform all reps on the same side before switching sides.

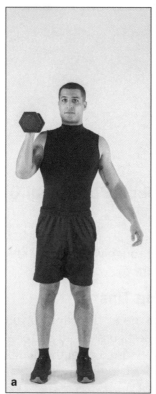
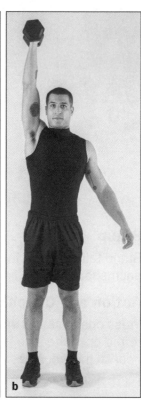

Machine Overhead Press

Setup

This exercise requires a specially designed machine that is available in most gyms. It allows you to push its handles vertically above your body. Sit tall with your back against the pad. Hold the handles at roughly shoulder level, with your elbows directly under the handles and your elbows bent (see figure *a*). Find a comfortable foot placement that allows you to perform the exercise with proper technique.

Action and Coaching Tips

Press the handles directly overhead until your arms are almost straight (see figure *b*). Slowly reverse the motion, lowering the handles to the starting position outside your shoulders. At the bottom of each repetition, your forearms should remain perpendicular to the floor. Do not allow your wrists to bend backward at any time.

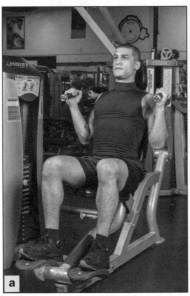 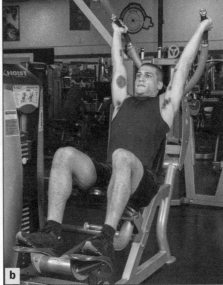

Best Middle-Delt Exercises in the Lengthened-to-Midrange Strength Zone

The exercises in this section help you maximize the strength and development of your middle (lateral) delts in the lengthened-to-midrange strength zone.

Cable Side Shoulder Raise

Setup

Stand tall, with your feet roughly hip-width apart next to a cable column. The handle is attached at your midshin-to-knee level. Grab the handle with your hand furthest away from the machine and move a few feet (about 60 cm) away from the cable to allow the arm that's holding the handle to reach across your body toward the cable's origin (see figure *a*). Your elbow should be slightly bent.

Action and Coaching Tips

Keeping your elbow slightly bent, raise your arm to the side at a roughly 30-degree angle in front of your torso until your elbow is just above your shoulder (see figure *b*). Do not overextend at your lower back or bend your torso to the side to raise the weight. Slowly lower the handle down and across your body to complete the rep. Perform all reps on the same side before switching sides.

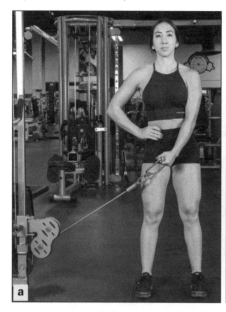
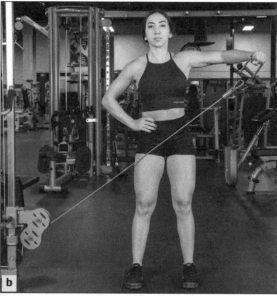

Dumbbell Side-Lying Side Shoulder Raise

Setup

Lie sideways on a flat bench or on the floor with your legs on either side of the bench or flat on the floor. Hold a dumbbell just in front of your bottom hip, with your elbow slightly bent. Place your other hand flat on the floor to support you (figure *a*).

Action and Coaching Tips

Keeping your elbow slightly bent, raise your arm toward the sky. Your arm moves out to the side of your torso until your elbow is just above your shoulder (see figure *b*). Slowly lower the dumbbell down and across your body to complete the rep. Do not allow the dumbbell to rest against your body, on the bench, or on the floor at the bottom of each rep. Perform all reps on the same side before switching sides.

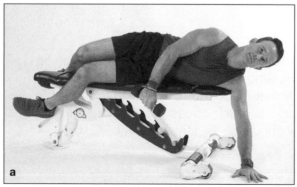
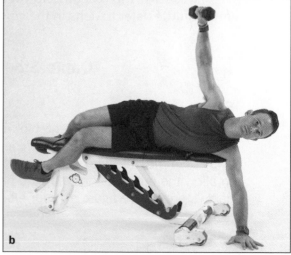

NT Loop Side Shoulder Raise

This exercise trains your middle deltoids in both the lengthened-to-midrange and the shortened-to-midrange strength zones. It's included in this section because it creates a significant challenge on the middle deltoids when the arms are by your sides, which is in the lengthened-to-midrange strength zone. This strength zone is missed by many of the middle deltoid exercises provided in the shortened-to-midrange strength zone category.

Setup

Stand tall with your feet roughly hip-width apart inside an NT Loop to securely anchor it; at your midshin-to-knee level cross over the NT Loop. Place your forearms inside the NT Loop so it's just below your elbows. Keep your elbows at a 90-degree angle by your side (see figure a).

Action and Coaching Tips

Keeping your elbows bent to 90 degrees, raise your arms until your elbows are just below your shoulders (see figure b). Do not overextend your lower back or bend your torso to the side to raise the weight. Slowly lower your arms to your sides to complete the rep.

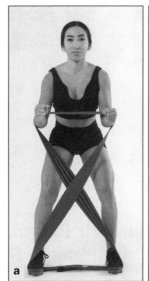
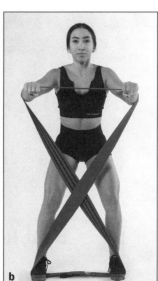

NT Loop Mini Side Shoulder Raise

You can perform this exercise with a regular rubber miniband, but I prefer using an NT Loop Mini, an exercise band I have designed to be more comfortable and stable when it is around the body.

This exercise trains your middle deltoids in both the lengthened-to-midrange and the shortened-to-midrange strength zones. It's included in this section because it creates a significant challenge on the middle deltoids when the arms are by your sides, which is in the lengthened-to-midrange strength zone. This strength zone is missed by many of the middle deltoid exercises provided in the shortened-to-midrange strength zone category.

Setup

Stand tall with your feet roughly hip-width apart and your arms inside the NT Loop Mini that is just below your elbow. Keep your elbows bent to 90 degrees and your arms at your sides (see figure a).

Action and Coaching Tips

Keeping your elbows bent to 90 degrees, raise one arm to the side of your torso until your elbow is roughly even with your shoulders (see figure b). Slowly lower your arm to your side to complete the rep. Alternate arms on each rep, so one arm is working isometrically (holding still against the resistance) while the other arm is moving against the resistance (see figure c).

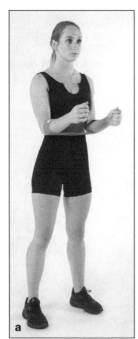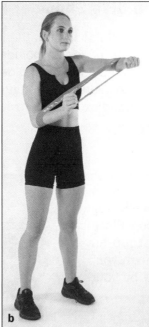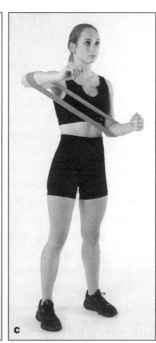

Best Rear-Delt Exercises in the Shortened-to-Midrange Strength Zone

The exercises in this section help you maximize the strength and development of your rear (posterior) deltoids in the shortened-to-midrange strength zone.

Dumbbell Rear-Delt Fly

Setup

Stand with your feet hip-width apart and hold a dumbbell in each hand. Bend forward at your hips, keeping your back straight so that your torso is roughly parallel to the floor and your knees are bent 15 to 20 degrees (see figure a).

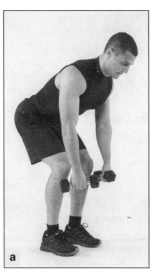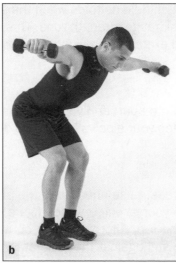

Action and Coaching Tips

Keeping a small bend in your elbows, raise your arms out to your sides (see figure b). Your arms should be at a 90-degree angle relative to your torso at the top of each repetition, thus forming a T shape with your torso at the top of each rep. Do not swing the dumbbells up. Pause for a second at the top of each repetition and pinch your shoulder blades together, then slowly lower the dumbbells in front of your torso. Do not allow your back to round at any time.

Dumbbell Face Pull

Setup

With your feet roughly shoulder-width apart and your knees slightly bent, stand with your torso at a 45-degree angle to the floor. Hold a dumbbell in each hand, with your arms straight below your shoulder and your palm facing your knees (see figure a).

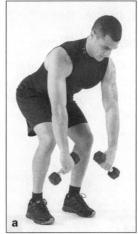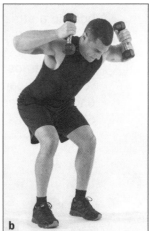

Action and Coaching Tips

Pull the dumbbells toward your face as you drive your arms apart so that your hands are just outside your ears and the dumbbells are perpendicular to the floor (see figure b). Slowly reverse the movement back to the starting position until your arms once again straighten to complete the rep. Do not jolt the weight up or overarch your lower back. Your elbows should be as high as your shoulders at the top of each repetition.

Cable Rope Face Pull

Setup

Stand in front of an adjustable cable column with a rope attached at or above your eye level. Hold one end of the rope in each hand, your palms facing down, and your elbows pointed out to the sides (see figure a).

Action and Coaching Tips

Pull the rope toward your face, without overarching your lower back, as you drive your arms apart so that your hands are just outside your ears (see figure b). At

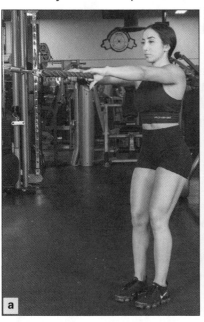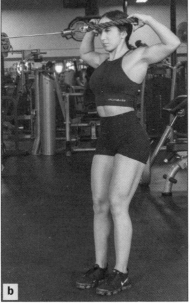

the end of each repetition, your elbows should be slightly higher than your shoulders, and the middle of the rope should be just in front of your forehead. Slowly reverse the movement to the starting position.

Suspension Trainer Face Pull

Setup

Using a suspension trainer, face the anchor and hold the straps, not the handles, using an overhand grip and your hands just outside of your shoulders. Keeping your arms straight and extended in front of your shoulders, lean back with your body in a straight line from head to toe (see figure *a*).

Action and Coaching Tips

Pull the straps toward your face, without overarching your lower back, as you drive your arms apart so that your hands are just outside your ears (see figure *b*). At the end of each repetition, your elbows should be slightly higher than your shoulders. Slowly reverse the movement to the starting position.

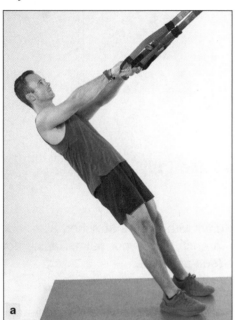 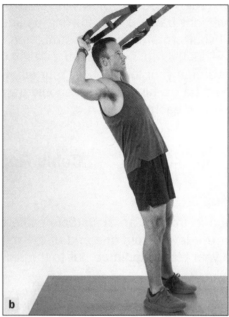

Suspension Trainer Wide-Grip Row

Setup

Using a suspension trainer, face the anchor and hold on to the handles with an overhand grip and your hands just outside of your shoulders. Keeping your arms straight and extended in front of your shoulders, lean back with your body in a straight line from head to toe (see figure *a*).

Action and Coaching Tips

Pull yourself up toward the anchor by bending at your elbows and performing a rowing motion while flaring out your elbows (see figure *b*). Do not allow your wrists to bend as you pull yourself up; keep your elbows directly behind your hands throughout. Your elbows should be at a 90-degree angle to your torso at the top of each repetition. Pause at the top for a second, then slowly lower yourself until your elbows are straight. Keep your body in a straight line; do not lead with your hips when pulling yourself up.

To increase the difficulty, start the exercise from a more severe backward lean by lowering the bar. This brings your body closer to the floor.

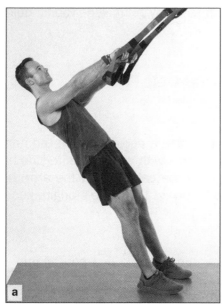
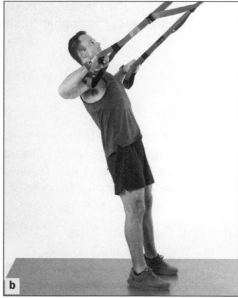

Best Rear-Delt Exercises in the Lengthened-to-Midrange Strength Zone

The exercises in this section help you maximize the strength and development of your rear (posterior) deltoids in the lengthened-to-midrange strength zone.

Dumbbell Side-Lying Rear-Delt Fly

Setup

Lie on your side on top of a bench and hold a dumbbell in your top hand. The lower hand is placed on the floor in front of the bench to stabilize the upper body. Reach your arm across your torso at shoulder height, keeping a slight bend in your elbow.

Action and Coaching Tips

Keeping a slight bend in your elbow and your hand in a neutral grip, lift your arm up and to the side until it's roughly above your torso (see figure b). Slowly reverse the motion, allowing your arm to reach down and across your body at the end of each rep. Complete all reps on the same side before

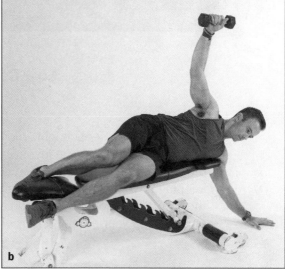

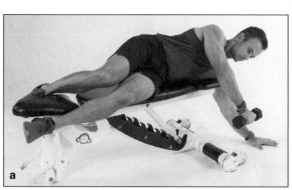

switching sides. Do not allow your torso to rotate at any point; keep your shoulders fairly perpendicular with the ground throughout.

Cable One-Arm Rear-Delt Fly

Setup
Stand with your feet roughly hip-width apart next to a cable column; the handle is attached at your shoulder level. Grab the handle with your opposite-side hand and move a few feet (about 60 cm) away from the cable. Allow the arm that's holding the handle to reach across your body toward the cable's origin, keeping your elbow slightly bent (see figure a).

Action and Coaching Tips
With a slight bend in your elbow and your hand positioned in a neutral grip, pull your arm to the outside while keeping it parallel to the floor so it forms a 90-degree angle with your torso (see figure b). Slowly reverse the motion, allowing your arm to reach across your body at the end of each rep. Complete all reps on the same side before switching sides. Do not allow your torso to rotate at any point; keep your shoulders fairly level with the ground throughout.

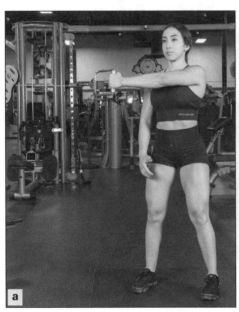 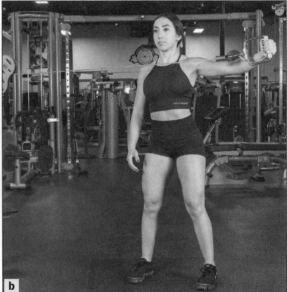

Low-Cable Rear-Delt Fly

Setup
Stand with your feet roughly hip-width apart next to a cable column that has a handle attached at ankle level. Grab the handle with your opposite-side hand and move a few feet (about 60 cm) away from the cable. Bend forward at your hips, keeping your back straight so that your torso is roughly parallel to the floor. Allow the arm that's holding the handle to reach across your body toward the cable's origin. Keep your elbow slightly bent (see figure a).

Action and Coaching Tips

With a slight bend in your elbow and your hand in a neutral grip, lift your arm to the outside until it's roughly parallel to the floor so that it forms a 90-degree angle with your torso (see figure *b*). Slowly reverse the motion, allowing your arm to reach across your body at the end of each rep. Complete all reps on the same side before switching sides. Do not allow your torso to rotate at any point; keep your shoulders fairly level with the ground throughout.

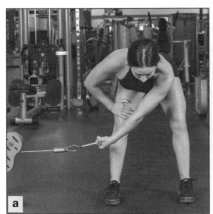
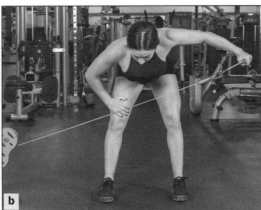

NT Loop Pull Apart

This exercise trains your rear deltoids in both the lengthened-to-midrange and the shortened-to-midrange strength zones. It's included in this section because this exercise creates a significant challenge on your middle deltoids when your arms are more in front of your body, which is in the lengthened-to-midrange strength zone. This strength zone is missed by many of the rear-delt exercises provided in the shortened-to-midrange strength zone category.

Setup

Stand tall while holding an NT Loop or rubber resistance band loop with both hands just outside shoulder width. Keep your arms extended in front of you at shoulder height (see figure *a*). There should be tension in the band to start each rep.

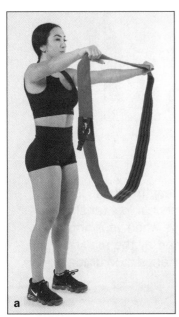
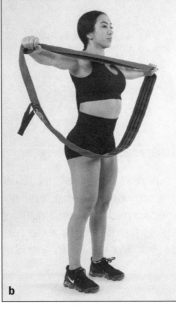

Action and Coaching Tips

With your elbows slightly bent, pull the band apart until it lightly touches the top of your chest (see figure *b*). As you pull the band apart, do not extend at your lower back or allow your shoulders to round forward. Slowly reverse the motion until your arms return to the width they started at. Keep tension in the band throughout.

To reduce the resistance, you can either begin with your hands positioned wider or hold one layer of the band instead of both layers as shown.

NT Loop Mini Rear-Delt Fly

This exercise trains your rear deltoids in both the lengthened-to-midrange and the shortened-to-midrange strength zones. It's included in this section because this exercise creates a significant challenge on your middle deltoids when your arms are more in front of your body, which is in the lengthened-to-midrange strength zone. This strength zone is missed by many of the rear-delt exercises provided in the shortened-to-midrange strength zone category.

Setup

Stand tall, with your feet roughly hip-width apart and your arms inside an NT Loop Mini that is just below your elbow. Keep your elbows bent to 90 degrees and your arms in front of your torso, just inside of your shoulder width. Your humerus (upper-arm bone) is parallel to the ground (see figure *a*).

Action and Coaching Tips

Keeping your elbows bent to 90 degrees and humerus parallel to the ground, drive one arm out to the side of your torso as far as you can without cheating by rotating your torso or extending at your lower back (see figure *b*). Slowly reverse the motion and bring your arm just inside of your same-side shoulder, and repeat the motion on the opposite arm (see figure *c*). Alternate arms on each rep so one arm is working isometrically (holding still against the resistance) while the other arm is moving against the resistance.

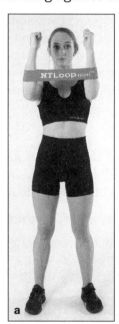
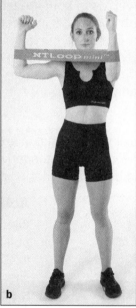
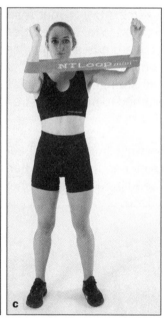

Machine Rear-Delt Fly

The machine rear-delt fly trains your rear deltoids in both strength zones. It is included in this category because it provides a great deal of mechanical tension on your rear delts in their lengthened-to-midrange strength zone when your arms are more in front of your body. This is the strength zone missed by the majority of the exercises in the Best Rear-Delt Exercises in the Shortened-to-Midrange Strength Zone section.

Setup

This exercise requires a specially designed machine that is available in most gyms. It allows you to pull its handles horizontally to the outside of your body. Sit tall with your chest in front of the pad. Hold the handles at shoulder height with either a neutral, overhand, or underhand grip, depending on the gripping options the machine allows (see figures *a* and *b* for an example using the neutral grip). Find a comfortable foot placement that allows you to perform the exercise with proper technique.

Action and Coaching Tips

Keeping your elbows slightly bent, open your arms out to the sides of your body (see figure *b*). Slowly reverse the movement. Be sure to keep a stable spine and minimize overarching in your lower back when performing this exercise.

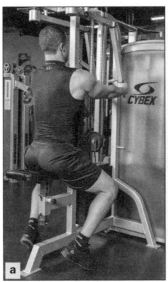 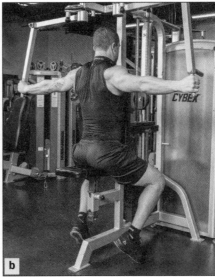

If you're looking to get bigger, stronger traps; the next chapter has your name on it! You'll find new moves for better trap pumps and better ways to do classic exercises for more complete trap development.

CHAPTER 6

The Best Trap Exercises

Training to develop trap strength through the true full range of motion involves performing at least one exercise for each of the following strength zones:

- Scapular elevation exercise
- Scapular retraction exercise

Picking at least one exercise from each category on this list maximizes your workout efficiency and helps you develop full-range strength in your traps.

Trap Exercise Mechanics

The trapezius is a large back muscle that is divided into three regions: upper, middle, and lower. The main role of all three regions of the trapezius is scapular (shoulder blade) stabilization, which occurs during all upper-body exercises and scapular retraction (pinching your shoulder blades together) (1, 2).

When talking about trap strengthening, it's common for people to mean the upper traps, which are addressed by exercises in the scapular elevation strength zone, such as barbell wide-grip shrugs (see figure 6.1).

Scapular retraction, which strengthens the mid and lower traps, is often neglected because it's the area of horizontal pulling exercises that many people cheat through; ensure you're strong by performing loaded scapular retraction exercises to train this strength zone, such as the dumbbell bent-over horizontal shrug (see figure 6.2). All loaded scapular retraction exercises can be performed immediately after performing a horizontal pulling exercise to maximize your workout time and efficiency.

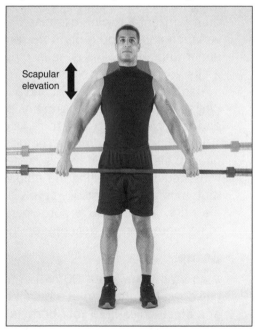

FIGURE 6.1 Barbell wide-grip shrug in the scapular elevation exercise strength zone.

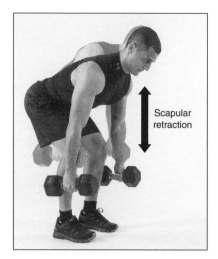

FIGURE 6.2 Dumbbell bent-over horizontal shrug in the scapular retraction exercise strength zone.

The general function of the upper trapezius is scapular upward rotation and elevation. So, loading those actions dynamically, like in all the scapular elevation exercises highlighted in this chapter, will build bigger upper traps that are full range strong. It's also important to note that exercises like barbell deadlifts isometrically load the upper traps.

Research has found that starting a shoulder shrug in 30 degrees of glenohumeral abduction (i.e., arms slightly out to the sides) generates greater upper-trapezius muscle activity than the shrug with the arms at the side (3). This is why the shoulder shrug exercises in this chapter keep your arms wider than the traditional position. When translated to the gym floor, performing barbell shrugs with something like a snatch grip might activate just a little more of the upper traps than when your hands are straight by your sides.

Best Trap Exercises for the Scapular Elevation Strength Zone

The exercises in this section help you maximize the strength and development of the upper trap musculature in the scapular elevation strength zone.

Cable Wide-Grip Angled Upright Row

Rowing exercises have long been recommended for strengthening the trapezius muscle, and the science backs up their effectiveness (4). But more specifically, upright rows have been shown to activate the upper traps to a greater degree than horizontal rowing exercises such as what bent-over rows do (5). And this variation allows you a bit more range of motion that you'll definitely feel in your upper traps. Plus, this is safer on your shoulders than a regular upright row, and it hits your upper traps better.

Use a relatively wide grip, and avoid pulling your elbows above shoulder height. Why these cues? A wider grip has been shown in studies to both increase deltoid and trapezius activity and to reduce biceps brachii activity (6).

In addition to maximizing recruitment of the muscle we're trying to develop, we need to also consider exercise safety and specifically shoulder safety. This is why you should avoid pulling the elbows above shoulder height. Research indicates that impingement typically peaks between 70 and 120 degrees of glenohumeral elevation. Even if you're not experiencing shoulder issues, keeping your elbows to no more than 90 degrees, or shoulder height, is a good idea (5,6).

Setup

Stand tall, a few feet (60 cm) in front of an adjustable cable column with a lat pull-down bar attached at a height below your knees. With your arms straight and at a small angle from your body, hold each side of the bar a few inches (about 5 cm) outside of shoulder width, with your palms facing down (see figure a).

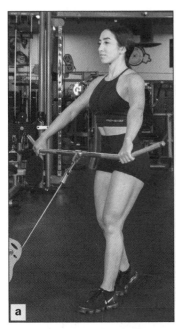
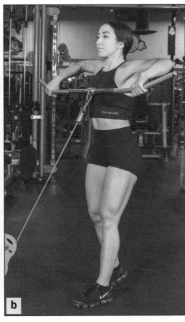

Action and Coaching Tips

Pull the bar up toward you at a 45-degree angle until your elbows reach just above shoulder height, and don't overarch at your lower back (see figure b). Pause at the top for one or two seconds before slowly reversing the motion. Do not allow your wrists to bend, and keep your elbows and forearms in line with the cable throughout.

Barbell Wide-Grip Shrug

Setup

Standing tall, with your feet hip-width apart, hold a barbell in front of your thighs. With your arms straight, grip the bar about 6 to 8 inches (15-20 cm) outside your hips (see figure a).

Action and Coaching Tips

Keeping your back straight, drive your shoulders up toward your ears (see figure b). Reverse the motion by lowering the barbell in a controlled manner. Keep the barbell close to your body throughout.

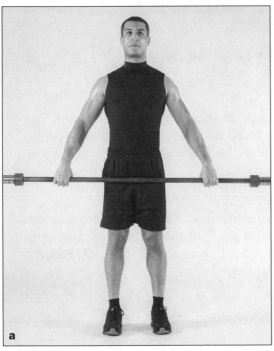
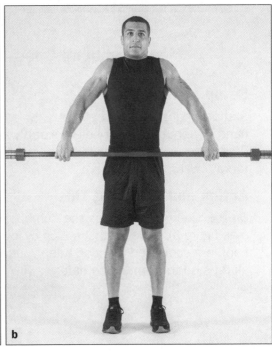

Cable One-Arm Shrug

Setup

With your right hand, grab the handle of a cable (or resistance band) that's attached at roughly ankle level. Stand tall, with your feet roughly shoulder-width apart and the cable at your right side (see figure a). Stand far enough away from the cable or band that it's at a roughly 45-degree angle to the floor.

Action and Coaching Tips

Keeping your back straight, drive your shoulder up toward your ear (see figure b). Reverse the motion by lowering your shoulder and hand back toward the cable in a controlled manner. Keep your arm out to your side throughout. Perform all reps on the same side before switching sides.

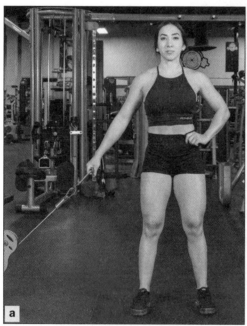 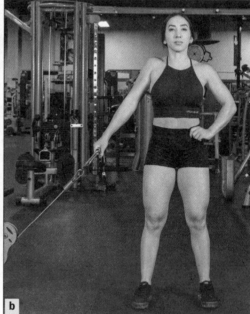

Dumbbell One-Arm Leaning Shrug

Setup

Stand upright and grab a stable pole that's at your side with your same-side hand at about shoulder height. Lean your torso away from that side at a roughly 30-degree angle while holding a dumbbell on the same side you're leaning your torso toward (see figure a).

Action and Coaching Tips

On the side you're holding the dumbbell on, drive your shoulder toward your ear (see figure b). Reverse the motion by lowering your shoulder and hand toward the floor in a controlled manner. Keep your arm out to your side throughout. Perform all reps on the same side before switching sides.

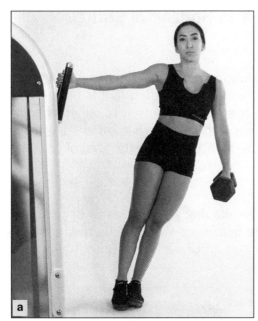
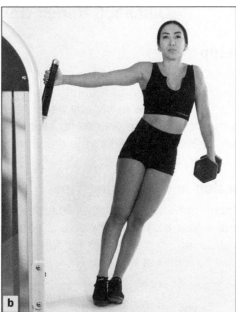

Best Trap Exercises for the Scapular Retraction Strength Zone

The exercises in this section help you maximize the strength and development of the mid- and lower-trap musculature in the scapular retraction strength zone.

Dumbbell Bent-Over Horizontal Shrug

Setup

Stand with your feet hip-width apart. Hold a dumbbell in each hand. Bend forward at the hips, keeping your back straight so that your torso is parallel to the floor (see figure a). Keep your knees bent 15 to 20 degrees.

Action and Coaching Tips

Pinch your shoulders blades together while allowing your elbows to bend slightly (see figure b). Pause for 2 to 3 sec-

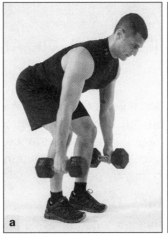
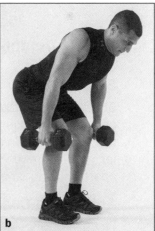

onds before slowly reversing the motion by protracting your shoulder blades (spreading them away from the spine) at the bottom of each rep. Do not allow your back to round at any time.

Dumbbell Bench One-Arm Horizontal Shrug

Setup

Stand parallel to a traditional weight bench with your right hand and right knee on top of the bench and a dumbbell in your left hand. Your left foot is on the floor, and the left knee is slightly bent. Keep a straight back that is roughly parallel to the floor. Rotate your torso slightly to the left so that your left shoulder—the same side you're holding the dumbbell on—is slightly below the level of your right shoulder (see figure *a*).

Action and Coaching Tips

Pinch your shoulder blades together while allowing your elbows to bend slightly (see figure *b*). Pause for 2 to 3 seconds before slowly reversing the motion by protracting your shoulder blades at the bottom of each rep. Do not allow your back to round at any time.

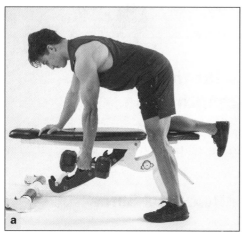 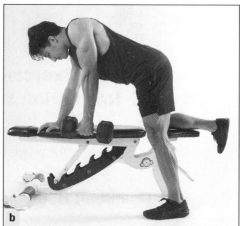

Dumbbell Off-Bench One-Arm Horizontal Shrug

Setup

Stand facing a traditional weight bench, with your right hand on top of the bench and a dumbbell in your left hand. Keep a straight back that is roughly parallel to the floor. Stand in a slightly staggered stance, with your left leg behind your right leg (see figure *a*). You can also stand in a parallel stance with your feet hip-width apart and your knees slightly bent.

Action and Coaching Tips

Pinch your shoulder blades together while allowing your elbows to bend slightly (see figure *b*). Pause for 2 to 3 seconds before slowly reversing the motion by protracting your shoulder blades at the bottom of each rep. Do not allow your back to round at any time.

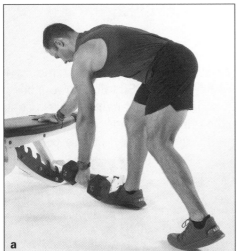
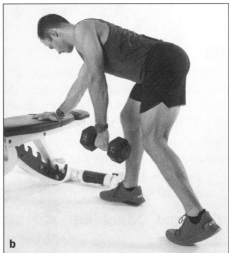

Cable One-Arm Horizontal Shrug

Setup

Stand tall, with your spine straight and your knees slightly bent while facing a cable column adjusted to roughly shoulder height. With your left hand, grab the handle in a neutral grip (i.e., with your palm facing the opposite side of your body) and split your stance so that your left leg is behind your right leg (see figure *a*). Keep your back heel raised off the ground to ensure that most of your weight is on your front leg.

Action and Coaching Tips

Pinch your shoulder blades together while allowing your elbows to bend slightly (see figure *b*). Pause for 2 to 3 seconds before slowly reversing the motion by protracting your shoulder blades at the bottom of each rep. Do not allow your back to round at any time.

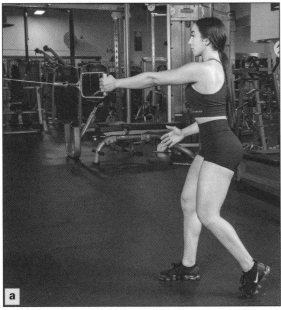
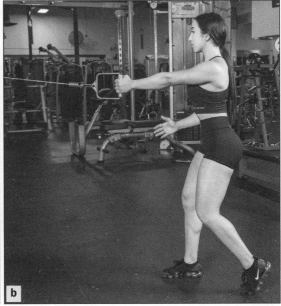

Machine Row Horizontal Shrug

Setup

This exercise requires a specially designed machine that is available in most gyms. It allows you to pull its handles horizontally into your body. Sit tall, with your chest in front of the pad. Hold the handles at about shoulder height using either a neutral, overhand, or underhand grip, depending on the gripping options the machine allows (see figures a and b for an example using the neutral grip). Find a comfortable foot placement that allows you to perform the exercise with proper technique.

Action and Coaching Tips

Keeping your arms almost straight, pinch (retract) your shoulder blades together and pause for a second or two (see figure b). Slowly reverse the movement by allowing your shoulder blades to separate (protract) as far as possible without rounding your spine.

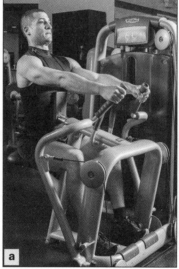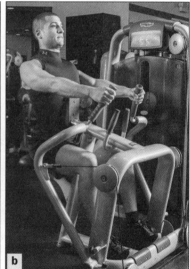

Suspension Trainer Horizontal Shrug

Setup

Using a suspension trainer, face the anchor point and hold the handles with your palms either facing each other or facing the sky and with your arms extended straight in front of your shoulders (see figure a for an example with the palms facing each other). Lean back with your body in a straight line from head to toe.

Action and Coaching Tips

Keeping your arms almost straight, pinch (retract) your shoulder blades together and pause for a second or two (see figure b). Slowly reverse the movement by allowing your shoulder blades to separate (protract) as far as possible without rounding your spine.

To increase the difficulty, start the exercise from a more severe backward lean, bringing your body closer to the floor.

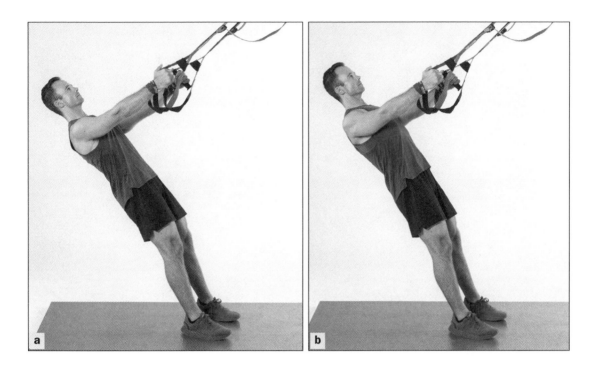

Training trends come and go, but biceps never go out of style! Let's look at the best exercises for your biceps.

CHAPTER 7

The Best Biceps Exercises

Training to develop biceps strength through the true full range of motion involves performing at least one exercise in each of the following strength zones:

- Lengthened-to-midrange strength zone: biceps exercise
- Shortened-to-midrange strength zone: biceps exercise

Picking at least one exercise from each category in this list maximizes your workout efficiency and helps you develop full-range biceps strength.

Biceps Exercise Mechanics

Biceps exercises in the lengthened-to-midrange strength zone generate the most mechanical tension on the biceps closer to the bottom of a biceps curl, when your elbow is closer to being straight. As an example, see the EZ-bar preacher curl in figure 7.1. Whereas biceps exercises in the shortened-to-mid-range strength zone create the most mechanical tension on your biceps closer to the top of the biceps curl, when your elbow is closer to being bent.

During any style of biceps curl, the point at which the musculature is maximally loaded is when the lever arm is at its longest. This occurs when your forearm is at a 90-degree angle to the line of force.

If you're using free weights, gravity is the line of force. Therefore, the point of maximal mechanical tension on your biceps is when your elbow reaches 90 degrees of flexion or when your forearm is parallel to the floor. As an example, see the EZ-bar biceps curl in figure 7.2. If you're doing biceps curls using a cable column, the cable itself is the line of

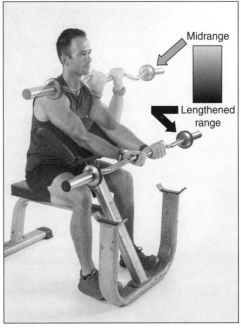

FIGURE 7.1 EZ-bar preacher curl in the lengthened-to-midrange strength zone.

force. In this case, the lever arm is at its longest when your forearm makes a 90-degree angle with the cable.

Although biceps exercises in each strength zone category involve the same motion of elbow flexion, they each train an important complementary aspect of biceps strength that is neglected by the other. Therefore, using the two strength zones as your biceps exercise checklist ensures you make smart exercise choices and get a better, more well-rounded biceps workout.

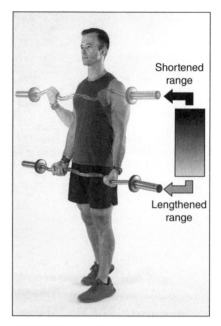

FIGURE 7.2 EZ-bar biceps curl in the shortened-to-midrange strength zone.

How to Target the Short Head and Long Head of Your Biceps

The bicep consists of two heads, which represent the two tendons that attach it to the shoulder blade bone: the long and the short head. Among bodybuilders, it's commonly thought that to emphasize the short head of your bicep, you need to do biceps curls while in shoulder flexion, which means with your elbows elevated at or near shoulder height.

The research shows the short head of the biceps gets loaded to a greater degree when your elbow is flexed to 90-degrees while the arm is at your side (1).

Practically, this suggests you don't need to do biceps curls while in shoulder flexion to effectively train the short head of your biceps, as it's worked effectively in basic biceps curls with the elbow by your side. So, all of the of biceps exercises listed in the shortened-to-midrange strength zone will effectively strengthen the short head of your biceps, and all of the exercises listed in the lengthened-to-midrange strength category will effectively strengthen the long head of your biceps.

Best Biceps Exercises in the Lengthened-to-Midrange Strength Zone

The exercises in this section help you maximize the strength and development of your biceps musculature while targeting the lengthened-to-midrange strength zone.

Cable One-Arm Face-Away Biceps Curl

Setup

Stand facing away from a cable column, with your feet roughly hip-width apart in a split stance and the handle attached to the column at ankle level. Hold the handle in one hand, with a slight bend in your elbow and your arm in line with your torso (see figure a).

Action and Coaching Tips

Curl the handle up toward your shoulder by bending at your elbow without allowing your elbow to move forward (see figure b). Do not cheat the weight up by overextending at your lower back. Once the cable lightly touches your outer forearm, reverse the motion by slowly lowering the handle until your elbow is straight. Perform all reps on the same side before switching sides. Do not allow your elbow to drift in front of or behind your torso throughout.

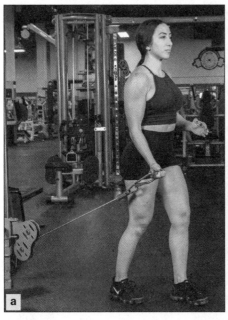 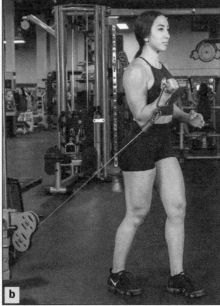

Band One-Arm Face-Away Biceps Curl

Setup

Anchor a resistance band securely around a stable object at your calf to knee level. Stand in front of the band, facing away from the anchor point with your feet in a split stance roughly hip-width apart. Hold the handle in one hand, with the anchor point in front of your working arm, keeping your arm straight and in line with your torso (see figure *a*).

Action and Coaching Tips

Curl the band up toward your shoulder by bending at your elbow without allowing your elbow to move forward (see figure *b*). Do not cheat the weight up by over-extending at your lower back.

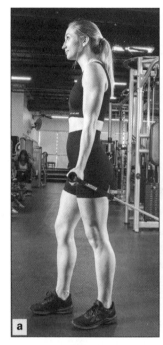
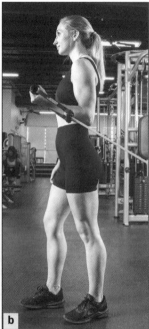

Once the band touches your forearm, reverse the motion by slowly lowering the band until your elbow is straight. Perform all reps on the same side before switching sides. Do not allow your elbow to drift in front of or behind your torso throughout.

You can increase the resistance by standing farther back from the anchor point, and decrease the resistance by standing closer to the anchor point. If you do move closer to the anchor point, make sure there is tension on the band to start each rep.

EZ-Bar Preacher Curl

Setup

To perform this exercise, use the apparatus that's commonly known as the preacher curl bench. Sit on the seat of the bench, with your spine upright and your feet hip-width apart. Place your chest and arms against the pad while holding an E-Z bar with both hands roughly shoulder-width apart and using an underhand grip (see figure *a*).

Action and Coaching Tips

Without allowing your shoulders to round forward, curl the bar up toward your shoulders by bending at your elbows (see figure *b*). Once your hands are above your elbows, reverse the motion by slowly lowering the bar. You can also perform this exercise with an overhand grip.

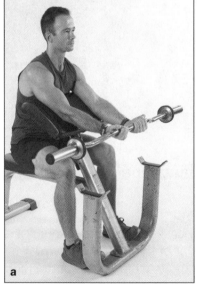
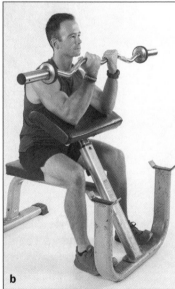

Dumbbell One-Arm Preacher Curl

Setup

To perform this exercise, use the apparatus that's commonly known as the preacher curl bench. Sit on the seat of the bench, with your spine upright and your feet roughly hip-width apart. Place your chest and arms against the pad while holding a dumbbell in one hand in front of your same-side shoulder and using an underhand grip (see figure *a*). You can place your nonworking arm on the bench or on your body wherever you feel most comfortable.

Action and Coaching Tips

Without allowing your shoulder to round forward, curl the dumbbell up toward your shoulder by bending at your elbow (see figure *b*). Once your hand is above your elbow, reverse the motion by slowly lowering the dumbbell until your elbow is straight. You can also perform this exercise with an overhand grip. Perform all reps on the same side before switching sides.

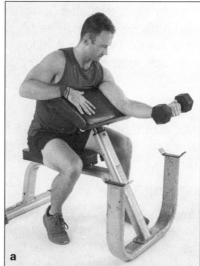
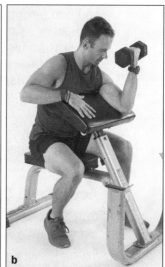

Dumbbell Incline Bench One-Arm Preacher Curl

Setup

Stand with your feet roughly shoulder-width apart behind an incline bench that's set to a roughly 45-degree angle. Position your armpit against the top of the bench and your arm resting on the bench while holding a dumbbell using an underhand grip (see figure *a*).

Action and Coaching Tips

Without allowing your shoulders to round forward, curl the dumbbell up toward your shoulder by bending at your elbow (see figure *b*). Once your forearm is above your elbow, reverse the motion by slowly lowering the dumbbell. Perform all reps on the same side before switching sides.

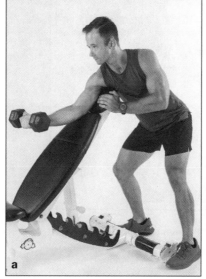
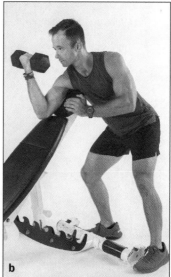

Best Biceps Exercises in the Shortened-to-Midrange Strength Zone

The exercises in this section help you maximize the strength and development of your biceps musculature while targeting the shortened-to-midrange strength zone.

EZ-Bar Biceps Curl

You can perform biceps curls with an EZ-bar, barbell, or dumbbells with your feet parallel or in a small staggered stance (as shown in this exercise). Some people prefer the staggered stance because it helps them to be less inclined to cheat by using their lower back. Both stances are effective options depending on your personal preference.

Setup

Stand tall, with your feet roughly hip-width apart, finding a comfortable stance. Using an underhand grip, hold an E-Z bar with both hands next to your hips (see figure a).

Action and Coaching Tips

Curl the bar up toward your shoulders by bending at your elbows without allowing your elbows to move forward (see figure b). Do not swing the weight up by overextending at your lower back. Once your hands are in front of your shoulders, reverse the motion by slowly lowering the bar.

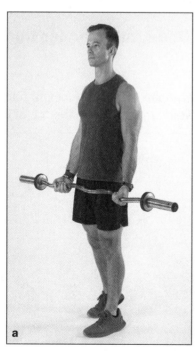 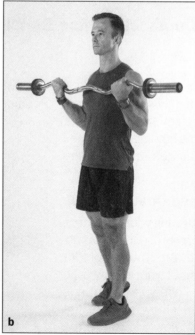

Dumbbell Standing Biceps Curl

Setup

Stand tall, with your feet hip-width apart. Hold a dumbbell in each hand in a neutral grip next to your hips (see figure *a*).

Action and Coaching Tips

Curl the dumbbells up toward your shoulders by bending at your elbows and turning your wrists so that your pinky fingers come closer to your shoulders without allowing your elbows to move forward or backward (see figure *b*). Do not swing the weight up by overextending at your lower back. Once your hands are in front of your shoulders, reverse the motion by slowly lowering the dumbbells back to your side.

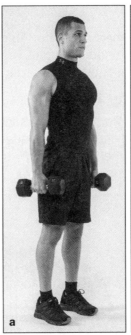
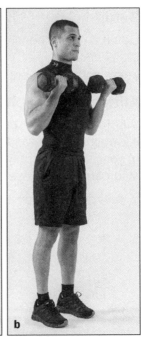

Dumbbell Concentration Biceps Curl

Setup

Sit on a bench with your feet wider than shoulder-width apart. Hold a dumbbell in one hand, and place the back of your arm against the inside of your same-side thigh with your arm straight. Do not allow the dumbbell to touch the floor (see figure *a*).

Action and Coaching Tips

Curl the dumbbell up toward your opposite-side shoulder by bending at your same-side elbow (see figure *b*). Do not swing the weight up by jerking your body. Once your hand is in front of your torso, reverse the motion by slowly lowering the dumb-bell until your arm is once again straight. Perform all reps on the same side before switching sides.

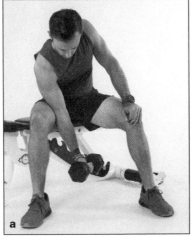
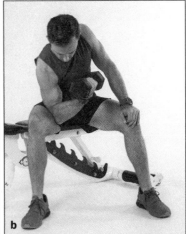

Dumbbell Incline Bench Biceps Curl

Setup

Lie on a weight bench angled at about 45 degrees, with your feet flat on the floor, pressing them firmly into the ground to keep you stable. Hold a pair of dumbbells below your shoulders and keep your arms straight (see figure *a*).

Action and Coaching Tips

Curl the dumbbells up toward your shoulders by bending at your elbows without allowing your elbows to move forward (see figure *b*). Once your hands are in front of your shoulders, reverse the motion by slowly lowering the dumbbells. You can also perform this exercise with a neutral grip.

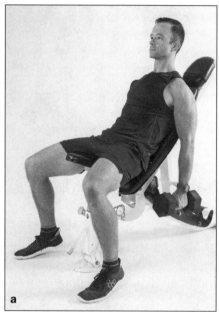 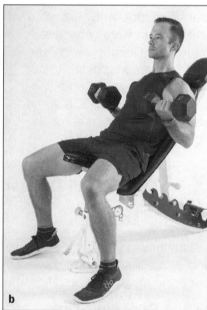

Cable EZ-Bar Biceps Curl

You can perform this exercise with your feet parallel or in a small staggered stance (as shown in this exercise). Some people prefer the staggered stance because it helps them to be less inclined to cheat by using their lower back. Both stances are effective options depending on your personal preference.

Setup

Stand tall in front of an adjustable cable column with an EZ-bar handle attached to the column below your knees. Hold each side of the handle with an underhand grip, using the angled grip portion of the bar (your palms turned slightly toward each other). Keep your arms by your sides and your elbows slightly bent (see figure a).

Action and Coaching Tips

Curl the EZ-bar handle up toward your shoulders by bending at your elbows without allowing them to move forward (see figure b). Once your hands are in front of your shoulders, reverse the motion by slowly lowering the EZ bar until your arms are almost straight.

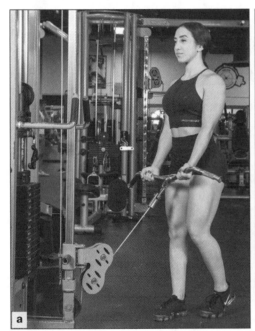
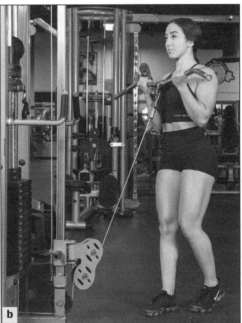

NT Loop Biceps Curl

Setup

Stand tall with your feet roughly shoulder-width apart and an NT Loop or a looped rubber resistance band securely anchored under your feet. Hold one side of the band with each hand with an underhand grip, with a slight bend in your elbows (see figure *a*).

Action and Coaching Tips

Curl the band up toward your shoulders by bending your elbows without allowing them to move upward (see figure *b*). Do not allow your lower back to overextend as you curl the band into you. Once you cannot bend your elbows any further, reverse the motion slowly until your elbows are straight again. You can make this exercise more difficult by grabbing the band farther down to create more tension.

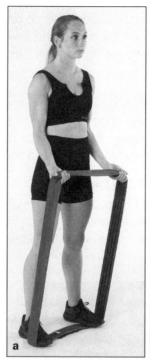
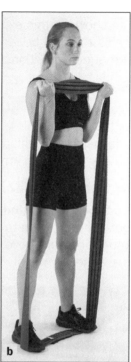

You don't just want stronger biceps—you want stronger arms. That means you also need to know how to get your triceps full-range strong, which is what the next chapter covers.

CHAPTER 8

The Best Triceps Exercises

Training to develop triceps strength through the true full range of motion involves performing at least one exercise for each of the following strength zones:

- Lengthened-to-midrange strength zone: triceps exercise
- Shortened-to-midrange strength zone: triceps exercise

Picking at least one exercise from each category in this list maximizes your workout efficiency and helps you develop full-range triceps strength.

Triceps Exercise Mechanics

During any style of triceps exercise, the point at which your triceps muscles experience the most mechanical tension is the point in the range of motion in which your forearm is at a 90-degree angle to the line of force.

If you're doing triceps exercises using a cable column or resistance band, the cable itself is the line of force. The point of maximal mechanical tension for your triceps here is when your forearm makes a 90-degree angle with the cable.

If you're using free weights, gravity is your line of force. So the point of maximal mechanical tension on your triceps is when your elbow reaches 90 degrees of extension or when your forearm is parallel to the floor.

During triceps exercises in the lengthened-to-midrange strength zone, your arms are above your head. These exercises create a loaded triceps stretch during the motion of bending your elbow. As an example, see the dumbbell behind-the-head triceps extension exercise in figure 8.1a.

During triceps exercises in the shortened-to-midrange strength zone your arms are in front of you or by your sides. These exercises create the most mechanical tension on the triceps between when your elbow is bent to 90 degrees and when your elbow is straightened. As an example, see the dumbbell triceps skull crusher exercise in figure 8.1b.

Although triceps exercises in both categories involve the same motion of elbow extension, they each train an important, complementary aspect of triceps strength that the other neglects. Therefore, using the two strength zones as your triceps exercise checklist ensures you will make smart exercise choices and get a better, more well-rounded triceps workout.

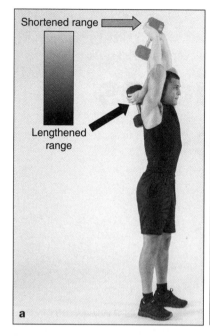
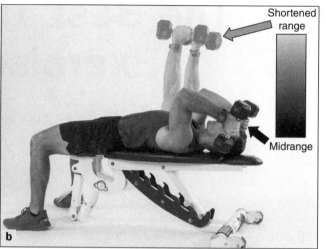

FIGURE 8.1 *(a)* Dumbbell behind-the-head triceps extension in lengthened-to-midrange strength zone; *(b)* dumbbell triceps skull crusher in shortened-to-midrange strength zone.

Arm Training Isn't Just For Looks!

Many sport coaches don't believe specific arm training protocols are functional or carry over to sport performance. I disagree.

Put simply, having strong triceps improves your ability to push something—such as an object or opponent—away from you, just as having strong biceps improves your ability to pull something—such as an object or opponent—toward you. This is why specific arm training for both the biceps and triceps can only help improve performance and prevent injury while also producing bigger arms in the process.

Best Triceps Exercises in the Lengthened-to-Midrange Strength Zone

The exercises in this section help you maximize the strength and development of the triceps musculature while targeting the lengthened-to-midrange strength zone.

Cable Rope Overhead Triceps Extension

Setup

Use an adjustable cable column to perform this exercise. The rope should be attached at mid-torso level. Stand in a split stance in front of the column, but face away from where the rope is attached. Lean your torso forward at a roughly 45-degree angle, and raise your rear heel off the ground. Hold each side of the band in each hand, with your palms facing each other. Your arms are by your ears, and your elbows are bent beyond 90 degrees (see figure *a*).

Action and Coaching Tips

Keeping your body in the starting position, extend your elbows until your arms are straight (see figure *b*). Do not drive your shoulders downward as you extend your arms on each rep. Slowly reverse the motion and repeat.

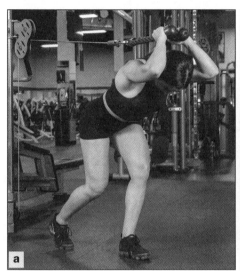 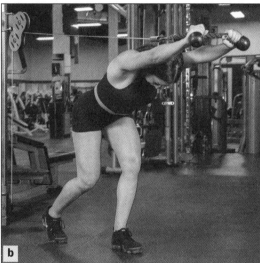

Kettlebell Behind-the-Head Triceps Extension

You can perform this exercise with your feet in a parallel or in a small staggered stance (as shown in this exercise). Some people prefer the staggered stance because it helps them to be less inclined to over arch at the lower back. Both stances are effective options depending on your personal preference.

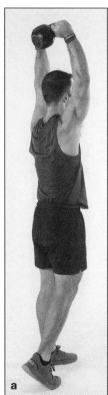 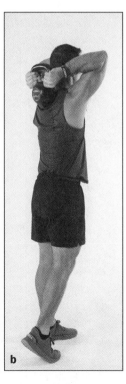

Setup

Stand with your feet hip-width apart in a split stance. Hold the handle of the kettlebell on each side, with your arms extended above your head and your elbows directly above your shoulder (see figure *a*).

Action and Coaching Tips

While keeping your elbows above your shoulders, bend your elbows and slowly lower the kettlebell behind your head until your elbow is fully bent (see figure *b*). Reverse the motion by extending at your elbows to press the kettlebell up and complete the rep.

Dumbbell Behind-the-Head Triceps Extension

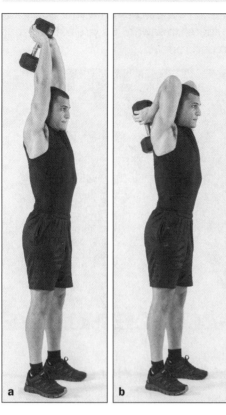

Setup

Stand with your feet hip-width apart. Hold a dumbbell with both hands overhead and your elbows directly above your shoulders. The handle is between your thumbs and forefingers, and the inside of the dumbbell is against the pinky side of your palms (see figure *a*).

Action and Coaching Tips

While keeping your elbows above your shoulders, bend your elbows and slowly lower the dumbbell behind your head until your elbows are fully bent (see figure *b*). Reverse the motion by extending at your elbows to press the dumbbell up and complete the rep.

Dumbbell One-Arm Behind-the-Head Triceps Extension

Setup

Stand with your feet hip-width apart. Hold a dumbbell with one arm extended above your head and your elbow directly above your shoulder (see figure *a*).

Action and Coaching Tips

While keeping your elbow above your shoulder, bend your elbow and slowly lower the dumbbell behind your head until your elbow is fully bent (see figure *b*). Reverse the motion by extending at your elbow to press the dumbbell up and complete the rep. Perform all reps on the same side before switching sides.

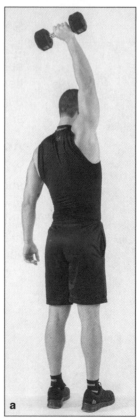
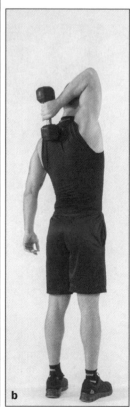

NT Loop Behind-the-Head Triceps Extension

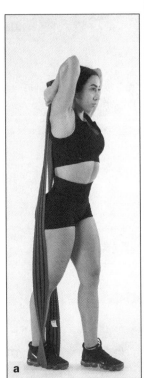
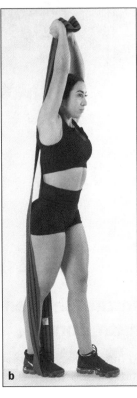

Setup

Stand in a split stance with an NT Loop anchored securely under your right foot. Hold the inside of the band with both hands roughly shoulder-width apart and palms facing up. Step your left foot through the band in front of your right foot and raise your arms above your head. Keeping your elbow bent, hold the band behind your head (see figure *a*).

Action and Coaching Tips

While keeping your elbows above your shoulders, extend your elbows until just before your arms are fully straight (see figure *b*). Slowly lower the band behind your head until your elbows are fully bent once again to complete the rep.

NT Loop Overhead Triceps Press

Setup

Anchor the NT Loop securely around a stable object at about your midtorso level. Stand in a split stance in front of the band, but face away from where the band is attached. Lean your torso forward at a roughly 45-degree angle, and raise your rear heel off the ground. Hold each side of the band in each hand, with your palms facing each other. Your arms are by your ears, and your elbows are bent beyond 90 degrees (see figure *a*).

Action and Coaching Tips

Keeping your body in the starting position, extend your elbows until your arms are straight (see figure *b*). Do not drive your shoulders downward as you extend your arms on each rep. Slowly reverse the motion and repeat.

You can increase the resistance by standing farther back from the anchor point, and decrease the resistance by standing closer to the anchor point. If you move closer to the anchor point, make sure there is tension on the band to start each rep.

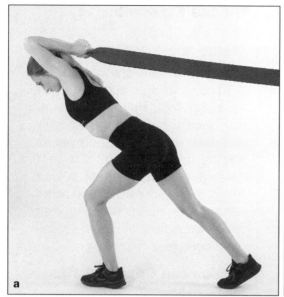
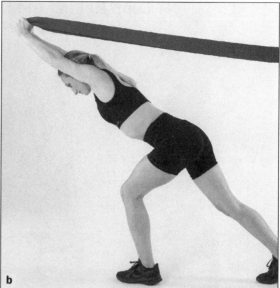

Best Triceps Exercises in the Shortened-to-Midrange Strength Zone

The exercises in this section help you maximize the strength and development of the triceps musculature while targeting the shortened-to-midrange strength zone.

Dumbbell Triceps Skull Crusher

Setup

Lie supine on a weight bench while holding a dumbbell in each hand. Your elbows are straight and arms at an angle above you so your elbows are about even with your eye line (see figure *a*).

Action and Coaching Tips

Bend your elbows, lowering the dumbbells toward each side of your forehead while keeping your palms facing one another (see figure *b*). Once your elbows

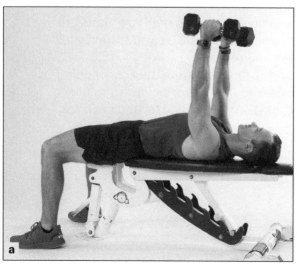
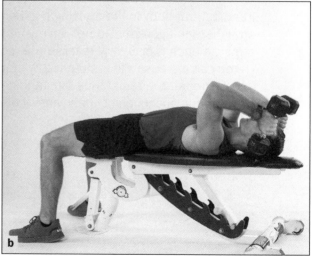

bend as much as possible without moving the lower part of your arm, reverse the motion and extend your elbows until they're almost straight again to complete the rep. To avoid getting hit in the head with the dumbbells, lower them slowly with deliberate control.

Dumbbell Triceps Saw Skull Crusher

Setup

Lie supine on a weight bench while holding a dumbbell in each hand. Your elbows are bent by your sides, and the dumbbells are just above your shoulders (see figure *a*).

Action and Coaching Tips

Drive your arms above you at a 45-degree angle until your elbows are straight and your arms are at roughly a 45-degree angle to your torso above your head (see figures *b* and *c*). Reverse the motion and return to the starting position to complete the rep. Keep the dumbbells from resting on the fronts of your shoulders at the start of each rep.

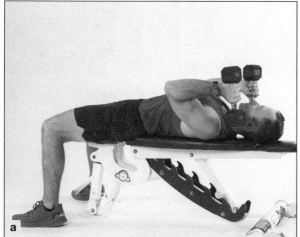

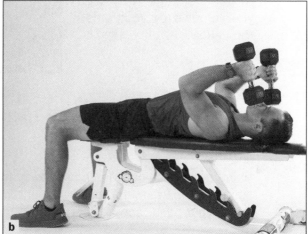

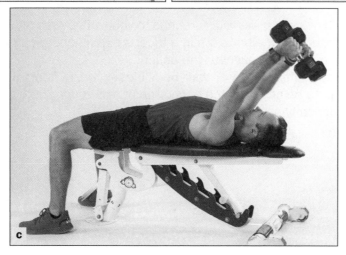

Cable Rope Triceps Extension

Setup

Stand in front of an adjustable cable column with a rope attached above your eye level. Hold one end of the rope in each hand, with your elbows bent above 90 degrees and your palms facing each other (see figure a).

Action and Coaching Tips

With your knees slightly bent, straighten your elbows until your arms are straight (see figure b). Do not allow your shoulders to round forward as you press the rope downward on each repetition. Slowly reverse the motion to complete the rep. Keep your elbows by your sides throughout.

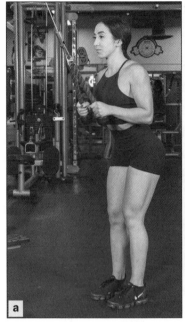 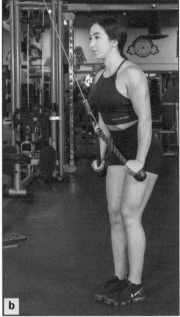

Suspension Trainer Skull Crusher

Setup

Using a suspension trainer, face away from the anchor point, grab the handles, and lean your weight forward with your arms extended at a roughly 45-degree angle above your head (see figure a).

Action and Coaching Tips

Bend at your elbows and lower your forehead to your wrists (see figure b). Reverse direction and extend your elbows, as in a triceps extension, to complete the rep. Keep your body straight throughout the action.

To increase the difficulty, lower your body closer to the floor; the closer your shoulders come to being under the anchor point, the tougher the exercise is. To decrease the difficulty use a higher body angle.

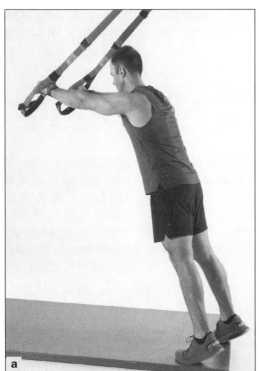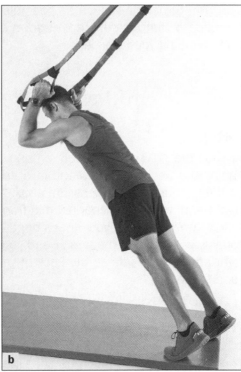

Cable One-Arm Triceps Kickback

Setup

Stand tall, facing a cable machine or a resistance band that's attached at roughly knee height. Hold the cable handle in your left hand with the cable's origin in front of your left arm. Stand with your feet roughly hip-width apart. Hinge at your hips and lean forward, keeping your knees bent 15 to 20 degrees until your torso becomes roughly parallel with the floor. Bend your left elbow above 90 degrees, with your left arm at your side so the back of your humerus is parallel to the floor (see figure *a*).

Action and Coaching Tips

Without allowing your torso to move or your shoulder to round forward, extend your elbow until it's fully straight (see figure *b*). Slowly reverse the motion by allowing

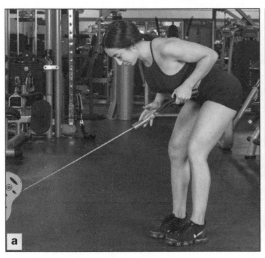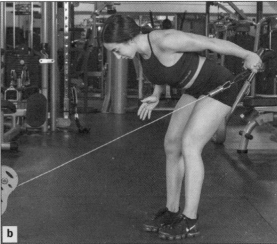

your arm to bend as much as possible while keeping your upper arm parallel to the floor to complete the rep. Perform all reps on the same side before switching and reversing your stance.

NT Loop One-Arm Triceps Kickback

Setup

Anchor the NT Loop securely around a stable object at about midthigh level. Facing the anchor point, stand in a split stance, with your right leg behind and your feet roughly shoulder-width apart in front of the band. Hold the band in your right hand, with the anchor point in front of your right arm. Hinge at your hips and lean forward, keeping your knees bent 15 to 20 degrees until your torso becomes roughly parallel with the floor. Bend your right elbow above 90 degrees, with your right arm at your side so the back of your humerus is roughly parallel to the floor (see figure *a*).

Action and Coaching Tips

Without allowing your torso to move or your shoulder to round forward, extend your elbow until it's fully straight (see figure *b*). Slowly reverse the motion by allowing your arm to bend as much as possible while keeping your upper arm parallel to the floor to complete the rep. Perform all reps on the same side before switching and reversing your stance.

You can increase the resistance by standing farther back from the anchor point and decrease the resistance by standing closer to the anchor point. If you move closer to the anchor point, make sure there is tension on the band to start each rep.

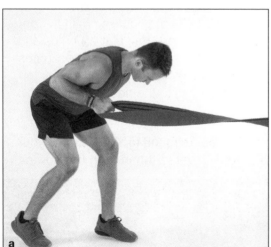
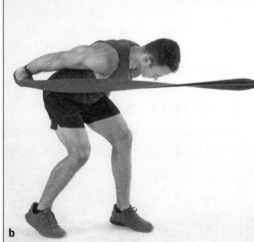

Machine Triceps Extension

Setup

This exercise requires a specially designed machine that is available in most gyms. Sit on the seat of the machine, with your spine upright and your feet hip-width apart. Place your chest and arms against the pad while holding the handles with both hands roughly shoulder-width apart in a neutral grip (see figure *a*).

Action and Coaching Tips

Without allowing your shoulders to round forward, push the handles down by extending your arm at your elbows (see figure *b*). Once your elbows are almost fully straight, slowly reverse the motion by bringing the handles up toward you.

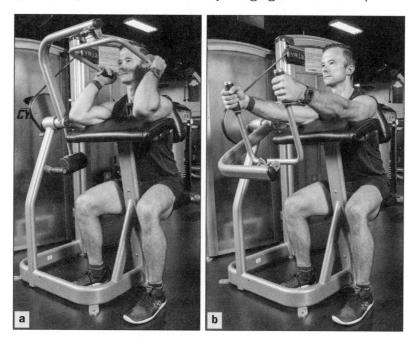

Now that we've covered the entire upper body, let's take a look at the lower body, starting with the hamstrings.

CHAPTER 9

The Best Hamstring Exercises

Training to develop your hamstring strength through the true full range of motion involves performing at least one exercise for each of the following strength zones:

- Lengthened-to-midrange strength zone: hip-hinging exercise
- Shortened-to-midrange strength zone: knee flexion exercise

Picking at least one exercise from each category in this list maximizes your workout efficiency and helps you develop full-range hamstring strength.

Hamstring Exercise Mechanics

Hip-hinge exercises are exercises like the dumbbell one-leg one-arm Romanian deadlift (see figure 9.1) or the dumbbell traveling Romanian deadlift lunge, where you keep a slight bend in your knees as you lower your torso until it's parallel to the floor while keeping a lordotic (inward) curve at your lower back.

Each week, include a focused knee-flexion exercise, such as a stability ball leg curl (single or double leg; see figure 9.2), Nordic hamstring curl, or machine leg curl (seated or lying).

Several studies have shown that when strength training programs include the Nordic hamstring curl incidences of hamstring strains are significantly reduced (1, 2, 3).

The research on leg curls is also compelling. One study separated elite soccer players into two groups. Although both groups used the same training programs, one group performed additional,

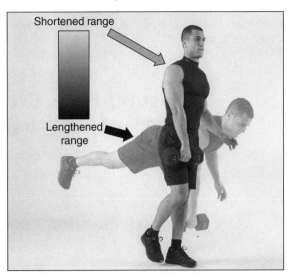

FIGURE 9.1 Dumbbell one-leg one-arm Romanian deadlift in lengthened-to-midrange strength zone: hip-hinging exercise.

specific hamstring training using the machine lying leg curl. The other group did not. The results showed that the addition of the machine lying leg curl increased sprint speed and decreased the risk of hamstring strain injury (4).

This supports the research showing that the machine lying leg curl (where movement originates at the knee joint) elicits significantly greater activation of the lower lateral and lower medial hamstrings than the Romanian deadlift, where movement originates at the hip joint, such as in the exercises in the hip-hinge strength zone category (5).

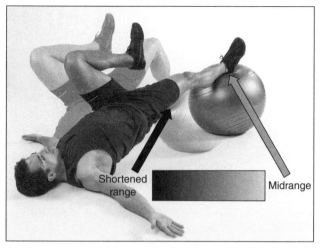

FIGURE 9.2   Stability ball one-leg curl in shortened-to-midrange strength zone: knee flexion exercise.

Misused Training Method: Standing on a Step for Romanian Deadlifts

The purpose of standing on an aerobic step (or some other slightly elevated surface) is to increase the range of motion beyond what is possible if you did the same exercise standing on the floor. That's why, when performing barbell elevated Romanian deadlifts, the goal is to make sure the weight plates lightly tap the floor on each rep.

But using a step to perform barbell elevated Romanian deadlifts misses the point when people don't perform the exercise with greater range of motion than they would if they were on the floor. So the exercise makes no sense.

Don't believe me? Think about barbell Romanian deadlifts. If you don't lower the plates below the level of whatever you're standing on, then the elevated surface does you no good. Standing on the floor would've been just fine. Although this should be obvious, there are countless instances of people in the gym failing to move through an increased range of motion while standing on an elevated surface because they're simply copying something they saw someone else do without understanding why they're doing it.

Best Hip-Hinge Exercises in the Lengthened-to-Midrange Strength Zone

The exercises in this section help you maximize the strength and development of the hamstrings in the lengthened-to-midrange strength zone via hip-hinge movements.

Barbell Elevated Romanian Deadlift

Setup

Stand tall on top of a small platform such as an aerobic step with your feet hip-width apart. Hold a barbell in front of your thighs with your arms straight; grip the bar just outside your hips (see figure a).

Action and Coaching Tips

Keeping your back straight, hinge at your hips and bend forward toward the floor; keep your knees bent at a 15- to 20-degree angle (see figure *b*). As you hinge forward, drive your hips backward, and do not allow your back to round. Once your torso is roughly parallel to the floor, drive your hips forward toward the barbell, reversing the motion to stand tall again without overextending at your lower back. Keep the barbell close to you throughout; it should touch your shins at the bottom and track against the fronts of your legs as you perform each repetition.

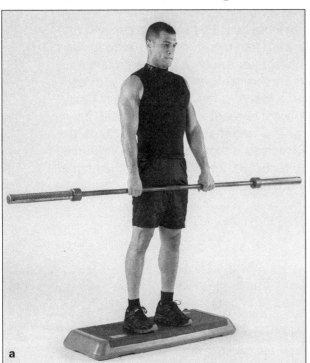

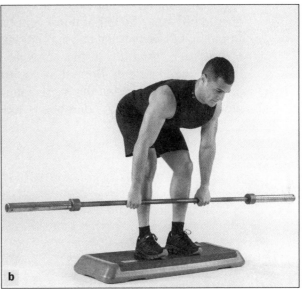

Dumbbell Romanian Deadlift

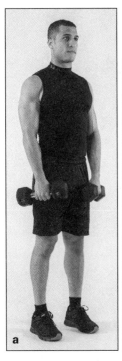

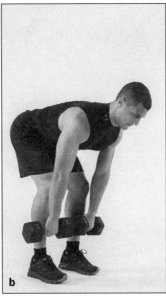

Setup

Stand tall with your feet hip-width apart (see figure *a*). Hold the dumbbells in front of your thighs.

Action and Coaching Tips

Keeping your back straight, hinge at your hips and bend forward toward the floor. Your knees are bent at a 15- to 20-degree angle (see figure *b*). As you hinge forward, drive your hips backward, and do not allow your back to round. Once your torso is roughly parallel to the floor, drive your hips forward toward the dumbbells, reversing the motion to stand tall again without overextending your lower back. Keep the dumbbells close to you throughout; they should touch your shins at the bottom and track against the fronts of your legs as you perform each repetition.

Dumbbell Traveling Romanian Deadlift Lunge

Setup

Stand tall, with your feet hip-width apart (see figure *a*). Hold a dumbbell in each hand at your sides in a new grip.

Action and Coaching Tips

Step forward with one leg, keeping your front knee bent 15 to 20 degrees and your back knee straight or slightly bent. As your front foot hits the ground, lean forward by hinging at your hips and allowing your rear heel to come off the ground (see figure *b*). Your torso should be no lower than parallel to the floor, and your back should be straight. Do not allow your back to round at the bottom of each lunge. Stand up tall while bringing your rear leg forward to meet your front leg (see figure *c*), and step forward with the opposite leg—the one that was behind you on the last rep (see figure *d*). Repeat as you travel across a room. Establish a rhythm by performing the step and the hip hinge simultaneously and by reversing the motion smoothly. Do not let the dumbbells touch the floor at any point.

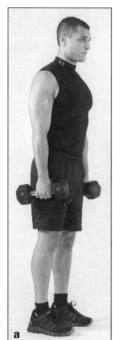
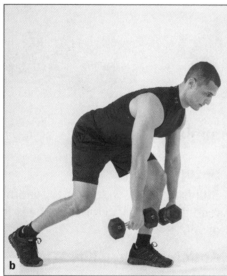
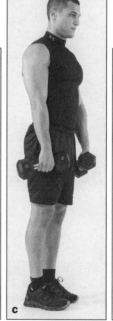
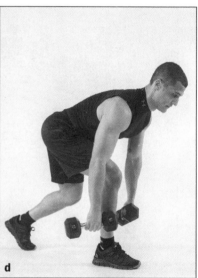

Dumbbell Lateral Romanian Deadlift Lunge

Setup

Stand tall while holding dumbbells in each hand against the outer front of the thighs, with your feet hip-width apart (see figure *a*).

Action and Coaching Tips

Step laterally with one leg just outside shoulder width, keeping your front knee bent 15 to 20 degrees and your back knee fairly straight. As your stepping foot hits the ground, shift your weight over your foot and hinge forward at your hips, allowing the dumbbells to track on each side of your leg (see figure *b*). Once your torso becomes parallel to the floor with your back straight—without allowing your back to round at the bottom of each lunge—reverse the motion by stepping back to the starting stance and return to an upright position. Perform the same motion by stepping laterally to the opposite side with the other leg (see figure *c*). Establish a rhythm by performing the step and the hip hinge simultaneously, and reverse the motion in the same smooth and coordinated manner. Do not let the dumbbells touch the floor at any point during this exercise.

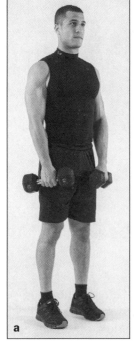 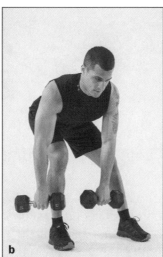 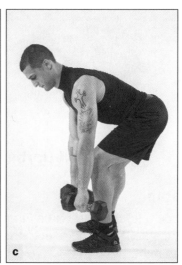

Dumbbell One-Leg One-Arm Romanian Deadlift

Setup

Stand on one leg and hold a dumbbell in the opposite hand at your hip (see figure *a*).

Action and Coaching Tips

Keeping your back and arm straight, hinge at your hip and bend forward; keep your weight-bearing knee bent at a 15- to 20-degree angle. As you hinge, allow your non-weight-bearing leg to elevate so that it remains in a straight line with your torso, and keep your hips and shoulders flat without allowing them to rotate (see figure *b*). Do not allow your lower back to round as you hinge your hips and lower your torso. Once your torso and non-weight-bearing leg are roughly parallel to the floor, reverse the motion by driving your hips forward to stand tall again, thus completing the rep. Perform all repetitions on one side before switching to the other side.

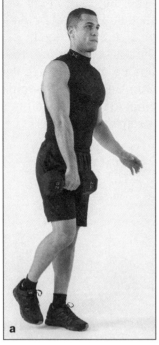

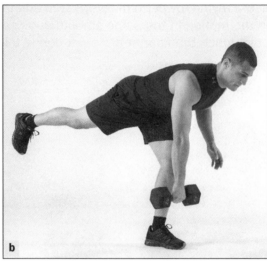

Angled-Barbell Leaning Romanian Deadlift

Setup

Place one end of a barbell in a corner or inside a landmine device that's on your right side. Stand parallel to the barbell in a split stance, with your left foot behind your right. Keep your left heel off the ground. Position the middle of your right foot so it's under the weighted end of the barbell. Keeping your back straight, hinge at your hips and bend forward; keep your knees bent at a 15- to 20-degree angle (see figure a). As you hinge forward, keep most of your weight on your right leg and drive your hips backward. Do not allow your back to round. Grab the end of the barbell with your left hand and keep your thumb on the top.

Action and Coaching Tips

Keeping your back straight, drive your hips toward the barbell as you lift the barbell and stand tall without overextending your lower back (see figure b). As you lift the barbell by pressing your right foot into the ground, simultaneously press yourself toward the anchor point of the barbell by leaning toward your left side so your body is at a slight angle at the top of each rep. Be sure to drive your hips toward the anchor point of the barbell, and don't lean with just your shoulders (see figure c). Reverse the motion and slowly lower the barbell to the starting position. Keep the barbell close to you throughout. Perform all the reps on the same side before switching sides.

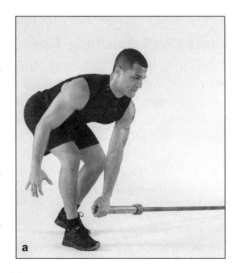

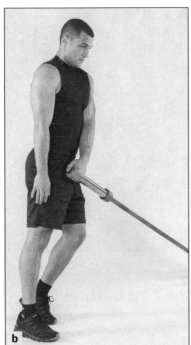
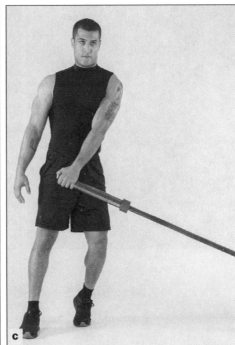

Best Knee Flexion Exercises in the Shortened-to-Midrange Strength Zone

The exercises in this section help you maximize the strength and development of the hamstrings in the shortened-to-midrange strength zone via the movement of knee flexion.

Machine Seated Leg Curl

Setup

For this exercise, use a seated hamstring curl (leg curl) machine. Sit tall and position the pad you'll be pushing against at the bottom of your calves. Position your legs hip-width apart and straight out, keeping the backs of your knees in contact with the seat pad (see figure a).

Action and Coaching Tips

Holding on to the handles, pull your calves against the pad by bending your knees to curl your legs under you as far as the machine will allow (see figure b). Slowly reverse the motion under control to complete the rep. Do not allow the portion of the weight stack that you're moving to rest on the other portion of the stack; rather, allow it to gently touch the rest of the stack at the end of each rep.

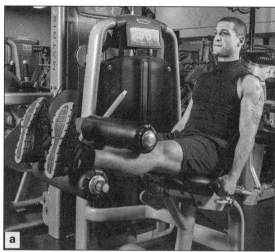
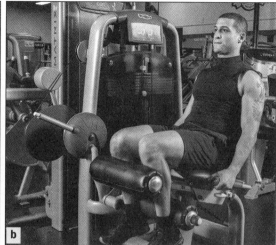

Machine Seated One-Leg Curl

Setup

For this exercise, use a seated hamstring curl (leg curl) machine. Sit tall and position the pad you'll be pushing against at the bottom of your calf. Position your leg straight out, keeping the back of your knee in contact with the seat pad (see figure a).

Action and Coaching Tips

Hold on to the handles, and using one leg, pull your calf against the pad by bending your knee to curl your leg under you as far as the machine will allow (see figure b). Slowly reverse the motion under control to complete the rep. Do not allow the portion of the weight stack that you're moving to rest on the other portion of the stack; rather, allow it to gently touch the rest of the stack at the end of each rep. Perform all reps on the same side before switching sides.

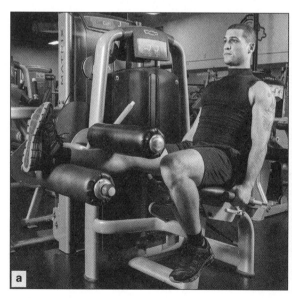
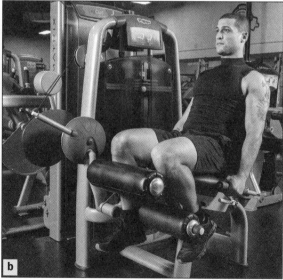

Machine Lying Leg Curl

Setup

For this exercise, use the machine that's commonly known as the lying hamstring curl or lying leg curl machine. Lie face down with your legs straight and your hip joint on top of the apex of the pads (see figure *a*). Adjust the pad you'll be pushing against so it's near the bottom of your calves.

Action and Coaching Tips

Hold on to the handles, and with your legs hip-width apart, pull your heels toward your glutes as far as possible (see figure *b*). Slowly reverse the motion under control. Do not allow the portion of the weight stack that you're moving to rest on the other portion of the stack; rather, allow it to gently touch the rest of the stack at the end of each rep.

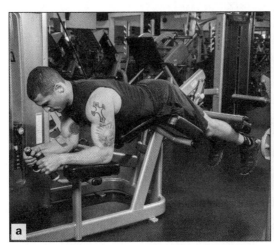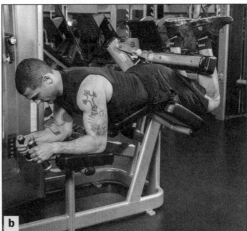

Machine Lying One-Leg Curl

Setup

For this exercise, use the machine that's commonly known as the lying hamstring curl or lying leg curl machine. Lie face down with your legs straight and your hip joint on top of the apex of the pads (see figure *a*). Adjust the pad you'll be pushing against so it's near the bottom of your calves.

Action and Coaching Tips

Hold on to the handles, and with your legs hip-width apart, pull one heel toward your glutes as far as possible while the other leg remains straight (see figure *b*). Slowly reverse the motion, under control. Do not allow the portion of the weight stack that you're moving to rest on the other portion of the stack; rather, allow it to gently touch the rest of the stack at the end of each rep. Perform all reps on the same side before switching sides.

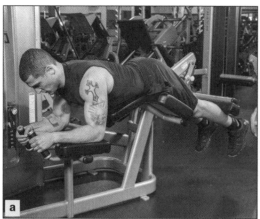
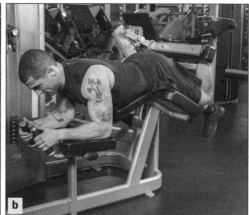

Nordic Hamstring Curl

Setup

This exercise requires either a partner or suitable gym equipment to securely lock your lower legs in place. Kneel tall, with your legs hip-width apart and your calves anchored (see figure *a*).

Action and Coaching Tips

Keeping your hips and back straight, slowly lower yourself toward the floor by extending at your knees. At the point where you can no longer lower yourself with control, allow your body to fall to the floor, using your hands to control your descent and landing in a position that resembles a kneeling push-up (see figure *b*). Use your hands to push back off the floor and help you reverse the motion so that you return to the tall kneeling position, thus completing the rep. Do not allow your hips to drift more than a few degrees behind you. Maintain a nearly straight line from your knees to your shoulders throughout.

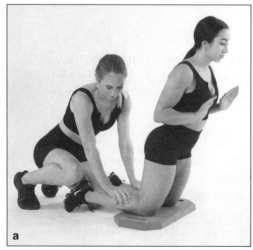
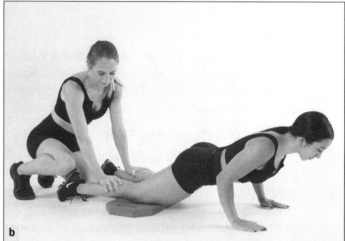

Stability Ball Leg Curl

Setup

Lie on your back on the floor, with your legs nearly hip-width apart, your heels resting on top of a 22- to 26-inch (55-65 cm) stability ball, and your arms out to the sides for balance. Raise your hips off the floor until your body forms a straight line (see figure a).

Action and Coaching Tips

Pull your heels toward your body while raising your hips toward the sky until your feet are under you (see figure b). Your body should form a straight line from your shoulders to your knees at the top of each rep. Slowly reverse the motion and repeat without allowing your hips to rest on the floor. Do not overextend your lower back at any time. If your feet drift lower on the ball while performing a set, adjust the foot position as needed.

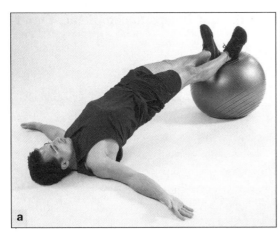 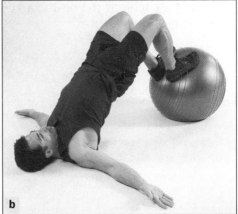

Stability Ball One-Leg Curl

Setup

Lie on your back on the floor, with your legs hip-width apart, your heels resting on top of an 18- to 22-inch (45-55 cm) stability ball, and your arms out to the side for balance. Raise your hips off the floor until your body forms a straight line, then raise one leg off the ball, flexing your hip and knee slightly above a 90-degree angle (see figure a).

Action and Coaching Tips

With one leg flexed, pull the ball toward your body with the heel that's on the ball while raising your hips toward the sky until your foot is under you (see figure b). Your body should form a straight line from your shoulders to your knee at the top of each rep. Slowly reverse the motion and repeat without allowing your hips to rest on the floor. Complete all repetitions on one side before switching to the other leg. Do not overextend your lower back at any time. If your feet drift lower on the ball while performing a set, adjust the foot position as needed.

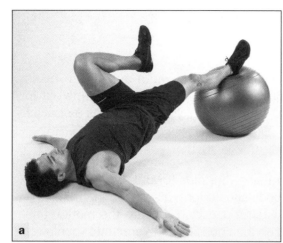 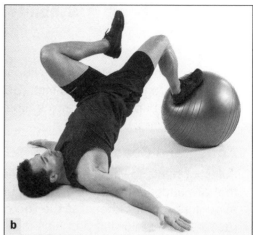

Now let's look at the best exercises for the quadriceps to complement your hamstring exercises.

CHAPTER 10

The Best Quadriceps Exercises

Training to develop your quadriceps strength through the true full range of motion involves performing at least one exercise for each of the following strength zones:

- Lengthened-to-midrange strength zone: Knee-bending exercise
- Shortened-to-midrange strength zone: Knee extension exercise

Picking at least one exercise from each category in this list maximizes your workout efficiency and helps you develop full-range quadriceps strength.

Quadriceps Exercise Mechanics

Squats and lunges are like horizontal chest presses in that they're most difficult at the bottom of the range of motion (see figure 10.1). This is where the lever arm is the longest and your knees are bent because your thigh is parallel or nearly parallel to the floor. As you get closer to the top and your knees extend, the lever arm shortens, and you gain a mechanical advantage on the weight as your thigh becomes vertical. So, even though the weight load you used was appropriate for the bottom part of the movement when your knees are bent, it's too light to create sufficient muscular overload on your quadriceps in the less difficult top ranges of motion when your knees are more extended. Therefore, full-range quadriceps strength is developed by using

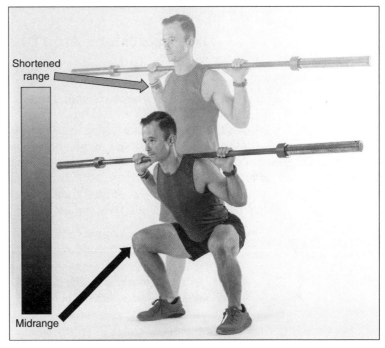

FIGURE 10.1 Barbell squat in lengthened-to-midrange strength zone: knee-bending exercise.

knee extension exercises (see figure 10.2) to strengthen your quads in the ranges missed by compound knee bend exercises like squats and lunges.

The quadriceps is made up of four muscles: rectus femoris, vastus lateralis, vastus medialis, and vastus intermedius. Research shows the machine leg extension creates much higher levels of activation in the rectus femoris of your quadriceps musculature than the squat does (1), which is likely why other research shows that the rectus femoris seems to grow more from knee extension exercises than the other three quadriceps muscles do (2).

Even if you're not motivated by that research, we can all agree that muscles

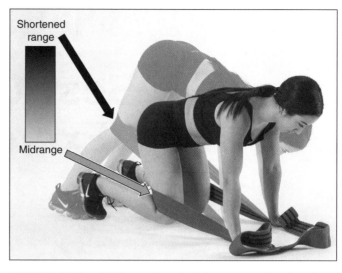

FIGURE 10.2 NT Loop inverted leg extension in shortened-to-midrange strength zone: knee extension exercise.

respond (make strength adaptations) to how they're loaded. In other words, to improve your strength in movements like backpedaling, decelerating forward momentum to change direction, or to walk downstairs or downhill, you need to train these actions with exercises such as reverse sled drags, NT Loop inverted leg extensions, and machine leg extensions, which are featured in the best knee extension exercises section of this chapter.

Additionally, a multitude of studies have shown that greater gains in quadriceps strength (even after anterior cruciate ligament reconstruction) occur when exercises like leg extensions are combined with exercises like squats and lunges than when using only exercises like squats and lunges (4).

Leg Extensions Aren't Bad or Dangerous!

Many trainers and lifters argue that the machine knee extension places tensile forces on the anterior cruciate ligament (ACL) and patellofemoral joint (PFJ). They say these exercises can be considered dangerous and instead recommend exercises like squats.

I had the honor of coauthoring with Andrew Vigotsky, a biomedical engineering PhD student, a peer-reviewed and highly referenced paper for a National Strength and Conditioning Association journal: "Are the Seated Leg Extension, Leg Curl, and Adduction Machine Exercises Non-Functional or Risky?" (6).

In our paper, we demonstrated that this perspective is not only shallow but is also logically inconsistent. Here are key points on leg extensions from our article:

- The tensile forces experienced by the ACL during the machine leg extension, using loads ranging from a dynamic 12 repetition maximum to a maximum voluntary isometric effort, are less than one-fifth of its ultimate strength. So, although tensile forces are placed on the ACL during the machine leg extension exercise, these forces are far below the threshold of the ACL. Thus, damage or injury from the leg extension to the ACL is not a concern.

- ACL forces during the knee extension are less than or equal to many other functional tasks, such as walking or landing. Therefore, machine leg extensions do not appear to be any more unsafe for the ACL than what's required for everyday activity.
- The recommendation of the squat being a safer exercise for knee ligament health is also logically inconsistent. For example, one study suggests that posterior cruciate ligament (PCL) forces in the squat are about 10 times greater than those placed on the ACL during the knee extension.
- When it comes to the PFJ, body weight squats to 90 degrees of knee flexion (knee bend) elicit greater peak PFJ stress than machine leg extensions when muscle activity amplitude is matched. Nevertheless, if someone has knee pain, exercise selection and range of motion should be tailored to the individual according to the recommendation of a medical professional; otherwise, the machine leg extension, like the squat, should not be considered universally contraindicated.

Best Knee-Bending Exercises in the Lengthened-to-Midrange Strength Zone

The exercises in this section help you maximize the strength and development of your quadriceps in the knee-bending strength zone.

Find Your Best Squat Stance

Many lifters think a proper squat is a shoulder-width stance with your feet pointed fairly straight forward. The new angle here is to not take such a one-size-fits-all approach to squatting.

Although the squat exercise descriptions I've provided here are general, you should adjust your stance (foot width and position) to best fit your body and to fit the way you move. Experiment with stances wider than parallel and turning your toes out slightly to find the stance that allows you to lower the deepest in the squat while maintaining an arch in your lower back.

The common and normal anatomical variations of the hip joint structure in addition to the length of one's torso, femur (thigh bone), and tibia (shin bone) determine function (7, 8, 9, 10). Therefore, an optimal squat is individual and comes in a variety of foot positions, stance widths, depths, and torso angles.

Barbell Squat

Setup

Place a barbell across your shoulders (not on your neck) and stand with your feet just farther than shoulder-width apart and your toes turned out 10 to 15 degrees (see figure a).

Action and Coaching Tips

Bend at your knees and hips and lower your body toward the floor; go as low as you can without losing the arch in your lower back (see figure b). Your heels should not lift off the ground, and avoid allowing your knees to drop in toward the midline of your body. Keep your knees tracking in the same direction as your toes. Once you've gone as deep as you can, reverse the motion and stand up.

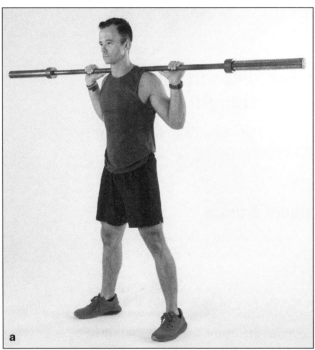
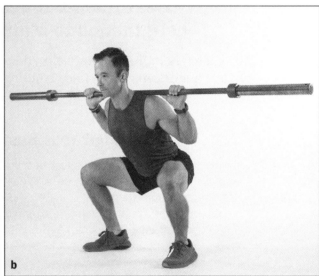

a   b

Barbell Heel-Raised Squat

Setup

Place a barbell across your shoulders (not on your neck) and stand with your feet just farther than shoulder-width apart and your toes turned out 10 to 15 degrees. Place your heels on top of small weight plates or a small wedge (see figure a).

Action and Coaching Tips

Bend at your knees and hips and lower your body toward the floor; go as low as you can without losing the arch in your lower back (see figure b). Your heels should not lift off the plates or wedge. Avoid allowing your knees to drop in toward the midline of your body; keep your knees tracking in the same direction as your toes. Once you've gone as low as you can, reverse the motion and stand up.

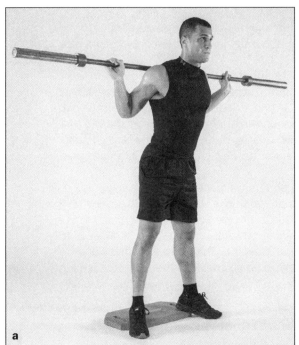
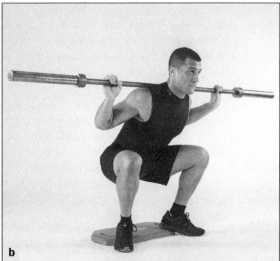

Heel-Raised Squats Aren't Bad

Lifters usually elevate their heels during barbell back squats for three reasons:

1. To increase their squat depth
2. Because it feels better to them
3. To keep their torso more upright, which increases demand on the quads

Although heel-elevated squats are a great exercise, some trainers and coaches say you shouldn't use them. These are the two most common reasons they give:

1. It reinforces dysfunctional movement, which could increase your injury risk.
2. It teaches your body how to squat wrong. Why not teach your body how to squat with your feet flat?

Are they right? No matter how good an exercise is, some trainers will claim it's bad for the two reasons listed. And although we're looking specifically at the heel-raised squat, the same points you'll see here can refute arguments against other "bad" exercises. So let's cut through the confusion, and then you can decide whether elevating your heels during squats is a thing you'd benefit from doing.

They Don't Reinforce Dysfunctional Movement

The reason some trainers say they reinforce dysfunctional movement is because squatting with your heels elevated eliminates ankle dorsiflexion (when you bend at the ankle). Whereas, squatting with your feet flat forces your ankles into dorsiflexion. This is why people with restricted ankle dorsiflexion feel like they can keep their knees and torso in better alignment when using a heel lift.

So in the case of someone with limited range of motion during ankle dorsiflexion, heel-raised squats do not increase their limitation but instead offer a technique that allows them to squat in a way that is more comfortable while working around their limitation. I agree with the concern about ignoring restricted range of motion during ankle dorsiflexion. It's been associated with issues such as ankle injuries (11) and knee injuries (12), and it may also lead to abnormal lower extremity biomechanics during multi-joint strengthening exercises (13).

It's important to work on improving ankle dorsiflexion if it's limited and to work on maintaining your current range of motion if it is not restricted. However, this in no way means heel-raised squats are a bad exercise that people must avoid, regardless of their available ankle dorsiflexion range of motion. It just means that they need to do other exercises that involve moving or loading their ankle complex in the ranges not accessed during heel-raised squats, such as the calf exercises highlighted in chapter 12.

In other words, it's not that heel-raised squats will cause you to lose your range of motion during ankle dorsiflexion. It's that you'll lose it if you don't do anything regularly that involves ankle dorsiflexion. This is why we do multiple exercises for all areas of the body in the strength zone training system: one exercise allows you to train in ranges of motion missed by another exercise. That said, go ahead and do heel-raised squats as you see fit. Just make sure you also do the calf exercises in chapter 12, which are designed to increase your range of motion and build strength throughout the chapter.

They Don't Make You Less Capable of Squatting Without a Lift

Some lifters who can do squats without the heel raised use an elevated heel to squat because it hits their quads more. Some do it because it involves less of the lower back, allowing them to go deep and still maintain a more upright torso.

But critics will argue against these reasons stating that the heel raise teaches your body to squat this way and, as a result, you'll lose your ability to squat well with heels on the ground. There are several problems with this line of thinking. Using their logic, I could say that trainers should never have clients or athletes ride a bike because it teaches them to move forward this way, therefore making them less able to walk or run properly. Each step you'd take would be in an (attempted) circular fashion if this were the case. We all know that just because the body learns how to ride a bike, that in no way causes the body to forget how to walk or run the way it normally does.

Learning how to do new things doesn't detract from other skills you've acquired because the human body is highly adaptable. It can learn lots of ways to move without one thing interfering with another. Multisport athletes are a shining example of this. In fact, they're more functional—not less—when they've exposed their bodies to many different forms of movement.

That said, it's a different story if all you ever do is squat with your heels raised. Then, yes, you'll get used to squatting that way. The best approach is to expose yourself to different squat variations to make your body more adaptable. That way, mixing in heel-raised squats won't reduce your ability to squat well when your feet are flat.

Trap Bar Squat

Although some people refer to this exercise as a deadlift rather than a squat, the torso and hip positions in this exercise more closely resemble that of a barbell squat than that of a barbell deadlift.

Setup

For this exercise you need a trap bar. Stand inside the bar, holding on to the handles. Your feet are roughly shoulder-width apart (see figure *a*).

Action and Coaching Tips

Slowly lower yourself so if you have loaded weight plates on the bar, they touch the floor. As you lower your body, keep your feet flat and your knees in line with your toes (see figure *b*). Maintain a strong inward arch in your lower back while lowering into a squatting position. Stand up tall so that your hands are directly outside of your hips. Slowly lower into the squat until the weight plates on the bar touch the floor.

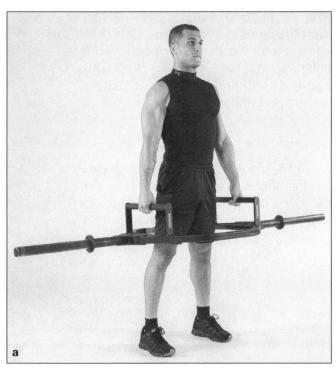
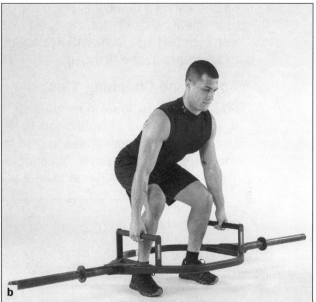

Dumbbell Goblet Squat

Setup

With both hands on one end of a dumbbell, place it against the top of your chest. Your forearms or elbows are clamped down on the bottom of the dumbbell. Stand with your feet just farther than shoulder-width apart and your toes turned out 10 to 15 degrees (see figure *a*).

Action and Coaching Tips

Bend at your knees and hips and lower your body toward the floor as low as you can without losing the arch in your lower back or allowing your heels to lift off the ground (see figure *b*). Once you've gone as deep as you can control in the squat, reverse the motion by extending your legs and returning to the standing position to

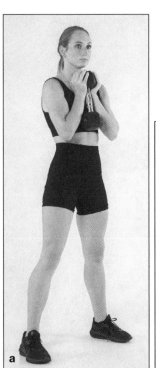
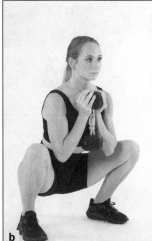

complete the rep. Keep your knees tracking in the same direction as your toes; do not allow your knees to drop in toward the midline of your body.

Dumbbell Goblet Squat With NT Loop Knee Resistance

Setup

Anchor an NT Loop band securely in front of you at knee height. Place both legs inside the NT Loop so it is near or just below the crook of your knees. Back away from the origin of the NT Loop to create tension on the band. With both hands on one end of a dumbbell, place the dumbbell against the top of your chest, with your forearms or elbows clamped down on the bottom of the dumbbell. Stand with your feet just farther than shoulder-width apart and your toes turned out 10 to 15 degrees (see figure a).

Action and Coaching Tips

Squat as low as you can by bending your knees and sitting your hips back (see figure b). Do not allow your heels to rise off the floor or your lower back to round. Also, do not allow your knees to drop in toward the midline of your body; keep your knees tracking in the same direction as your toes. Reverse the motion by extending your legs against the band until your knees are straight to complete a rep.

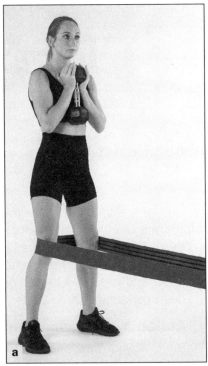
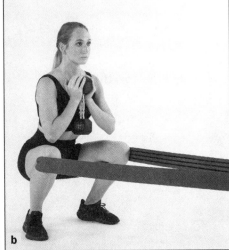

Dumbbell Traveling Lunge

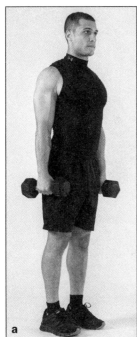

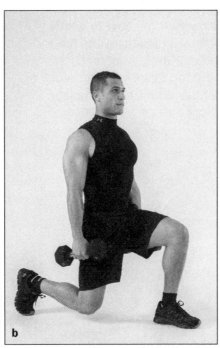

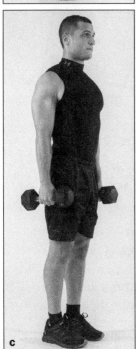

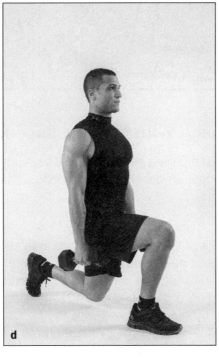

Using a shorter stride length that allows for a slightly forward shin angle at the bottom of each rep, as opposed to a longer stride with a more vertical shin angle, focuses this exercise more on your quads.

Setup

Stand tall, with your feet around hip-width apart. Hold a dumbbell in each hand at your sides using a neutral grip (see figure a). You can also do this exercise using only body weight by allowing your hands to hang at your sides or by interlacing your fingers behind your head.

Action and Coaching Tips

Take a step forward and drop your body so that your back knee lightly touches the floor as you keep your torso upright (see figure b). Stand up tall while bringing your rear leg forward to meet your front leg (see figure c) and step forward with the opposite leg—the one that was behind you on the last rep (see figure d). Do not step so far out on each lunge that you're unable to do this exercise smoothly and with control. Repeat as you walk down the room.

Dumbbell Step-Up

Setup

Stand facing a weight bench or platform and put your right foot on the platform. Hold a dumbbell in each hand by your hips (see figure a). You can also do this exercise using only body weight by allowing your hands to hang at your sides or by interlacing your fingers behind your head.

Action and Coaching Tips

Step up by straightening your right knee (see figure *b*). Once you're on top of the platform, allow your left foot to gently touch the platform to help maintain your balance, and then reverse the motion by stepping down with your left foot first. Bring your right foot down to the floor. Place your left foot on top of the platform and repeat the exercise to complete one rep. Switch the working leg (i.e., the stepping leg) on the ground, not when you're on top of the platform. Move smoothly and with control; avoid jerking your torso forward to initiate each rep. Lean slightly forward while keeping most of your weight on the front leg throughout.

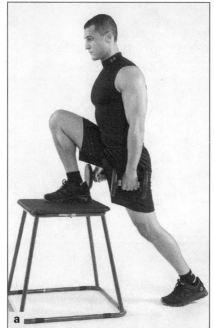

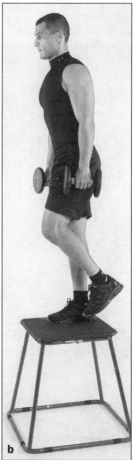

Dumbbell Reverse Lunge With NT Loop Knee Resistance

Using a shorter stride length that allows a slightly forward shin angle at the bottom of each rep, as opposed to a longer stride with a more vertical shin angle, focuses this exercise more on the quads.

Setup

Anchor an NT Loop securely in front of you at your knee height. Place your right leg inside the NT Loop so it is just below the crook of your knee. Back away from the origin of the NT Loop to create tension on the band and stand tall with your legs hip-width apart while holding a dumbbell in each hand at your sides (see figure *a*). Your right leg should be directly in line with the band. You can also do this exercise using only body weight by allowing your hands to hang at your sides or by interlacing your fingers behind your head.

Action and Coaching Tips

Keeping your torso upright, lower your body toward the floor by taking a step back with your left leg until your back knee lightly touches the floor without allowing your left knee to rest on the floor (see figure *b*). As you lower your body, keep your back straight and torso upright. Drive your right heel into the ground to raise your body to the starting position, and step your left leg up so it's next to your right

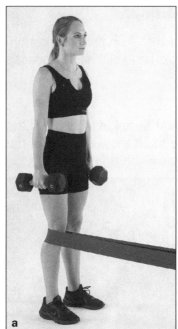

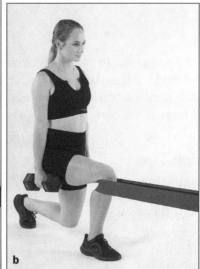

to complete the rep. Perform all reps on one side before switching to the other leg. Keep the majority of your weight on your front foot throughout the exercise.

Dumbbell Elevated Split Squat

Using a shorter stride length that allows a slightly forward shin angle at the bottom of each rep, as opposed to a longer stride with a more vertical shin angle, focuses this exercise more on the quads.

Setup

Stand tall while holding a dumbbell in each hand at your sides. Stand in a split stance with each foot on top of a small platform or weight plate. Your front foot should be far enough in front of your back foot that your front shin can stay nearly vertical as you drop into each rep (see figure *a*). You can also do this exercise using only body weight by allowing your hands to hang at your sides or by interlacing your fingers behind your head.

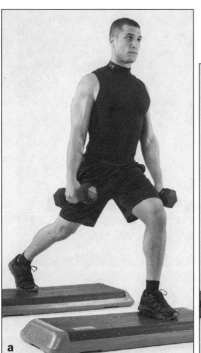

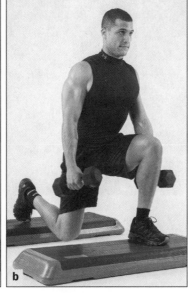

Action and Coaching Tips

Keeping your torso upright, lower your body toward the floor without allowing your back knee to rest on the floor (see figure *b*). As you lower your body, keep your back straight and torso upright. Drive your front heel into the ground to raise your body to the starting position, thus completing the rep. Perform all reps on one side before switching to the other leg. Keep your weight mostly on your front foot throughout the exercise.

Cable Front-to-Back Split Squat

Using a shorter stride length that allows a slightly forward shin angle at the bottom of each rep, as opposed to a longer stride with a more vertical shin angle, focuses this exercise more on the quads.

Setup

Stand in front of a cable column with a handle attached at ankle level. Hold the handle in your left hand and back away from the cable to lift the weight off of the weight stack. Stand in a split stance with your legs hip-width apart. The left leg is back, and your left heel is off the ground (see figure a).

Action and Coaching Tips

Keeping your torso upright, lower your body toward the floor as you simultaneously shift your body toward the cable. Lower as far down and forward as you can while keeping your front foot flat on the ground (see figure b). As you lower your body, keep your back straight and torso upright. Drive your front foot into the ground to raise your body as you simultaneously shift your body backward, away from the cable until your front knee is straight. Perform all reps on one side before switching to the other leg (see figure c).

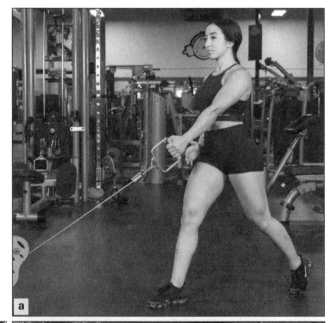

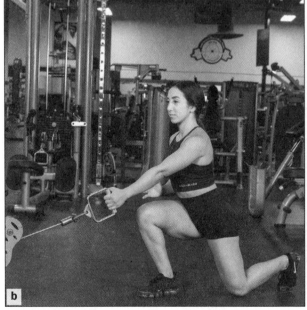

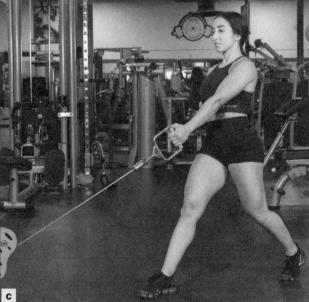

Machine Leg Press

Placing your feet at the middle or lower on the platform rather than closer to the top of the platform allows a slightly forward shin angle at the bottom of each rep, which focuses this exercise more on the quads.

Setup

For this exercise, use the machine that's commonly known as the leg press machine. Sit with a tall torso and place your feet roughly shoulder-width apart and flat on the platform (see figure *a*).

Action and Coaching Tips

Bend at your knees and hips as far as you can while keeping your feet flat on the platform and maintaining your starting alignment (see figure *b*). Once you've gone as deep as you can control, reverse the motion by extending your legs and finishing each rep without locking out your knees. Keep your knees tracking in the same direction as your toes, and do not allow your knees to drop in toward the midline of your body as you perform the action.

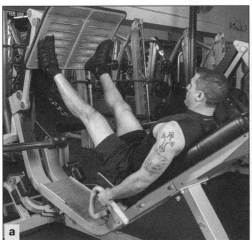 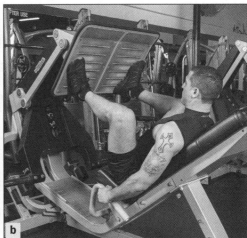

Dumbbell Stability Ball Wall Squat

Setup

Stand with your feet shoulder-width apart and your toes pointed straight as you lean against a 22- to 26-inch (55-65 cm) stability ball that's on the wall at your lower back. Your toes should be 12 to 20 inches (30-50 cm) in front of your hips, and your knees should be slightly bent. Hold a dumbbell in each hand by your hips (see figure *a*). You can also do this exercise using only body weight by allowing your hands to hang at your sides or by interlacing your fingers behind your head.

Action and Coaching Tips

Keeping your torso upright, bend at your knees and hips and lower your body toward the floor as much as you can by rolling the ball down the wall along your back without losing the arch in your lower back (see figure *b*). Once you've gone as deep as you can control in the squat, reverse the motion by extending your legs, rolling the ball up the wall along your back, and returning to the standing position to complete the rep. Keep your knees tracking in the same direction as your toes; do not allow your knees to drop in toward the midline of your body throughout.

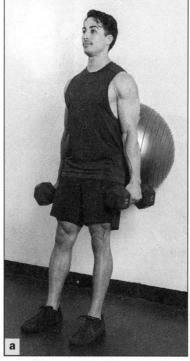
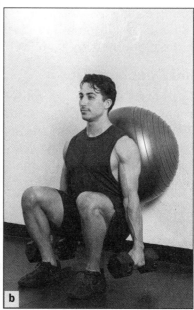

Zombie Squat With NT Loop Knee Resistance

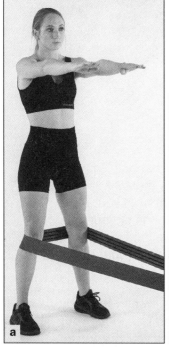

Setup

Anchor an NT Loop securely in front of you at knee height. Place both legs inside the NT Loop so it is just at or below the crook of your knees. Back away from the origin of the NT Loop to create tension on the band. Stand tall with your feet shoulder-width apart and your toes turned out about 10 degrees. Extend your arms in front of you at shoulder height (see figure a). Keeping your arms extended in front of you at shoulder height serves as a counterbalance to help keep your torso upright as you lower yourself on each rep.

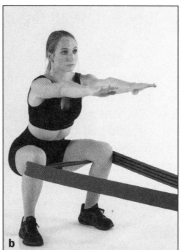

Action and Coaching Tips

Squat by bending your knees and sitting back at your hips. Lower so your thighs are almost parallel to the floor without allowing your lower back to round (see figure b). As you squat, do not allow your heels to come off the ground or your knees to come together toward the midline of your body. Your knees should track in the same direction as your toes. Reverse and stand up to complete the rep.

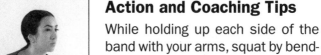

NT Loop Squat

Setup

Stand inside an NT Loop, with your feet on top of the band slightly wider than shoulder-width apart and your toes turned out about 10 degrees. Bend at your torso and bring the top end of the band behind your head so it rests comfortably at the bottom of your neck when you stand up tall (see figure *a*). Grab each side of the band and lift up on the band to create resistance. The lower you grab on to the band to lift it up, the more resistance you create.

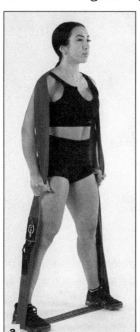

Action and Coaching Tips

While holding up each side of the band with your arms, squat by bending your knees and sitting back at your hips. Lower so your thighs are roughly parallel to the floor without allowing your lower back to round (see figure *b*). As you squat, do not allow your heels to come off the ground or your knees to come together toward the midline of your body. Your knees should track in the same direction as your toes. Reverse and stand up to complete the rep.

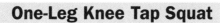

One-Leg Knee Tap Squat

Setup

Stand facing away from a pad that is 3 to 5 inches (about 8-13 cm) thick, a small stack of weight plates with a mat on top, or a workout step. Shift your weight to your left leg and lift the right foot off the floor, with the knee bent to around 90 degrees and slightly behind your left leg. Your hands are outstretched in front of you to serve as a counterbalance (see figure *a*). You can also perform the exercise while holding a dumbbell at each shoulder.

Action and Coaching Tips

Slowly lower yourself toward the floor by bending your weight-bearing knee and sitting back at your hips until you lightly tap your back knee on the object (see figure *b*). Do not allow your back (non-weight-bearing) foot to touch the floor. Reverse the motion and stand up again. Perform all reps on the same side before switching sides.

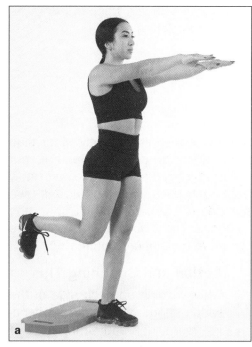

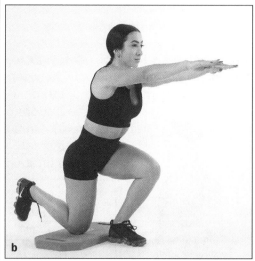

NT Loop Zercher Reverse Lunge

Setup

Stand in a split stance with your front foot on top of the middle of both layers of an NT Loop. Place each side of the NT Loop around your arms so it remains near the crooks of your elbows. Clasp your hands together, palm to palm, with your elbows bent to at least 90 degrees, and pull your arms into your torso. Keep your hands directly above your front leg and your torso upright (see figure a).

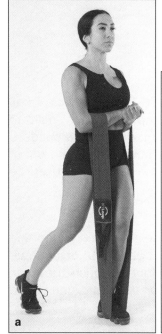

Action and Coaching Tips

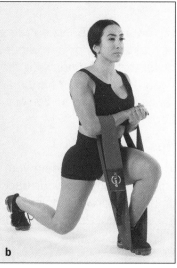

Step back with your back leg, and lower your body toward the floor until your back knee lightly touches the floor without allowing your back knee to rest on the floor (see figure b). Reverse the motion by driving your front foot into the ground and standing up by straightening your front knee as you bring your back leg next to your front leg with your heel elevated. Perform all reps on one side before switching to the other leg. Keep the majority of your weight on your front foot throughout the exercise.

Best Knee Extension Exercises in the Shortened-to-Midrange Strength Zone

The exercises in this section help you maximize the strength and development of your quadriceps in the knee extension strength zone.

Machine Leg Extension

Setup

Sit tall on the leg extension machine, with the pad for your legs at low-shin level, your legs hip-width apart, and the backs of your knees in contact with the seat pad (see figure a).

Action and Coaching Tips

Holding on to the handles, push your shins into the pad and extend your legs, keeping your ankles dorsiflexed until just before your knees are fully straight (see figure b). Slowly reverse the motion to complete one rep. Do not allow the weight stack you are moving to rest on the stack, instead allow it to gently touch at the end of each rep.

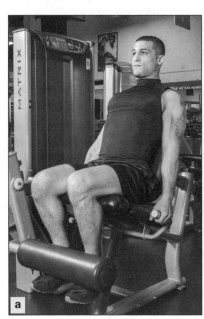 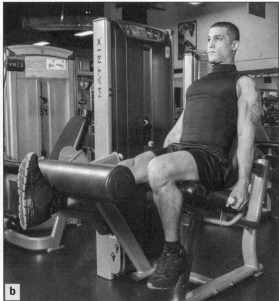

Machine Unilateral Leg Extension

Setup

For this exercise, use the machine that's commonly known as the leg extension machine. Sit tall, with the pad for your legs at the low-shin level, your legs hip-width apart, and the backs of your knees in contact with the seat pad (see figure *a*).

Action and Coaching Tips

Hold on to the handles and using one leg at a time, push your shin into the pad and extend your leg, keeping your ankle dorsiflexed until just before your knee is almost straight (see figure *b*). Slowly reverse the motion to complete the rep. Do not allow the weight stack you are moving to rest on the stack, instead allow it to gently touch at the end of each rep. Perform all reps on the same leg before switching legs.

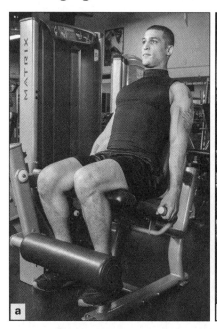 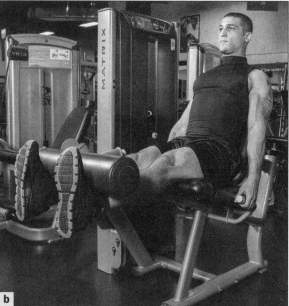

Reverse Sled Drag

Setup

Use a weight sled with strap handles to perform this exercise. Stand with the sled about 2 yards (1.8 m) in front of you while holding the strap handles in your hands at roughly hip height and your arms straight. Assume a partial split squat position so your thighs are at a roughly 45-degree angle to the floor (see figure *a*).

Action and Coaching Tips

Drive your legs into the ground and move backward by stepping one leg after the other (see figure *b*). Do not round your upper back at any time; keep your torso and arms straight throughout. Use a weight load that's neither light enough for you to run with nor heavy enough that you have to lean your body backward at a 45-degree angle. Instead, find a load at which you can move the sled in a smooth, deliberate manner with each step.

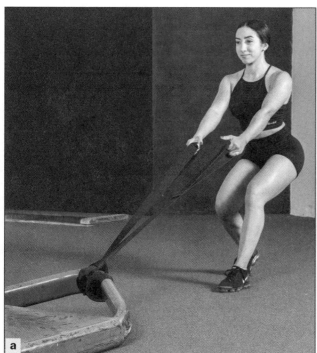 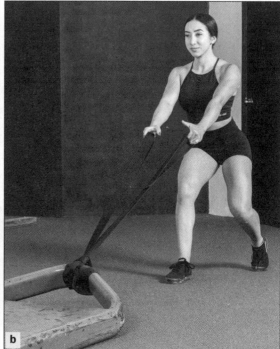

Unilateral Reverse Sled Drag

This is the same exercise as the reverse sled drag except here you're focusing on using one leg at a time instead of alternating legs. This allows you to concentrate on using each side individually to make sure you have balanced strength between your left and right sides.

Setup

Use a weight sled with strap handles to perform this exercise. Stand with the sled about 2 yards (1.8 m) in front of you while holding the strap handles in your hands at hip height and your arms straight. Assume a partial squat position so your thighs are at a roughly 45-degree angle to the floor.

Action and Coaching Tips

Drive your right leg into the ground and move backward by stepping your left leg backward (see figure *a*). Then place your right leg next to your left (see figure *b*) and repeat as you drag the sled down the room (see figure *c*). Do not round your upper back at any time; keep your torso and arms straight throughout. Be sure to use a weight load at which you can move the sled in a smooth, deliberate manner with each step. Perform all reps on one side before switching sides.

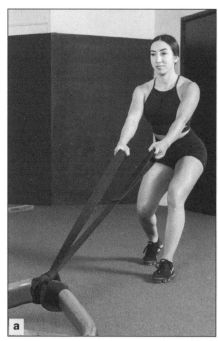
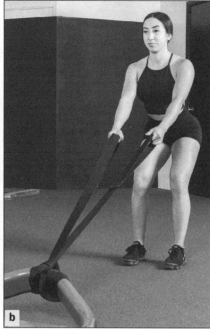
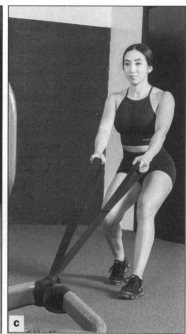

Weight Plate Push

Setup

Place a heavy weight plate—try 35 to 45 pounds (about 15-20 kg)—on top of a towel or on a turf surface so that it glides. For an additional challenge, you can also place a set of dumbbells (25-35 lb, or about 11-15 kg) inside of the weight plate. Get into a push-up position, with your hands on top of the weight plate or the dumbbells.

Action and Coaching Tips

Drive with your legs by bringing your knees up toward your chest in alternating fashion to push the plate quickly across the floor for 40 to 50 yards (35-46 m) (see figures *a* and *b*). As you improve, increase the load challenge by placing a pair of heavier dumbbells inside the weight plate.

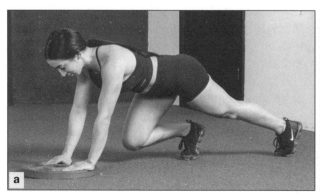
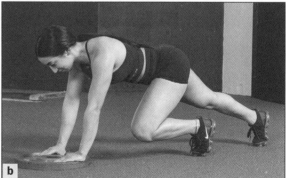

NT Loop Inverted Leg Extension

Setup

Step inside an NT Loop and place it behind your knees, with your legs roughly hip-width apart. Assume an all-fours position on the floor, with each side of the NT Loop under each hand. Take as much slack out of the band as needed to match your strength level. The lower you grab the band, the more resistance you create. With your hands on the floor holding the band under your shoulders, slightly lift your knees off the ground (see figure *a*).

Action and Coaching Tips

Extend your legs by pushing your knees against the band until your legs are straight (see figure *b*). Slowly reverse the motion by bending your knees, stopping just before your knees touch the ground to complete the rep.

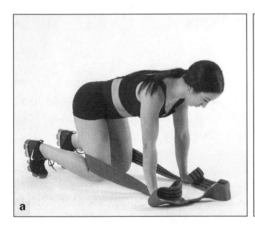
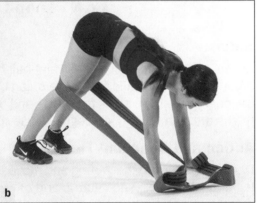

NT Loop Feet-Elevated Inverted Leg Extension

Setup

Step inside an NT Loop and place it behind your knees, with your legs hip-width apart. Assume an all-fours position on the floor, with each side of the NT Loop under each hand. Take as much slack out of the band as needed to match your strength level. The lower you grab the band, the more resistance you create. With your hands on the floor holding the band under your shoulders, place your feet on top of a bench or platform that's roughly the same height as your head. Lift your knees just off the floor, keeping your knees bent (see figure *a*).

Action and Coaching Tips

Extend your legs by pushing the back of your knees against the band until your legs are straight (see figure *b*). Slowly reverse the motion by bending your knees, stopping just before your knees touch the ground to complete the rep.

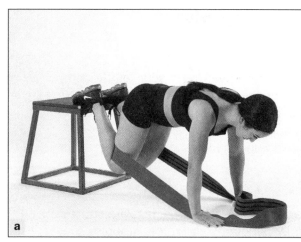
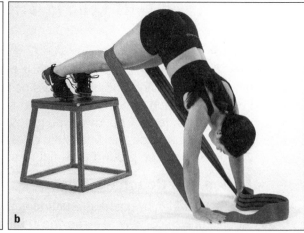

NT Loop Low Walk

Setup

Anchor an NT Loop securely at waist height. Stand inside the NT Loop so it wraps around your waist while facing the origin of the band. Stand far enough back from the origin to remove slack from the band. Assume a partial squat position so your thighs are at a roughly 45-degree angle to the floor (see figure *a*).

Action and Coaching Tips

Drive your legs into the ground and move backward by taking small steps with one leg after the other (see figure *b* and *c*). Walk backward for four to six steps, then reverse the action by walking forward for four to six steps without allowing slack in the band. Stay low in a squat stance throughout.

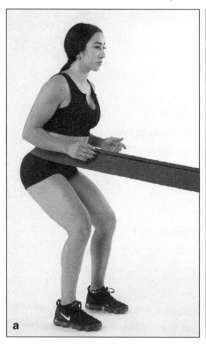
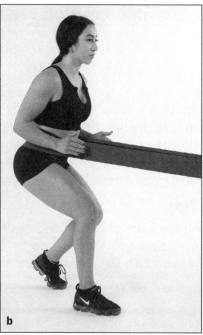
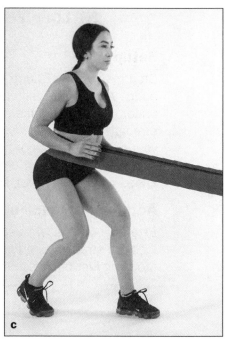

Even if you perform deadlifts and squats, you might be missing exercises that will help you develop athletic glutes and hips. That's what the next chapter is all about.

CHAPTER 11

The Best Glute and Hip Exercises

Training to develop your glute and hip strength through the true full range of motion involves performing at least one exercise for each of the following strength zones:

- Lengthened-to-midrange range strength zone: hip-hinging exercise
- Shortened-to-midrange range strength zone: hip extension exercise
- Hip abduction exercises
- Hip adduction exercises

Picking at least one exercise from each category on this list maximizes your workout efficiency and helps you develop full-range glute and hip strength.

Training the Inner Thigh

Some trainers may argue that compound and single-leg exercises like wide-stance squats, lunges, and single-leg squats train the adductors effectively enough to offset the need for additional adductor isolation exercises. However, the highest hip adductor muscle activity values for the wide-stance squat (5), along with those found during a single-leg squat and a lunge, are relatively low compared to exercises that focus primarily on the hip adduction movement (6). So, with respect to reaching greater levels of muscle activity in the adductors, isolation exercises are superior to squats and lunges.

Additionally, it's important to see how the scientific evidence falls in line with the principle of specificity. Research demonstrates that strength gains are highly specific to the part of the movement one trains in, with limited transfer to the rest of the untrained ranges of the movement that may not be addressed in a given exercise (7, 8).

With this in mind, exercises developed to train the hip adductors directly—such as the bent-knee Copenhagen hip adduction exercise, the NT Loop quadruped hip adduction, and the machine hip adduction—move through larger ranges of motion of hip adduction than exercises such as squats, single-leg squats, and lunges. Therefore, when training the adductor musculature, it makes sense to add such exercises into a program to train in ranges of motions that may not be sufficiently addressed by compound exercises (9).

Glute and Hip Exercise Mechanics

It's important to understand that there are quad-focused lunges and split squats, and there are glute-focused lunges and split squats. The beauty of the lunge exercise is that you can manipulate the stride length and torso position to change the lower-body training stimulus. A forward torso lean and longer stride hit the glutes and hamstrings more (1), which is what you'll see demonstrated in this chapter, whereas we discussed the opposite in the previous chapter that focused on the quads. That's why the lunges in chapter 10 use a shorter stride, the shoulders stay over hips by keeping an upright torso, and the shin angles slightly forward. All this emphasizes the quads (2).

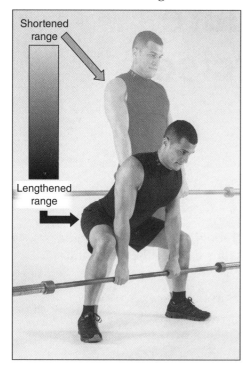

FIGURE 11.1 Barbell hybrid deadlift in lengthened-to-midrange range strength zone: hip-hinging exercise.

The same is true for split squat variations. The lunges and split squat variations in this chapter are done with a longer stride and a forward leaning torso to load the glutes to a greater degree than the exercises in chapter 10. By leaning your torso slightly forward and extending your stride a bit, you can make lunges and deadlifts work the glutes more while still working the quads (see figure 11.1).

It's also important to understand that exercises such as squats, Romanian deadlifts, lunges, and many variations of those exercises provided in chapters 9 and 10 load your glutes when they're closer to a lengthened (stretched) range. The additional deadlift and lunge variations provided in this chapter focus on strengthening the glutes in their lengthened-to-midrange zone.

In addition to the exercises featured in this chapter, the hip-hinging exercises in chapter 9 and knee-bending exercises in chapter 10 strengthen your glutes in their lengthened-to-midrange strength zone. However, these exercises don't do a great job of loading the glutes when they're in a shortened range. In other words, Romanian deadlifts, squats, and lunges create the greatest load on the glutes when your hips are flexed (at the bottom), but there's little load on the glutes at the top when your hips are extended.

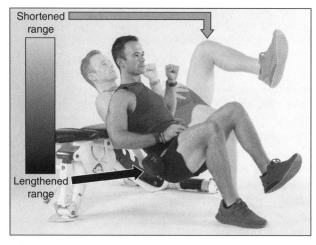

FIGURE 11.2 Dumbbell one-leg hip thrust in shortened-to-midrange range strength zone: hip extension exercise.

Because strength is position specific, it's important to regularly perform shortened-to-midrange hip extension exercises such as hip thrusts, reverse hip extensions, hip lifts, 45-degree hip extensions, and cable one-leg Romanian deadlifts to train the glutes in the more shortened ranges of hip extension that are neglected by most squat, deadlift, and lunge variations (see figure 11.2).

In regard to the hips, much has been made about hip abduction exercises such as pushing your knees out against a band loop while you hip thrust or squat and doing band lateral hip shuffles (see figure 11.3). And yes, they should be a weekly component of a comprehensive lower-body strength program.

You often see "booty builders" place a big training emphasis on hip abduction by pushing the knees out against a band loop. They do this during a variety of exercises when it's not necessary or beneficial. This doesn't create a complementary ratio to their regular hip adduction exercises. And the imbalance is risky.

Here's a reminder: Hip abduction is what you do when pushing your legs apart. Hip adduction is what you do when drawing them together.

Research on professional hockey players found that they were 17 times more likely to sustain an adductor muscle strain (groin injury) if their adductor strength (muscles that move the leg toward the body's midline) was less than 80 percent of their abductor strength (muscles that move the leg away from the body's midline) (3). Although that strength ratio is based on one study, another systematic review (a study of studies) found that hip adductor strength was one of the most common risk factors for groin injury in sport (4). In other words, an emphasis on hip abduction exercises that's not complemented with hip adduction exercises may put you at an increased risk of injury. This is one reason why your lower-body strength training programs should include at least one hip adduction exercise each week, such as machine seated hip adduction, side-lying hip adduction (see figure 11.4), NT Loop quadruped hip adduction, and the bent-knee Copenhagen hip adduction.

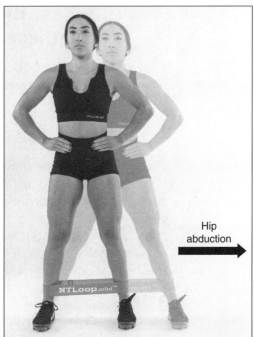

FIGURE 11.3 Band lateral hip shuffle in hip abduction exercises.

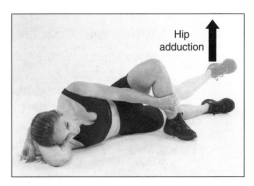

FIGURE 11.4 Side-lying hip adduction in hip adduction exercises.

The Hip Exercise That Trainers Hate That Isn't Bad: Machine Hip Adduction

This exercise is often used in the false belief that it will spot reduce the inner thighs. Add in the notion that many trainers hold that seated, single-joint (isolation) exercises are nonfunctional or that any benefits from isolation exercise can also be gained from multi-joint exercises, and you can see why the machine hip adduction is commonly on a trainer's hit list.

Why the Machine Hip Adduction Isn't Bad

You can't spot reduce, but you sure as heck can spot enhance! Squats, deadlifts, and their variations, along with hip abduction and hip extension exercises in the shortened-to-midrange strength zone are great exercises for spot enhancing (i.e., building) your glutes, but no hip adduction exercise will slim your inner thighs. That said, isolated hip adductor training exercises offer potential performance benefits and reduction of injury risk, as I've shown previously.

Best Hip-Hinging Exercises in the Lengthened-to-Midrange Strength Zone

The exercises in this section help you maximize the strength of your glutes in the lengthened-to-midrange strength zone via hip-hinging movements.

Barbell Hybrid Deadlift

This lift combines the Romanian and sumo deadlifts, which you'd do with a wider stance and a more upright torso. For many, the barbell hybrid deadlift is a smart substitute for traditional deadlifts for two reasons. First, the wider stance is easier and more natural for most lifters to do while maintaining the alignment cues. Second, this starting position keeps the barbell closer to the hips than the conventional style, which provides a shorter lever arm. This gives you a greater mechanical advantage while placing less overall stress on the lower back.

Setup

Stand in front of a barbell, with your feet slightly farther than shoulder-width apart and turned out 15 degrees. Keeping your back straight and maintaining an arch in your lower back, hinge at your hips and bend your knees. Lower your torso to about a 45-degree angle and grab the bar; your hands are shoulder-width apart (see figure a).

Action and Coaching Tips

Keeping your back straight, drive your hips forward toward the barbell and lift it off the ground while straightening your legs (see figure b). Reverse the motion and slowly lower the barbell back to the floor to complete the rep. As you hinge forward, drive your hips backward and do not allow your back to round. Lift the bar by extending your hips, not by overextending your lower back. Keep the barbell close to you throughout; it

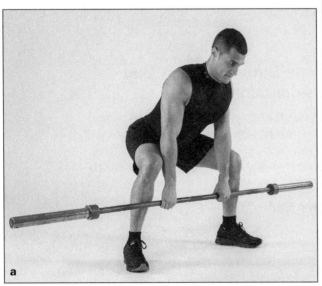

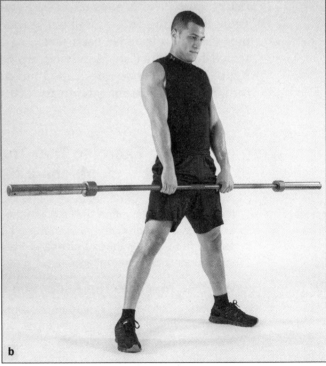

should touch your shins and track against the front of your legs as you perform each repetition. Your arms should be close to touching the insides of your legs at the bottom of each lift.

Dumbbell Hybrid Deadlift

Setup

Stand with a vertical dumbbell on the floor between your legs. Your feet are slightly farther than shoulder-width apart and turned out 15 degrees. Keeping your back straight and maintaining an arch in your lower back, hinge at your hips and bend your knees. Lower your torso to about a 45-degree angle and grab the top of the dumbbell.

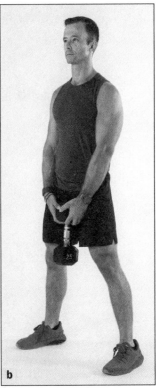
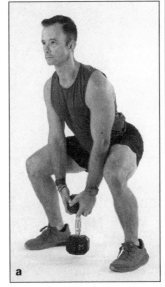

Action and Coaching Tips

Keeping your back straight, drive your hips forward toward the dumbbell and lift it off the ground while straightening your legs (see figures *a* and *b*). Reverse the motion and slowly lower the dumbbell back to the floor to complete the rep. As you hinge forward, drive your hips backward and do not allow your back to round. Lift the dumbbell by extending your hips, not by overextending your lower back.

Dumbbell Romanian Deadlift with NT Loop Hip Resistance

Adding the NT Loop around your hips loads the exercise at the portion of the range of motion that doesn't otherwise get as much work—the top. This allows you to train your glutes in both their lengthened and shortened ranges. To more effectively hit the top of the range of motion, place the band below your hip bones; this prevents it from rolling up as you hinge, and it gives you more direct tension in line with your glutes to drive your hips forward. This increases the demand on the glutes at the top.

Setup

Anchor an NT Loop securely behind you at hip height. Place both legs inside the NT Loop so it is around the top of your thighs just below your hip bones. Walk away from the origin of the NT Loop to create tension on the band. Stand tall with your feet hip-width apart. Hold the dumbbells in front of your thighs (see figure *a*).

Action and Coaching Tips

Keeping your back straight, hinge at your hips and bend forward toward the floor, with your knees bent at a 15- to 20-degree angle (see figure *b*). As you hinge forward, drive your hips backward and do not allow your back to round. Once your torso is roughly parallel to the floor, drive your hips forward toward the dumbbells,

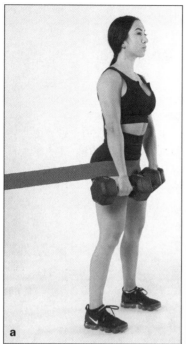

reversing the motion to stand tall again without overextending your lower back. Keep the dumbbells close to you throughout; they should touch your shins at the bottom and track against the front of your legs as you perform each repetition.

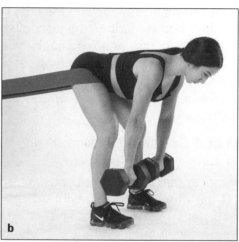

Dumbbell One-Leg Romanian Deadlift With NT Loop Thigh Resistance

By adding the NT Loop around your thigh, you load the portion of the range of motion that doesn't get as much work—the top. This allows you to train your glutes in both their lengthened and shortened ranges.

This single-leg version is better than the more common double-leg version. The split stance provides a great base of support to resist the pull of the band, which means you'll be able to work against more band tension without being pulled off your feet. And that means a better training effect. Plus, having the band wrapped high around your working thigh—your front leg—allows you to concentrate all of the band's tension on the side you're working. Placing the band somewhat in line with your glutes more effectively trains them than when the band is around your waist.

Setup

Anchor an NT Loop securely behind you at midthigh height. Place one leg inside the NT Loop so it is around the top of your thigh. Walk away from the origin of the loop to create tension on the band. Stand tall in a staggered stance with your legs hip-width apart and the leg that's inside the NT Loop in front. Keep a slight bend in your rear knee and keep your rear heel off the ground so all your weight is on your front leg. Hold a dumbbell in one hand on the same side as your back leg (see figure *a*).

Action and Coaching Tips

Keeping your back straight, hinge at your hips and bend forward toward the floor, with your front knee bent at a 15- to 20-degree angle (see figure *b*). As you hinge forward, drive your hips backward and do not allow your back to round or your rear heel to touch the ground. Once your torso is roughly parallel to the floor, drive your hips forward toward the dumbbell, reversing the motion to stand tall again without overextending your lower back. Perform all reps on the same side before switching sides.

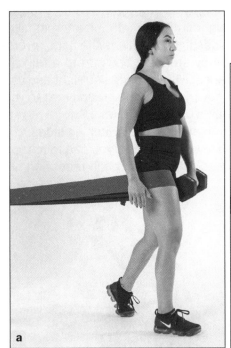
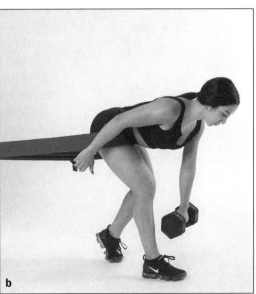

Dumbbell Glute Destroyer Lunge

Here's the scientific foundation for why I developed the glute destroyer lunge. If you want to maximize glute recruitment when doing lunges, you need to do three things:

1. Lean your torso forward at a roughly 45-degree angle, which increases glute and hamstring recruitment over an upright stance (10).
2. Take a long stride if doing walking lunges or perform them atop an elevated platform if performing reverse lunges. This recruits more glute than a narrow or level stance (11, 12).
3. Use an offset load that's heavier on the back-leg side (e.g., hold a single dumbbell or two unevenly loaded dumbbells), which has been shown to recruit more gluteus medius than loading the front-leg side (13).

Put them all together and you have the best lunge variation for glutes.

Setup

With your feet roughly hip-width apart, stand on the flat side of an Olympic-type weight plate or on an aerobic step platform, with your left foot on the platform and right foot hovering over the floor. Hold a dumbbell in your hand next to your right thigh (see figure *a*).

You can also perform this exercise holding two unevenly loaded dumbbells, with the heavier dumbbell in your right hand.

Action and Coaching Tips

Take a large step backward with your right leg, placing the toes and the ball of your foot on the floor while bending both knees and lowering your body into a lunge. As your knees bend, hinge at your hips and lean your torso forward at a roughly 45-degree angle while keeping your back straight until your left ribs are resting on your left thigh (see figure *b)*. Once your back knee lightly touches the floor, reverse

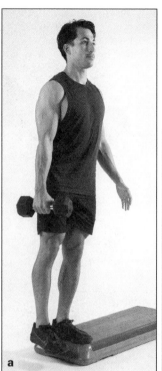

the motion by stepping back up to a tall, single-leg stance, with your legs straight and your right foot hovering over the ground next to your left foot that's on the platform. Perform all reps on the same side before switching sides. Use a platform low enough that you can touch your back knee to the floor on each repetition.

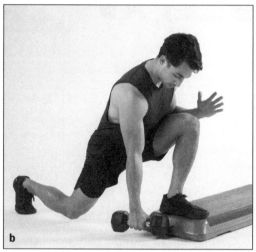

Dumbbell Traveling Glute Destroyer Lunge

Make sure you read the scientific foundation for the glute destroyer lunge in the previous exercise to learn why this is one the best lunge variations for the glutes.

Setup

Stand tall, with your feet hip-width apart while holding a dumbbell in your right hand outside of your right thigh (see figure *a*). You can also perform this exercise holding two unevenly loaded dumbbells, with the heavier dumbbell in your right hand.

Action and Coaching Tips

Take a large step forward with your left leg and drop your body so that your back knee lightly touches the floor. As your knees bend, hinge at your hips and lean your torso forward at a roughly 45-degree angle while keeping your back straight until your left ribs are resting on your left thigh. Once your back knee lightly touches the floor (see figure *b*), stand up tall while bringing your rear leg forward to meet your front leg and repeat this action by lunging forward again with your left leg. Perform all reps on the same leg while traveling down the room before switching sides.

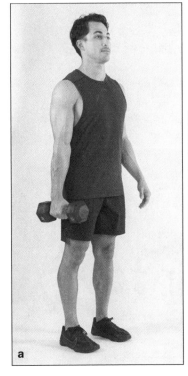
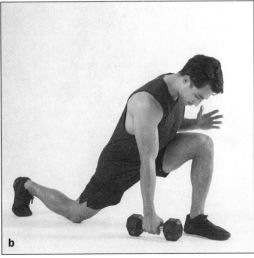

Dumbbell Leaning Bulgarian Split Squat

Setup

Stand tall while holding a dumbbell in each hand by your sides. Assume a split squat stance by placing your right foot on top of a bench or platform behind you. Your front leg should be far enough in front of the platform that your shin can stay fairly vertical as you drop into each rep (see figure *a*). You can also perform this exercise using only body weight by allowing your hands to hang by your sides or by interlacing your fingers behind your head.

Action and Coaching Tips

Lower your body toward the floor without allowing your back knee to rest on the floor. As you lower your body, keep your back straight and lean your torso forward at about a 45-degree angle (see figure *b*). Drive your heel into the ground to raise your body to the starting position, thus completing the rep. Perform all reps on one side before switching to the other leg. Keep your weight on your front foot throughout the exercise.

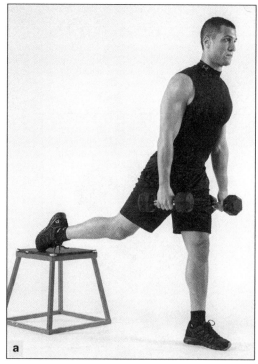

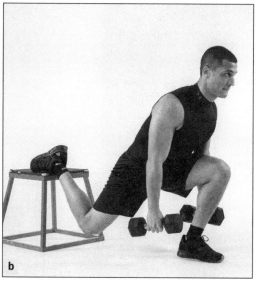

Band Loop Hybrid Deadlift

Setup

First, step your left foot inside one end of the resistance band loop and your right foot on top of the band with your feet just outside of shoulder-width apart and turned out 15 degrees. Second, grab the other end of the band that's on the outside of your right foot, pull it over your right foot, and loop the end around your left foot the way you did in the first step. Third, lower your torso to about a 45-degree angle and grab the middle of the band with your hands roughly shoulder-width apart by hinging at your hips and bending your knees while keeping your back straight and maintaining an arch in your lower back (see figure *a*).

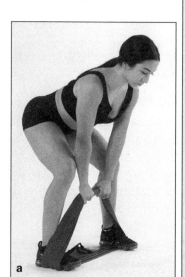

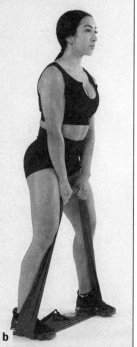

Action and Coaching Tips

Keeping your back straight, begin performing this exercise in a fairly fast manner by driving your hips forward while straightening your legs and standing tall (see figure *b*). Be sure to extend at your hips, and don't overextend your lower back. Reverse the motion and slowly lower yourself to the starting position to complete the rep.

Best Hip Extension Exercises in the Shortened-to-Midrange Strength Zone

The exercises in this section help you maximize the strength of your glutes in the shortened-to-midrange strength zone via hip extension movements.

Cable One-Leg Romanian Deadlift

Unlike the one-leg one-arm Romanian deadlift with a dumbbell, this exercise uses a cable column on the low setting to change the vector of resistance to a 45-degree angle. The dumbbell pulls you toward the floor; the cable pulls you toward its anchor point at a 45-degree angle.

Setup

Stand tall in a staggered stance with the back heel lifted while holding the cable handle in your opposite hand (see figure *a*). You can also perform this exercise with a resistance band that is anchored low, no higher than ankle level.

Action and Coaching Tips

Keeping your back and arm straight, hinge at your hips and bend forward toward the floor; keep your weight-bearing knee bent at a 15- to 20-degree angle (see figure *b*). Do not allow your lower back to round as you hinge your hips and lower your torso. At the bottom position, keep your hips and shoulders flat and do not allow them to rotate; the foot of your non-weight-bearing leg should point at the floor. Once your torso and non-weight-bearing leg are just above parallel to the floor, reverse the motion by driving your hips forward toward the cable to stand tall again, thus completing the rep. Perform all repetitions on one side before switching sides. The range of motion is shorter when using the cable than when using the dumbbell because the force you're working against is at a higher point.

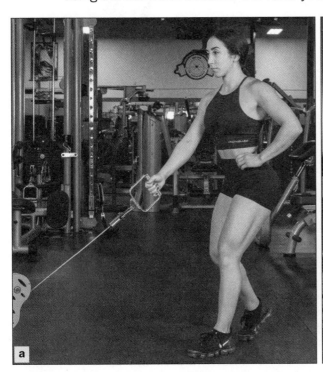
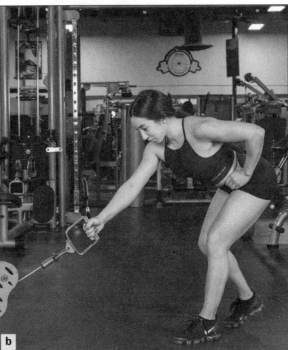

NT Loop Hip Thrust

Setup

Sit on the floor in front of a bench and anchor an NT loop under both feet, with the other end around your thighs. Pull the middle of the band that's between your feet between your legs and stretch it around your thighs so both layers of the band are just below your hips and running down the outside of your calves. Rest your shoulders on a weight bench or chair while keeping your knees bent so your heels are directly under your knees (see figure a).

Action and Coaching Tips

Drive your heels into the floor and lift your hips as high as possible without pushing your belly outward or overarching at your lower back. Do not lift the heels off of the ground at the top. Pause for 1 or 2 seconds at the top of each repetition (see figure b). Slowly lower your hips toward the floor until you either lightly contact the floor or can't go any deeper. Keep your head and face forward throughout. This helps you better extend from your hips and avoid using your lower back. Your hips may not rise as high as your shoulders at the top of each rep.

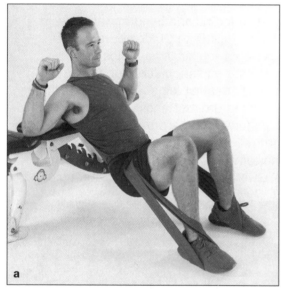 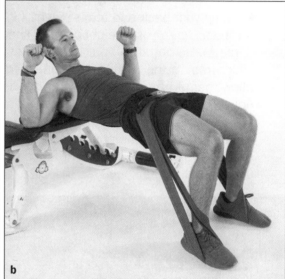

One-Leg Hip Thrust

Setup

Sit on the floor with your shoulders elevated on a weight bench or chair and your elbows resting on the bench. Position your arms to the sides across the bench. Position your legs so that your knees are bent about 90 degrees and your feet are directly below your knees. Keeping your right knee bent 90 degrees, lift your left knee above your hip and lift your hips so that your body makes a straight line from knee to nose (see figure a).

Action and Coaching Tips

Keeping your right leg lifted, lower your hips toward the floor until you either lightly contact the floor or can't go any deeper (see figure b). Drive your hips up to the top position, making sure to extend from your hips, not your lower back, thus completing the rep. Push through your heel on each repetition; do not lift the heel off the ground at the top. Pause for 1 or 2 seconds at the top of each repetition. Complete all repetitions on one side before switching to the other leg. Complete all repetitions on one side before switching to the other leg.

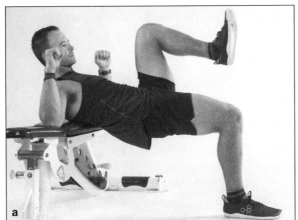 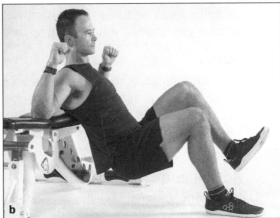

Dumbbell One-Leg Hip Thrust

Setup

Sit on the floor with your shoulders elevated on a weight bench or chair and the shoulders resting on the bench. Position the left arm to the side across the bench; hold a dumbbell in your right hand in front of your right hip. Position the dumbbell over your hip in a way that feels comfortable. Position your legs so that your knees are bent about 90 degrees and your feet are directly below your knees. Keeping your left knee bent 90 degrees, lift it above your hip and lift your hips so that your body makes a straight line from right knee to nose (see figure *a*).

Action and Coaching Tips

Keeping your left leg lifted, lower your hips toward the floor until you either lightly contact the floor or can't go any deeper (see figure *b*). Drive your hips up to the top position, making sure to extend from your hips, not your lower back, thus completing the rep. Push through your heel on each repetition; do not lift the heel off the ground at the top. Pause for 1 or 2 seconds at the top of each repetition. Complete all repetitions on one side before switching to the other leg.

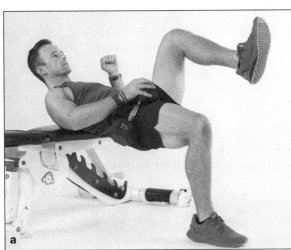 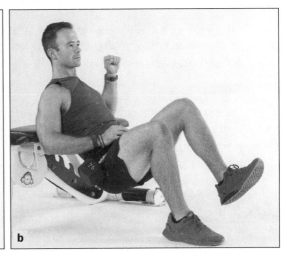

45-Degree Hip Extension

Although this exercise is commonly referred to as a 45-degree back extension, the focus of this version is to create the extension motion via *hip* extension—hence, the name used here. Keeping your spine straight while you perform the motion at your hip joints ensures the maximal involvement from your glute and hamstring muscles instead of your lower-back muscles.

Setup

Use an apparatus known as a back extension machine, which is found in most gyms. With your feet hip-width apart, rest your thighs against the pad, which is positioned below your hip bones so you're able to hinge at your hips without rounding out at your lower back. Keep your back straight. Cross your arms in front of your chest.

Action and Coaching Tips

Hinge at your hips, keeping your back straight, and lower yourself (see figure *a*). Reverse the motion by extending at your hips without arching your lower back too much. Pull yourself up so that your body forms a straight line from shoulders to hips to ankles (see figure *b*). To make the exercise more difficult, hold a weight plate at your belly or chest.

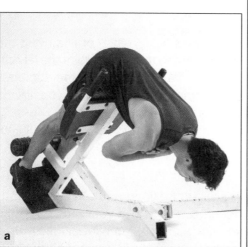
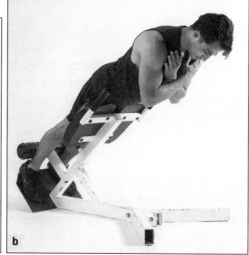

Weight Plate One-Leg Hip Lift

Although you'll feel this exercise mostly at the bottom of your hamstring, just above your knee, you're still using your glutes to drive your hips up and off the ground on each rep.

Setup

Lie on your back with your legs together, your knees bent 15 degrees, and your feet resting on top of a weight bench or chair. Raise one leg off the bench or chair, flexing your hip and knee a little beyond a 90-degree angle. With both hands, hold a weight plate at the shin of the flexed leg (see figure *a*). This exercise can also be done with body weight only.

Action and Coaching Tips

With one leg flexed, raise your hips straight up as high as you can while keeping a slight bend in your knee (see figure b). Do not overextend your lower back at any time; don't allow your hips to rotate during the exercise. Slowly reverse the motion, allowing your hips to lightly touch the floor. Complete all repetitions on one side before switching to the other leg.

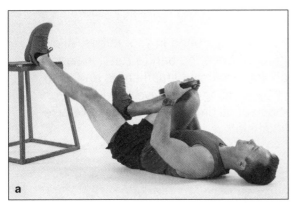
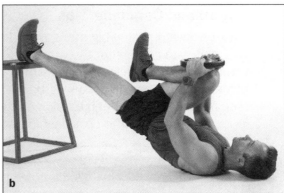

Weight Plate One-Leg Hip Bridge

Setup

Lie on your back (supine) on the floor, with your knees bent and heels on the floor. Lift your right knee above your hip so your knee is in front of your rib and chest area. Hold a weight plate at your shin of the flexed leg with both hands (see figure a). This exercise can also be done with body weight only.

Action and Coaching Tips

Keeping your right leg lifted, drive your hips up as high as you can without overextending your lower back (see figure b). Pause for 2 or 3 seconds at the top position before slowly lowering yourself to the floor. Repeat all reps on the same side before switching legs.

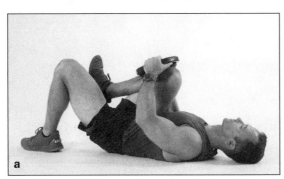
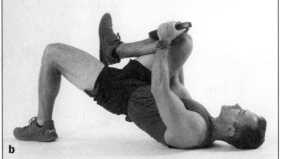

NT Loop Glute Walk

Setup

Anchor an NT Loop or rubber resistance band loop at ankle level to something stable. Place the band around the backs of your calves and stand facing the anchor point, with your feet shoulder-width apart (see figure *a*).

Action and Coaching Tips

Walk backward, taking big steps while keeping a slight bend in your knees. Allow your glutes to do most of the work (see figure *b*). Once the band's tension keeps you from walking backward any farther, walk forward using small steps and keep the same form as when walking backward by avoiding excessive pelvic rotation (see figures *c* and *d*). Keep tension on the band at all times. Perform this exercise in increments of four to six steps in each direction.

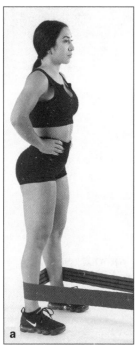 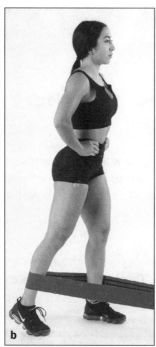 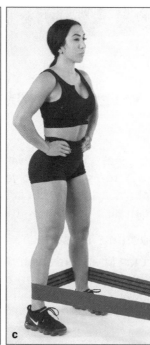 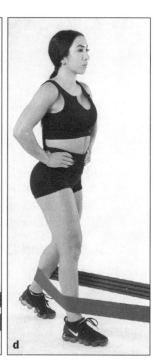

Stability Ball Reverse Hip Extension

Setup

Lie facedown on a 22-inch (55 cm) stability ball, with the ball under your belly and hips. Rest your forearms on the floor at shoulder width, with your torso angled toward the floor and your head just above your hands. Keep your legs straight and your toes just above the ground just wider than shoulder width (see figure *a*).

Action and Coaching Tips

Keeping your feet wide apart, hinge at your hips and lift your legs so that your body forms a straight line (see figure *b*). As you raise your legs, also allow your feet to move farther apart while keeping your legs straight. Do not overextend at your lower back or allow the ball to roll at any point. Keep the weight on your forearms throughout.

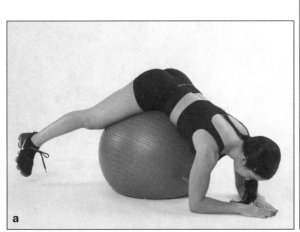
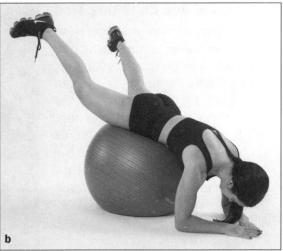

What About Cable Pull-Throughs and Barbell Hip Thrusts?

Sure, cable or band pull-throughs also load your glutes closer to their shortened-to-mid-range (hips extended) position, but they're not featured in this book because of their awkward nature and their limited ability to continuously add progressive overload. I prefer to use the options listed in the hip extension in the shortened-to-midrange section of this chapter. With pull-throughs you're not limited by the weight your hips can extend against; you're limited by how much you can hold without getting pulled backward, which has much more to do with your body weight than your strength level.

The barbell hip thrust exercise has become a mainstay on social media among fitness influencers. Although they may be experts in taking gym selfies, they might be severely unqualified to provide safe and reliable training info. Some coaches have argued that hip thrusts can be risky if you go too heavy relative to your strength level or substitute lumbar extension for hip extension. This is true, but none of these points apply exclusively to the hip thrust. Any exercise becomes riskier when you lift beyond your strength capacity or use poor technique.

That said, if you trained with me, we wouldn't do barbell hip thrusts, but not because I think it's a bad exercise. I simply prefer and recommend single-leg hip thrusts because they don't take nearly as much time and equipment to set up.

Best Exercises in the Hip Abduction Strength Zone

The exercises in this section help you maximize the strength and development of your hip abductor musculature in the hip abduction strength zone.

Machine Seated Hip Abduction

Setup

For this exercise, you'll use equipment commonly known as the hip abduction machine. Sit tall with your legs together so you can press against the pads with the outsides of your legs (see figure *a*).

Action and Coaching Tips

Holding on to the handles, push the outsides of your thighs into the pads and drive your legs apart as far as you can (see figure *b*). Slowly reverse the motion to complete one rep. Do not allow the weight stack you're moving to rest on the stack. Instead, allow it to gently touch at the end of each rep.

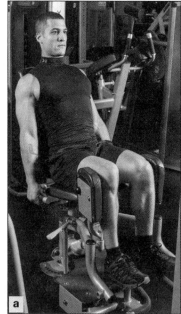
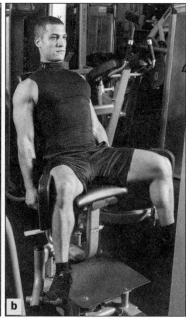

Band Lateral Hip Shuffle

Setup

Place a mini band around your legs just above your ankles. Keep your legs straight, your hands on your hips, and your feet positioned hip-width apart (see figure *a*).

Action and Coaching Tips

Take small lateral steps to your left, maintaining tension in the band (see figures *b* and *c*), then sidestep back to your right in the same manner. Do not allow your torso to wobble from side to side; keep your spine and pelvis stable throughout the exercise. Do not allow your knees to give in to the band and drop toward the midline.

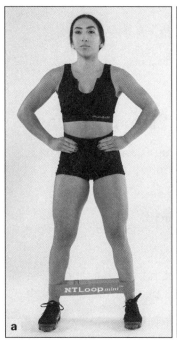
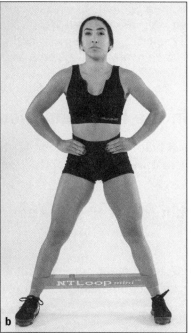
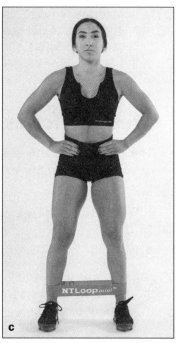

Band Low Lateral Hip Shuffle

Setup

Place a mini band around your legs just above your knees. Keep your hands on your hips and your feet positioned hip-width apart. Squat until your knees are bent roughly 45 degrees (see figure *a*).

Action and Coaching Tips

Take small lateral steps to your left, maintaining tension in the band (see figures *b* and *c*), then sidestep back to your right in the same manner. Do not allow your torso to wobble from side to side; keep your spine and pelvis stable throughout the exercise. Do not allow your knees to give in to the band and drop toward the midline. Keep your knees in line with your feet throughout.

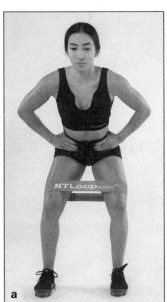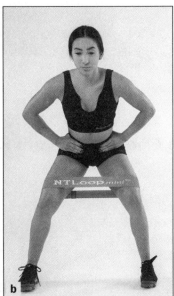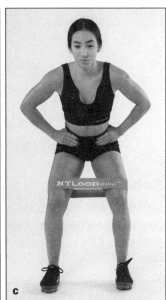

Weight Plate Side-Lying Hip Abduction

Setup

Lie on your left side, with your head resting on your left arm (your bottom arm), which is extended on the floor at a roughly 45-degree angle under your head. Your legs are straight, with your right foot internally rotated downward and just behind your left heel. Hold a weight-plate in your right hand on top of your right thigh, with your arm fairly straight (see figure *a*). You can also perform this exercise with only body weight.

Action and Coaching Tips

Keeping your legs straight and your right foot turned slightly downward, lift your right leg off the ground as a high as you can without allowing your foot to externally rotate toward the sky (see figure *b*). Your legs should stay roughly in line with your torso, and do not allow your torso to roll at any point; keep your shoulders and hips perpendicular to the floor. Pause for 2 to 3 seconds at the top. Slowly reverse the motion, allowing your leg to return to the floor. Perform all reps on one side before switching sides.

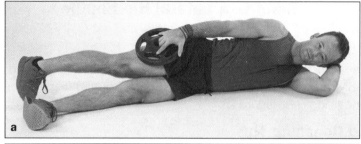

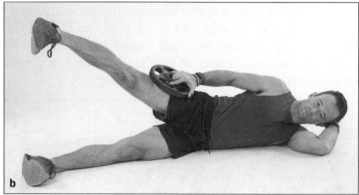

Dynamic Side Elbow Plank With Hip Abduction

Setup

Lie on your right side, with your right forearm on the floor and your elbow directly under your shoulder. Place your left foot on top with of your right foot, keeping your hips and knees straight. Use a pad or a rolled towel under your elbow for comfort if necessary (see figure *a*).

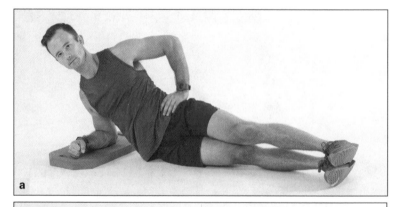

Action and Coaching Tips

Lift your right hip off the ground while simultaneously raising your top (left) leg toward the sky as high as possible. Keep your left foot parallel to the ground (see figure *b*) and your body in a straight line throughout. Pause for a second at the top and slowly reverse the motion to complete the rep. Perform all reps on the same side before switching to the other side.

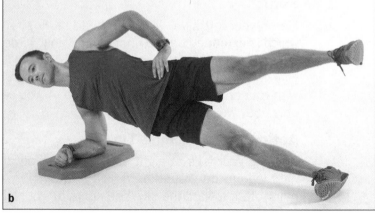

Dynamic Bent-Knee Side Elbow Plank With Hip Abduction

Setup

Lie on your right side, with your right forearm on the floor and your elbow directly under your shoulder. Place your left leg on top of your right leg, keeping your hips bent and knees bent so your ankles are below your hips. Use a pad or a rolled towel under your elbow for comfort if necessary (see figure *a*).

Action and Coaching Tips

Lift your right hip off the ground while driving your hips forward and simultaneously raising your top (left) leg toward the sky as high as possible and keeping your left knee bent (see figure *b*). At the top of each rep, keep your body in a straight line from your knees to your hips to your shoulders. Pause for a second and slowly reverse the motion to complete the rep. Perform all reps on the same side before switching to the other side.

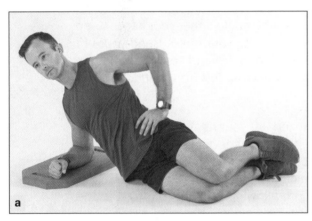
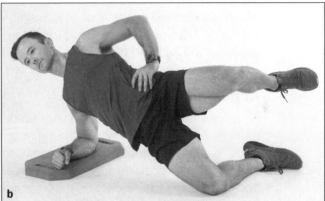

Best Exercises in the Hip Adduction Strength Zone

The exercises in this section help you maximize the strength and development of your adductor musculature in the hip adduction strength zone.

Side-Lying Hip Adduction Leg Scissors

Setup

Lie on your right side, with your head resting on your right arm (your bottom arm), which is extended on the floor at a roughly 45-degree angle under your head. Keep both legs straight and in line with your torso. Lift your top leg and hold it 12 to 16 inches (about 30-40 cm) above your bottom leg (see figure *a*).

Action and Coaching Tips

Keeping your knee straight and your ankle flexed, lift your right leg off the ground as high as you can without allowing your hip to flex (see figure *b*). Your bottom leg should stay in line with your torso. Do not allow your torso to roll at any point, and keep your shoulders and hips perpendicular to the floor. Pause for 2 to 3 seconds at the top. Slowly reverse the motion, allowing your leg to return to the floor. Perform all reps on one side before switching sides.

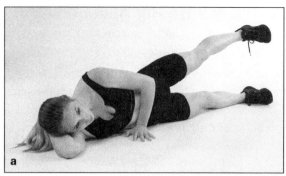
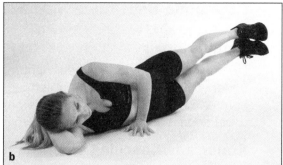

Side-Lying Hip Adduction

Setup

Lie on your right side, with your head resting on your right arm (your bottom arm), which is extended on the floor at a roughly 45-degree angle under your head. Keep your right leg (your bottom leg) straight and in line with your torso. Bend your left leg (your top leg) and place your foot flat on the floor in front of your bottom knee to thigh area (see figure a). Grab your left shin with your left (top) hand.

Action and Coaching Tips

Keeping your knee straight and your ankle flexed, lift your right leg off the ground as high as you can without allowing your hip to flex (see figure b). Your bottom leg should stay in line with your torso. Do not allow your torso to roll at any point, and keep your shoulders and hips perpendicular to the floor. Pause for 2 to 3 seconds at the top. Slowly reverse the motion, allowing your leg to return to the floor. Perform all reps on one side before switching sides.

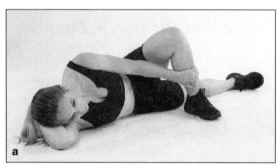
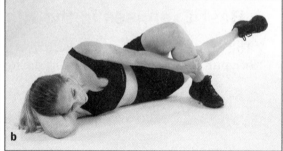

Bent-Knee Copenhagen Hip Adduction

Setup

Lie on the floor on your right side, with your elbow directly under your right shoulder, your right leg straight, and your left leg bent 90 degrees. Rest your left knee and calf on a bench or plyometric box that's roughly 17 to 20 inches (43-50 cm) high while your right leg is under the box platform (see figure a). Place a rolled-up towel or mat under your left leg and right elbow for comfort.

Action and Coaching Tips

Keeping your right leg straight and your body in a straight line from your left knee to your hips to your shoulders, press your left leg into the top of the platform as you elevate your right hip off the ground. Simultaneously lift your right leg to squeeze the inside of your right thigh against the inside of your left thigh or until your thighs are roughly parallel with each other (see figure *b*). Pause for 1 or 2 seconds at the top before reversing the action and lowering your right leg and hip back to the floor to complete the rep. Do all reps on the same side before switching sides and performing this exercise with your right leg on top of the platform.

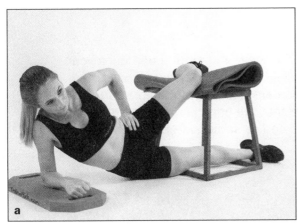
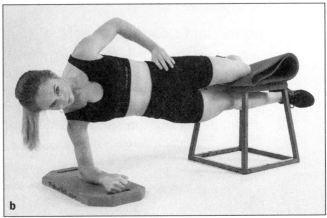

Machine Seated Hip Adduction

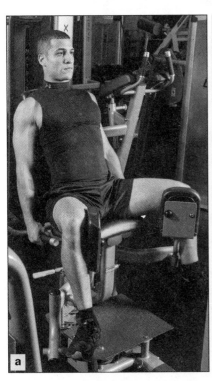
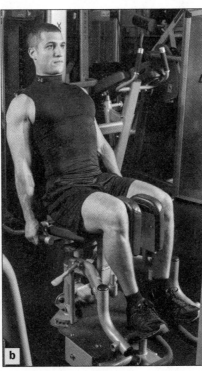

Setup

For this exercise, use the machine that's commonly known as the hip adduction machine. Sit tall, with the insides of your thighs against the pads. Position the pads as wide as you're able to manage without discomfort (see figure *a*).

Action and Coaching Tips

Holding on to the handles, push the insides of your thighs into the pads and drive your legs together until the pads touch or until your thighs are roughly parallel with each other (see figure *b*).

Slowly reverse the motion to complete the rep. Do not allow the weight stack you're moving to rest on the stack. Instead, allow it to gently touch at the end of each rep.

NT Loop Quadruped Hip Adduction

Setup

Anchor an NT Loop around a stable object at mid-shin height. Place your right leg inside the band just above your knee, with its anchor point on your right side. Move away from the anchor point to create tension on the band. Assume a quadruped position on your hands and knees, with your arms straight and knees bent to 90 degrees. Place a rolled-up towel or mat under your left knee for comfort. Place your hands just outside of shoulder width and your knees as far apart as possible (see figure *a*).

Action and Coaching Tips

Keeping your back flat, lift your right knee just above the ground and bring your right knee to your left knee, squeezing your legs together for a second (see figure *b*). Slowly reverse the motion until your knees are again spread apart as far as possible to complete the rep. Keep the knee that the band is attached to off the ground throughout the set. Perform all reps on the same side before switching

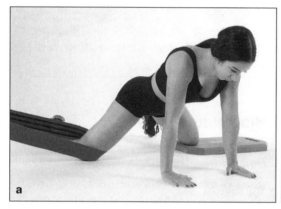
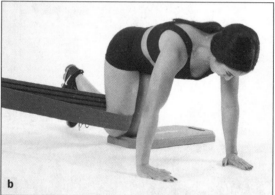

sides.

To round out your lower body, the next chapter covers the best exercises for the back of the lower leg: the calves.

CHAPTER 12

The Best Calf Exercises

Training to develop calf strength through the true full range of motion involves performing at least one exercise for each of the following strength zones:

- Straight-knee calf exercise
- Bent-knee calf exercise

Picking at least one exercise from each category on this list maximizes your workout efficiency and helps you develop full-range calf strength.

Calves Exercise Mechanics

Your calves are made up of the gastrocnemius and the soleus. Research shows that performing calf raises (ankle plantarflexion) with a straight knee creates superior gastrocnemius muscle activity and doing calf raises with a bent knee creates superior soleus muscle activity (2, 3, 4, 5). So it makes sense to perform at least one calf exercise in each knee position to maximize your training time and efficiency.

Also, unlike when doing exercises for most other areas of your body, doing calf raises through the full range of motion builds full-range strength during plantarflexion at the ankle. This is because of the mechanics involved and the relatively smaller range of motion at the ankle joint compared to other joints such as the hip, shoulder, and elbow. So, when performing the calf exercises provided in this chapter, you're building strength from their shortened range through the lengthened range, such as in the barbell ankles-together calf raise (see figure 12.1) and the dumbbell half-kneeling calf raise (see figure 12.2).

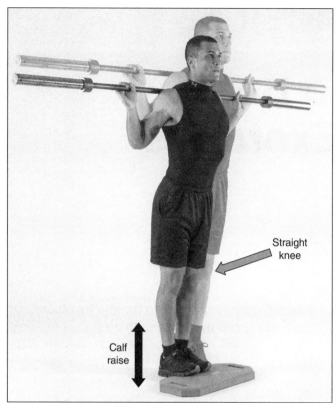

FIGURE 12.1   Barbell ankles-together calf raise exercise in straight-knee strength zone.

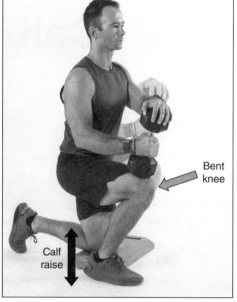

FIGURE 12.2   Dumbbell half-kneeling calf raise exercise in bent-knee strength zone.

How to Build Athletic Calves

People who train mainly for aesthetics focus on calf growth, but it's far less common to see athletes working on their calves. And that's a shame because it could be what gives them an advantage.

Research has shown significant correlation between strength in a calf raise and sprint performance. Researchers concluded that the dynamic maximum strength of the calves is a basic prerequisite for short sprints and should be regarded as a performance reserve (1). These results come as no surprise given that ankle plantarflexion (pointing your toes) is involved in actions like sprinting, jumping, and cutting. So calf training should be a no-brainer for athletes and people who want to perform well. But if your mind goes straight to the traditional calf machines, you need an update. There are powerful calf strengtheners that you should add to your arsenal.

The main issue with traditional calf raises is that you roll more weight toward your pinky toes as you raise your heels. Do a standing body weight calf raise right now and see for yourself. But that's not what happens when you're walking and running. As your back foot propels you forward, you roll more of your weight toward your big toe as you plantarflex.

This doesn't mean tossing out your standard calf raises; they offer performance benefits too, as the research mentioned earlier shows. But for a more comprehensive approach, try adding exercises like the barbell ankles-together calf raise, dumbbell one-leg leaning calf raise, and dumbbell traveling calf raise because they'll better replicate the way your foot presses into the ground when you walk or run.

Best Calf Exercises in the Straight-Knee Strength Zone

The exercises in this section help you maximize the strength and development of your calves in the straight-knee strength zone.

Barbell Ankles-Together Calf Raise

Setup

Place small weight plates or a pad under the front of your feet. Stand tall, with the insides of your feet and ankle bones together, and place a barbell across the tops of your shoulders behind your head (see figure *a*).

Action and Coaching Tips

Push your toes into the pad and lift your heels as high as you can off the floor while keeping the insides of your ankle bones touching (see figure *b*). You should be on the balls of your feet (see figure *c*). Slowly lower yourself until your heels touch the floor to complete the rep. Do not bounce; control the lowering (eccentric) portion of each rep by allowing your heels to touch the floor gently—not fully resting on the floor—until all reps have been completed.

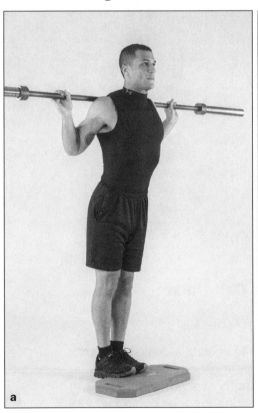

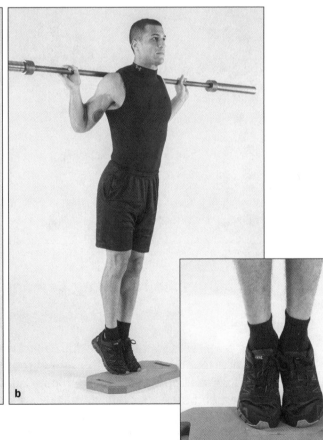

Dumbbell Traveling Calf Raise

Setup

As the name implies, this exercise combines a dumbbell farmers walk with a calf raise. Stand at one end of the room and hold a heavy dumbbell in each hand, with your palms facing your body by your hips (see figure *a*).

Action and Coaching Tips

Walk to the other end of the room. On each step, as soon as your foot hits the ground, quickly drive your toes into the floor and lift your heels as high as you can off of the floor so you are on the balls of your feet (see figures *b* and *c*). Lower yourself after each step with control until your heel touches the floor to complete the rep. Perform this heel raise action in a smooth and coordinated action with each step.

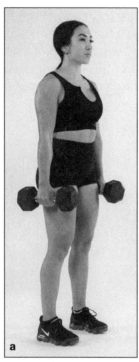
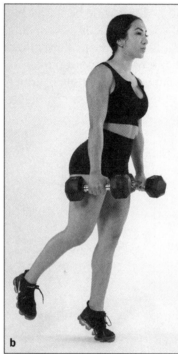
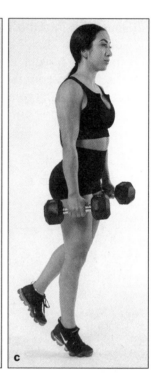

Dumbbell One-Leg Leaning Calf Raise

Setup

Stand facing a wall with your feet hip-width apart while holding a dumbbell in your left hand. Place your right hand on the wall at roughly chest height and lean your body forward while keeping your torso, hips, and knees in a straight line. Bend your right knee and step your left leg backward, placing it as far behind you as possible while keeping your heel on the ground and your left foot pointed at the wall. Your left knee, hip, and torso should form a straight line. Lift your right foot off the floor while keeping your right knee bent at about a 90-degree angle (see figure *a*).

Action and Coaching Tips

While maintaining your body position, lift your left heel as high as you can off the floor so you're on the ball of your foot (see figure *b*). Slowly lower yourself until your heel touches the floor to complete the rep. Do not allow your left foot to rotate outward at any point; keep it straight and pointed at the wall throughout. Do not bounce; control the lowering (eccentric) portion of each rep by allowing your heel to touch the floor gently—not fully resting on the floor—until all reps have been completed. Perform all the reps on the same side before switching sides.

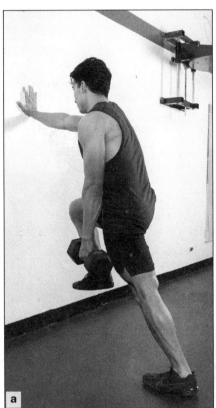 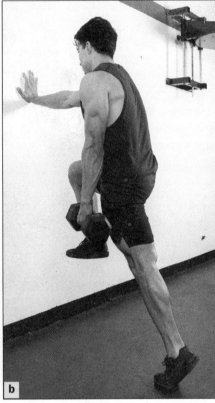

Dumbbell Foot-Elevated Calf Raise

Setup

Stand facing a plyometric box or stable surface that's at roughly knee to midthigh height, with your feet hip-width apart while holding a dumbbell in each hand. Place one foot on the platform and lean your hips forward while keeping your torso upright and your bottom knee straight. Your back leg, which is on the ground, should be behind your torso as far behind you as possible while keeping your heel on the ground and your left foot pointed straight ahead (see figure *a*). If the front of your bottom foot is more than 2 to 3 inches (5-8 cm) behind your same-side hip, use a higher platform to elevate your front foot.

Action and Coaching Tips

While maintaining your body position with the right leg that's on the floor, lift your heel as high as you can off the floor so you are on the ball of your foot (see figure b). Slowly lower yourself until your heel touches the floor to complete the rep. Do not allow your foot to rotate outward at any point; keep it straight throughout. Do not bounce; control the lowering (eccentric) portion of each rep by allowing your heel to touch the floor gently— not fully resting on the floor—until all reps have been completed. Perform all the reps on the same side before switching sides.

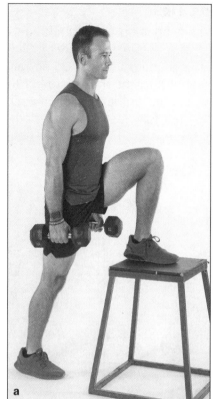
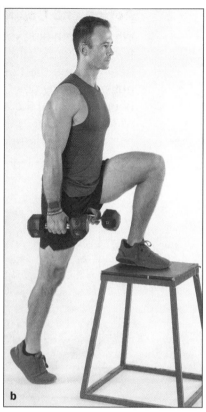

Machine Ankles-Together Calf Raise

Setup

To perform this exercise, use equipment that's known as the calf raise machine. Place the balls of your feet on the platform and your feet hip-width apart. Stand tall and move the insides of your feet and ankle bones together; place the pads across the tops of your shoulders on either side your head.

Action and Coaching Tips

Push your toes into the platform and lift your heels as high as you can so you are on the balls of your feet. Keep the insides of your ankle bones touching (see figure a). Slowly lower your heels as far as possible to complete the rep (see figure b). Do not bounce; control the lowering (eccentric) portion of each rep.

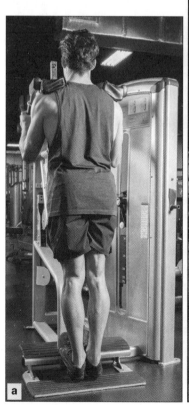
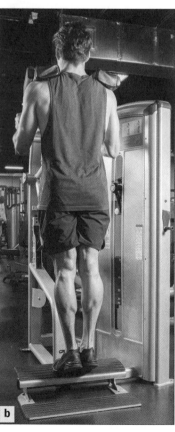

Best Calf Exercises in the Bent-Knee Strength Zone

The exercises in this section help you maximize the strength and development of your calves in the bent-knee strength zone.

Dumbbell Half-Kneeling Calf Raise

It's important to position your working-side foot closer to your body. This increases the range of motion, making it more productive. You can also use a kettlebell for this exercise.

Setup

Using a mat or rolled towel underneath your down knee for comfort, assume a half-kneeling position on the floor, with your torso straight and both knees bent at roughly 90 degrees. Step one leg forward and place your foot flat on the ground. Move your front foot back as far as you can while keeping your heel on the floor and your foot straight. Place either a vertical dumbbell or the bottom of a kettlebell on your front thigh just above the knee (see figure a).

Action and Coaching Tips

Push the toes of your front foot into the ground and lift your heel as high as you can off the floor so you're on the ball of your foot (see figure b). Slowly lower your heel until it touches the floor to complete the rep. Do not bounce; control the lowering (eccentric) portion of each rep by allowing your heel to touch the floor gently—not fully resting on the floor—until all reps have been completed. Perform all the reps on the same side before switching sides. Positioning your front foot closer to you by bending your knee more than 90 degrees increases the range of motion of this exercise, which makes it more productive.

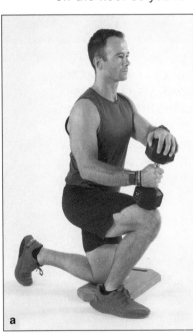
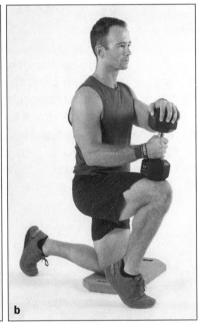

Dumbbell One-Leg Seated Calf Raise

It's important to position your working-side foot closer to your body. This increases the range of motion, which makes it more productive. You can also use a kettlebell for this exercise.

Setup

Sit tall on a weight bench, with your feet roughly hip-width apart. Move one of your feet under you as far as you can while keeping your heel on the floor and your foot straight. Place either the side of a dumbbell or the bottom of a kettlebell on your thigh just above the knee (not at midthigh) of the leg you just moved (see figure a).

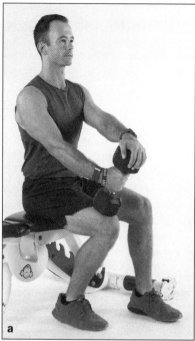 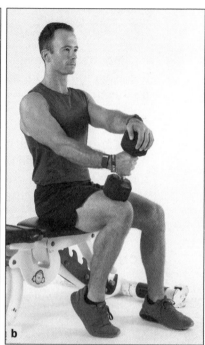

Action and Coaching Tips

Push your toes into the ground and lift your heel as high as you can off of the floor so you're on the ball of your foot (see figure b). Slowly lower your heel until it touches the floor to complete the rep. Do not bounce; control the lowering (eccentric) portion of each rep by allowing your heel to touch the floor gently—not fully resting on the floor—until all reps have been completed. Perform all the reps on the same side before switching sides. Positioning your working-side foot closer to you by bending your knee more than 90 degrees increases the range of motion demand on this exercise, which makes it more productive.

Machine Seated Calf Raise

Setup

To perform this exercise, use the seated calf raise machine. Place the balls of your feet of the platform, with your feet hip-width apart. Sit tall, with your knees bent roughly 90 degrees and place the pads across the tops of your knees (see figure *a*).

Action and Coaching Tips

Push your toes into the platform and lift your heels as high as you can so that you are on the balls of your feet (see figure *b*). Slowly lower your heels as far as possible to complete the rep. Do not bounce; control the lowering (eccentric) portion of each rep.

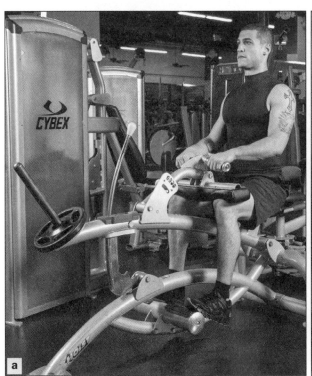
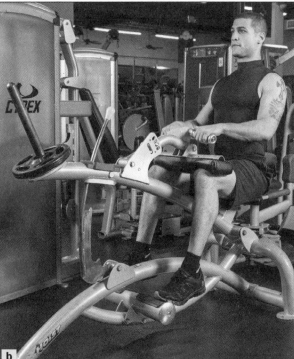

The next chapter covers the training zones that will build core strength and will provide you with plenty of exercises for improving core strength and performance. It also clarifies common myths and misconceptions about core exercises.

CHAPTER 13

The Best Core Exercises

Training to develop core strength through the true full range of motion involves performing at least one exercise for each of the following strength zones:

- Linear core exercise
- Lateral core exercise
- Rotational core exercise

Picking at least one exercise from each category on this list maximizes your workout efficiency and helps you develop full-range core strength.

Core Exercise Mechanics

It's commonly said among trainers and lifters that "abs are built in the kitchen." In reality, abs are *revealed* in the kitchen (with your diet), but they're built in the gym. The exercises presented in this chapter focus on helping you maximize the strength of your abdominals and obliques. They also help you improve your rotational strength and power.

Many trainers and lifters believe that this is a complete ab training program:

- Anti-spinal-extension exercises, such as planks or stability ball rollouts
- Anti-spinal-lateral-flexion exercises, such as side planks
- Anti-spinal-rotation exercises, such as antirotation presses or dumbbell plank rows

Anti-spinal-movement exercises are great for improving the function of your core musculature, which is why they're included in this book. They improve the ability of your core muscles to remain stiff so the spine can bear greater loads (1) and transfer force between the hips and the shoulders. However, anti-spinal movement exercises are just isomeric exercises. And isometric exercises (planks, side planks, cable anti-rotation presses) are only half of a complete core-strengthening puzzle. Why? Because your core musculature doesn't just transfer force and reduce force by limiting torso movement (through isometric action), it also helps to produce force by creating motion or dynamic movement (2).

From mixed martial arts to golf, you can't deny the obvious active movement role the core plays in power production during sporting events. Try to imagine

Serena Williams serving a ball without moving her torso. You can also appreciate the active movement contribution the torso makes in power production by trying a simple experiment performing an overhead throw with a medicine ball weighing four to six pounds (1.8-2.7 kg). First perform an overhead throw in the standard athletic fashion by extending at your spine and hips a bit (don't go to end range) to allow your anterior torso musculature to eccentrically load. Then compare that to an anti-extension soccer-style throw where you don't allow your spine to move at all. You already know which of the two throws will be more powerful, not to mention which throw will feel more natural and athletic.

So based on what the principle of specificity dictates (and barring injury), it makes the most sense to train both anti-spinal movements and active spinal movements in order to maximize your core strength and performance. Put simply, if you want to do all you can to improve the ability of your core muscles to transfer force by limiting trunk movement, you have to use isometric core exercises. And if you want to do all you can to improve core strength, you have to add dynamic core exercises. That's why this chapter includes both types of core-training exercises for each of the three core-training strength zones.

Your core-training routine must hit each of these categories in order to be comprehensive. A well-rounded routine covers the major types of movement performed by your torso and coordinates the muscles that make those movements possible. Those movements are to resist as well as create torso or linear flexion (see figure 13.1), lateral flexion (see figure 13.2), and rotation (see figure 13.3).

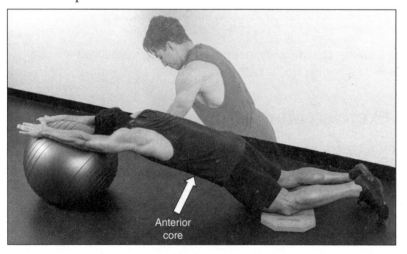

FIGURE 13.1 Stability ball rollout exercise in linear core strength zone.

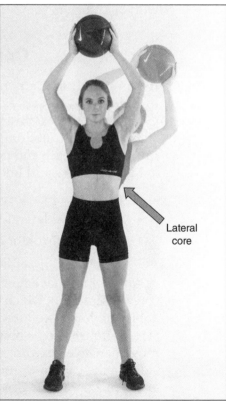

FIGURE 13.2 Medicine ball side lean exercise in lateral core strength zone.

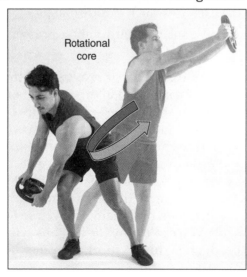

FIGURE 13.3 Weight plate chop exercise in the rotational core strength zone.

The Four Ab Exercises You're Doing Wrong: How to Do Them Right

These four ab exercises are commonly done in a much less effective way than they should be. Here's how to avoid the common mistakes and get the most out of them. This will help you to better understand the descriptions provided for how to properly perform these exercises in their corresponding strength zone categories following this section. Photos with an X in this section show the improper technique while photos with a check mark show the proper technique.

1. Dumbbell side bend: You see this exercise all the time in the gym, but it doesn't make biomechanical sense. And many people do it by holding two dumbbells, one on each side. But the weight on one side offsets the weight on the other, making this exercise ineffective at loading the lateral flexors of the torso.

The reasoning for the right way (p. 204): There's not much resistance when you're standing upright holding a dumbbell because the dumbbell is very close to your body, giving you a huge mechanical advantage over the weight. But when doing them with a cable or stretch band, the angle of the cable forces you to work hard to stay upright and maintain that position between reps, giving you more time under tension through the range of motion. Now, you could hold very heavy dumbbells, but they may exceed your grip strength. You can create the same training effect with a cable and use much lower loads.

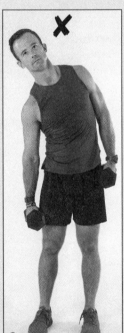
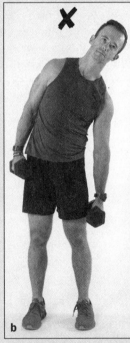
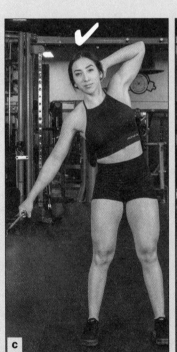
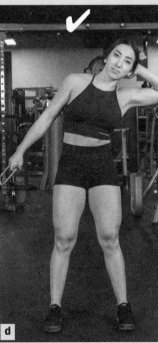

a   b   c   d

2. Hanging knee raise: Whether you're hanging from a pull-up bar, have your elbows in ab straps, or you're on a machine, the leg raise is a great exercise if you do it right. But most people don't. They start with their legs hanging straight down and then flex at their hips. That's mostly a hip flexor exercise, not an ab exercise.

The reasoning for the right way (p. 199): Although the way this exercises is usually performed involves the abs, the degree of involvement is negligible because the focus is on tucking the legs instead of tucking the pelvis. By keeping your knees up towards your chest, the movement becomes tucking your pelvis, which targets the abs far better.

> continued

> *continued*

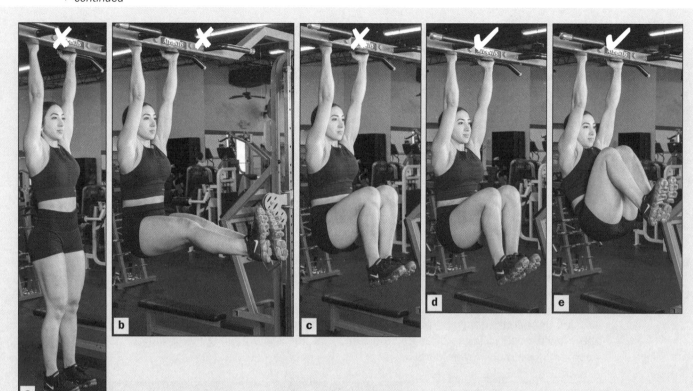

3. Leg lowering: You see it all the time: Someone's lying on the floor on their back with their legs in the air and they're raising and lowering them. Sometimes they've got their hands under their bottom and other times they're holding a partner's ankles.

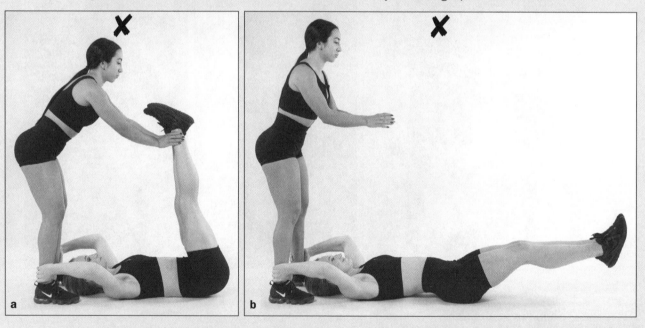

The reasoning for the right way (p. 192): Allowing your lower back to arch off the floor reduces the involvement of your abs in resisting spinal extension. It also places more stress on the lower back, which may increase to the point of discomfort and injury.

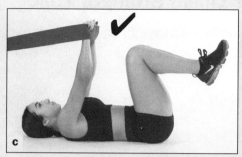

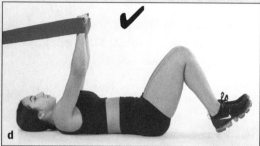

4. Stability ball crunch: Another thing you often see is someone lying on a stability ball doing noncrunches by bending and extending at their knees while the ball rolls back and forth under them.

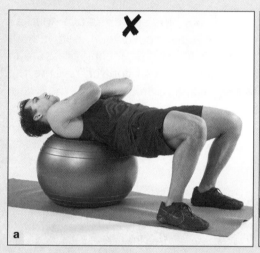

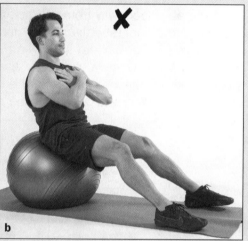

The reasoning for the right way (p. 196): To focus on your abs when doing ball crunches, the ball shouldn't move under you at all. Instead, keep your knees bent at a roughly 90-degree angle throughout, and flex and extend your spine over the ball in a controlled manner. If the ball rolls back and forth, it's primarily your knees (bending and extending) that drives the motion, not your abs.

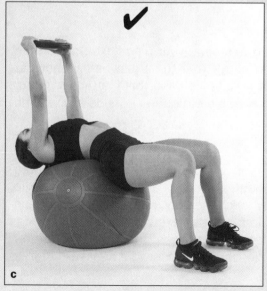

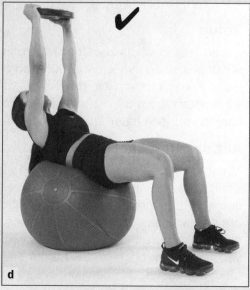

Best Core Exercises in the Linear Strength Zone

The exercises in this section help you maximize the strength and development of your core in the linear strength zone.

Ab Wheel Rollout

Setup

Kneel with your hands on the handles of an ab wheel device, your wrists just under your shoulders, and your arms straight (see figure a). You may also need to place a pad, pillow, or folded towel under your knees for comfort.

Action and Coaching Tips

Drive the ab wheel away from you by extending your hips and arms overhead as if diving into a pool (see figure b). Push the wheel just above your head without allowing your lower back to sag toward the floor and without feeling pressure in your lower back. Once you've gone as far as you can with control, reverse the motion and pull the wheel back to the starting position, finishing with the wheel under your shoulders to complete one rep.

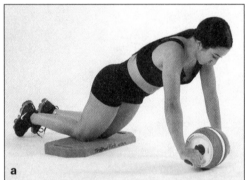
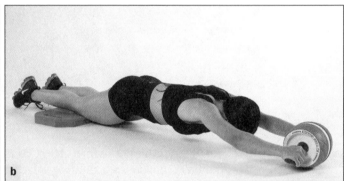

Band Leg Lowering

Setup

Lie on your back on the floor with your knees bent, your hips flexed more than 90 degrees, and your arms outstretched above your torso just below shoulder level. In each hand, hold the handle of a resistance band that's attached about 12 inches (about 30 cm) off the floor to a stable structure or inside a doorjamb behind you (see figure a).

Action and Coaching Tips

Maintaining tension against the band with your arms, slowly lower your legs toward the floor (see figure b). Keep your knees bent, and do not allow your lower back to come off the floor. Once your heels lightly touch the floor, reverse the motion and bring your knees back above your hips. To make this exercise more challenging, simply extend your legs farther as you lower them toward the floor—the farther you straighten your legs, the harder the exercise; the closer your heels are to your hips, the easier the exercise.

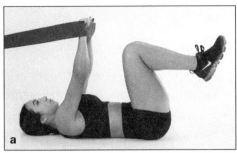 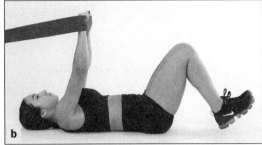

Stability Ball Arc

Setup

Place both forearms on top of a 22- to 26-inch (55-65 cm) stability ball and get into a plank position, with your body in a straight line and your feet just farther than shoulder-width apart (see figure a). Contract your glutes and posteriorly rotate your pelvis by bringing your front hip bones toward your head and your tailbone toward your feet. In other words, if you imagine your pelvis as a bucket of water, the posterior pelvic tilt will tip the bucket so that water would spill out of your back, whereas an anterior pelvic tilt would make water spill out from the front.

Action and Coaching Tips

Move your arms in small arcs from where your elbows are under the left side of your torso, to straightening your arms as you reach out above your head, to bringing your arms back under the left side of your torso (see figure b). Alternate between left-to-right arcs and right-to-left arcs (see figures c and d) without allowing your head or hips to sag toward the floor. On each arc, squeeze your glutes tightly each time you reach your arms out. Reach your arms as far as you can without feeling discomfort in your lower back.

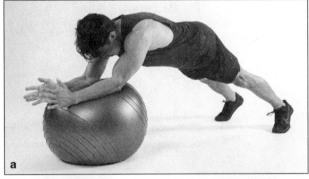

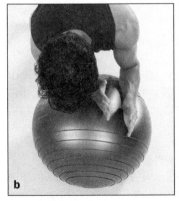 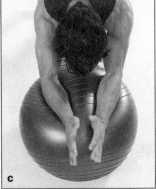 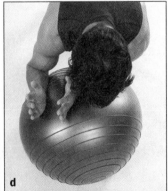

Stability Ball Rollout

Setup

Kneel on the floor or a pad with your hands on a 22- to 26-inch (55-65 cm) stability ball, with your knees hip-width apart, your arms straight, and your palms shoulder-width apart (see figure *a*).

Action and Coaching Tips

Drive the ball away from you by reaching your arms overhead as if diving into a pool. Roll the ball out as far as you can without allowing your head or lower back to sag toward the floor (see figure *b*). Once you've gone as far as you can or your arms are completely overhead in a straight line with your torso, reverse the motion by driving your arms downward into the ball and pull it back to the starting position without allowing your hips to flex.

To make this exercise more difficult, use a smaller ball. Use a larger ball to make this exercise easier.

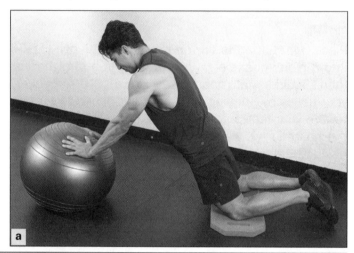

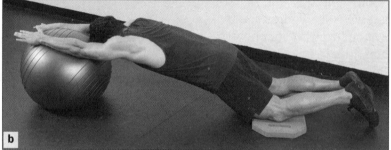

Arm Walkout

Setup

Kneel, keeping your hands flat on the floor just above your shoulders and your arms straight under your shoulders. Your torso should form a nearly straight line from your head to your knees. You may also need to place a pad, pillow, or folded towel under your knees for comfort (see figure *a*).

Action and Coaching Tips

Walk your arms out in front of you as far as possible without feeling discomfort in your lower back and while keeping your body in a straight line (see figures *b-d*); do not allow your hips or head to sag toward the floor. Squeeze your glutes tightly each time you walk your hands out to the long position. Reverse the motion, walking your hands back so that they end up just in front of your shoulders.

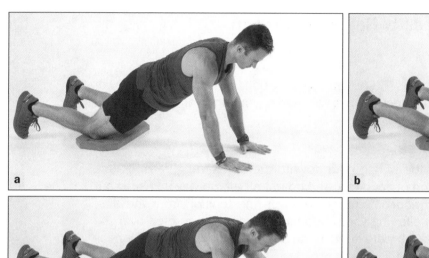

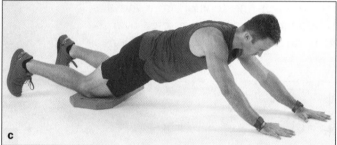

Suspension Trainer Arm Fallout

Setup

Facing away from the anchor point of a suspension trainer, grab the handles and lean your weight forward with your elbows slightly bent and arms shoulder-width apart at a roughly 45-degree angle to the floor (see figure a).

Action and Coaching Tips

Without bending your elbows, reach your arms above your head as if diving into a pool (see figure b). Pull your arms back in to complete the rep. Do not

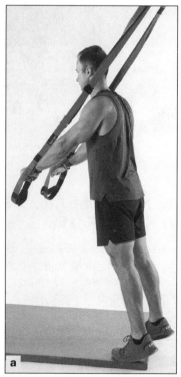

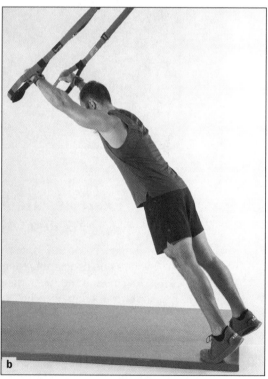

allow your hips to sag toward the floor. To increase the difficulty, start the exercise from a more severe forward lean, which brings your body closer to the floor.

Stability Ball Plate Crunch

Setup

Lie faceup with a 22- to 26-inch (55-65 cm) stability ball in the arch of your lower back and hold a weight plate directly above your chest; your arms are outstretched (see figure a).

Action and Coaching Tips

Perform a crunch, keeping the weight plate toward the sky (see figure b). Pause for 1 or 2 seconds at the top of each rep, and do not sit all the way up (with your torso perpendicular to the floor); doing so removes the tension from the abs. Slowly reverse the motion, allowing your abdominal muscles to stretch over the ball. Do not allow your neck to hyperextend in the bottom position; keep your neck in a neutral position throughout.

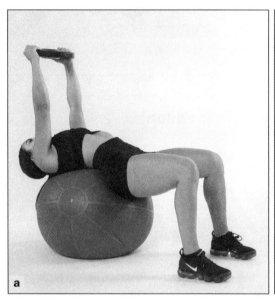
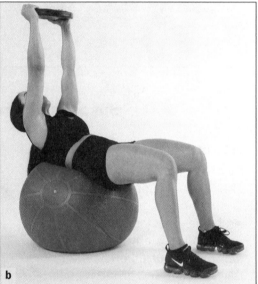

Exercises Trainers Hate That Aren't Bad: Crunches and Other Spinal Flexion Exercises

Mention crunches, a common spinal flexion exercise, and many trainers assume you're hoping to spot reduce belly fat. They think that people believe feeling a muscle burn means they're burning fat, and they know it's not possible. Many trainers also hate crunches because they represent inefficient training and simply not knowing what you're doing. You can't go into a gym and not see people flailing around on the ground for endless reps while yanking their head forward and thinking they know how to exercise.

Stack all that on top of the fact that people sit in a forward flexed position all day and then come to the gym and repeatedly flex forward doing crunches and you can see why many trainers cringe when they hear the word "crunches."

In short, crunches, in one exercise, represent almost everything many trainers think is wrong with mainstream fitness practices.

I don't program standard crunches; that is why they're not in this book. But it's not because I think they're bad; I just prefer spinal flexion exercises like stability ball plate crunches and reverse crunches. They are more time efficient because they provide a sufficient training stimulus without the endless reps. I also use spinal flexion exercises in conjunction with anti-spinal-movement exercises, which is why you see both kinds of exercises in this book.

Many trainers are against any sort of spinal flexion exercises and exclusively use anti-spinal-movement exercises. They take this approach because they believe that spinal flexion exercises are, among other things, inherently dangerous, bad for your posture, and nonfunctional. Many coaches and trainers also believe that spinal flexion exercises like stability ball plate crunches and reverse crunches are dangerous. They base this idea on research from spine expert Dr. Stuart McGill. But I believe they have misinterpreted his findings. In 2017, Dr. McGill coauthored a paper on spinal flexion exercises (1). The following are core-training recommendations taken from this paper:

- "If the ability to bear heavy loads is important to a client, it may be better to choose abdominal exercises with high muscular loads such as push-up position walkouts, rollout planks, or stir the pot."
- "If flexibility is more important to the client, the personal trainer may want to select full-range curl-ups and crunches, and reduce heavy loading."
- "If maximal muscular development is the primary goal, including the crunch and/or its numerous variations, together with other exercises, may help to enhance desired results."

So you can see that spinal flexion exercises are no different than any other resistance training exercise. Sure, spinal flexion exercises like crunches may be problematic if you overuse them or apply them in a way that exceeds your physical capacity, but you could say that about any exercise. The issue is not with the exercise itself but with poor application, such as doing endless reps.

You can train smart and add spinal flexion exercises to the programs in this book. In fact, research has shown that spinal flexion exercises can help promote nutrient delivery to the intervertebral discs (3).

But the arguments against crunches don't end there. Many trainers believe that spinal flexion exercises like stability-ball plate crunches will harm your posture. First off, if you believe doing crunches will cause you to have a more flexed posture because that's the movement involved in the exercise, then you must also believe that doing Romanian deadlifts will lock you into spinal extension because that's the posture involved in the exercise.

Secondly, spinal flexion exercises like stability ball plate crunches allow for greater abdominal muscle stretch than floor crunches do. This is important because strength training at longer (stretched) muscle lengths, which includes an eccentric component, not only causes muscles to be stronger at long lengths but also promotes flexibility by causing muscle fibers to produce new sarcomeres in series within a muscle, which allows the muscle to lengthen more (4, 5). In other words, full-range resistance training regimens, which train the muscles at long (stretched) lengths and include an eccentric component, can improve flexibility as well as, if not better than, typical static stretching.

Reverse Crunch

Setup

Lie on your back on a weight bench, with your knees bent and your hips flexed into your belly. With your elbows bent, hold on to the bench just behind and above your head (see figure *a*). This exercise can be made more difficult if you lie on an incline bench with your head higher than your legs.

Action and Coaching Tips

Smoothly and with control, do a reverse crunch by rolling your lower back up off the bench and bringing your knees toward your chin (see figure *b*). Do not use momentum or jerk your body. Slowly reverse this motion, lowering your spine back toward the bench, one vertebra at a time. Do not allow your legs to extend or your head to lift off the bench at any point.

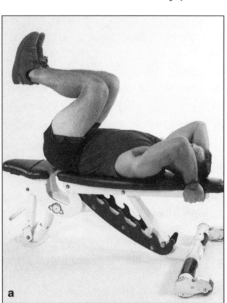
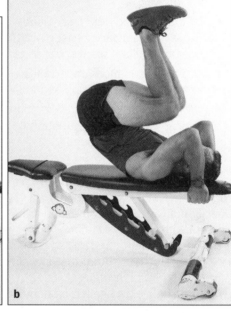

Incline Bench Reverse Crunch

You can make the reverse crunch more difficult by lying on an incline bench, with your head higher than your legs.

Setup

Lie on your back on a weight bench that's at an incline, with your knees bent and your hips flexed into your belly. With your elbows bent, hold on to the bench just behind and above your head (see figure *a*). The higher the incline, the harder you make the exercise.

Action and Coaching Tips

Smoothly and with control, do a reverse crunch by rolling your lower back off the bench and bringing your knees toward your chin (see figure *b*). Do not use momentum or jerk your body. Slowly reverse this motion, lowering your spine back toward the bench, one vertebra at a time. Do not allow your legs to extend or your head to lift off the bench at any point.

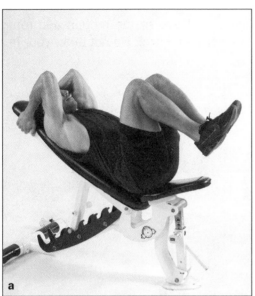
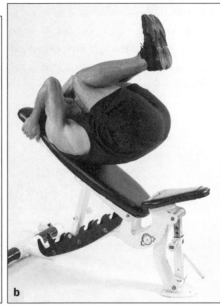

Hanging Knee Raise

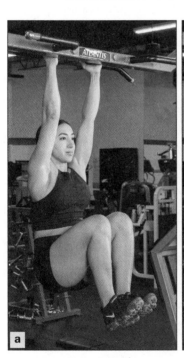
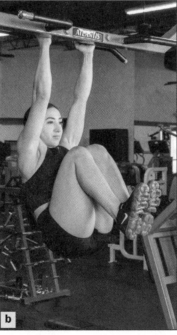

Setup

Hang from a pull-up bar with an overhand grip and your hands roughly shoulder-width apart. Flex your hips and bend your knees, holding them above your hips in front of your torso (see figure *a*).

Action and Coaching Tips

In a controlled fashion, roll your torso upward, bringing your knees toward your chin (see figure *b*). Slowly reverse this motion without untucking your knees from your body. Don't allow your knees to drop below your hips at any point. Do not use momentum or jerk your body at any point.

Stability Ball Knee Tuck

Setup

Hold yourself in a push-up position, with your hands directly under your shoulders and your feet and shins resting on top of a 22- to 26-inch (55-65 cm) stability ball (see figure *a*). Keep your legs hip-width apart.

Action and Coaching Tips

Pull your knees into your chest (see figure b). Reverse the motion and repeat, performing the exercise smoothly with deliberate control. Do not allow your head or lower back to sag toward the floor.

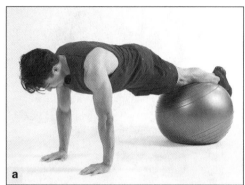
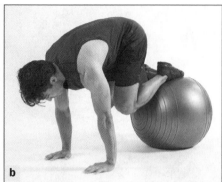

Stability Ball Pike Rollout

Setup

This exercise combines the ball pike and the ball rollout into one abdominal exercise. Hold yourself in a push-up position, with your hands directly under your shoulders and your feet hip-width apart on top of a 22- to 26-inch (55-65 cm) ball (see figure a).

Action and Coaching Tips

Keep your legs straight and perform the pike portion by pushing your hips toward the ceiling while keeping your back nearly flat (see figure b). During the pike portion of the exer-

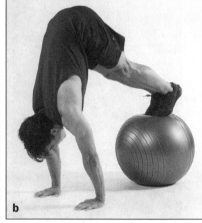

cise, raise your hips until just before they reach above your shoulders. After straightening your hips and coming back to the starting position, perform the rollback portion by pushing your body

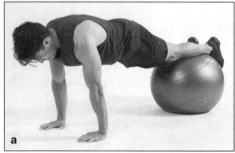

backward on the ball until your arms are fully extended in front of you and your legs are fully extended behind you (see figure c). Do not allow your hips or head to sag toward the floor as you extend your arms into the rollback portion of the exercise. Reverse the motion, then repeat.

To make the exercise easier, start with the ball closer to your belly button.

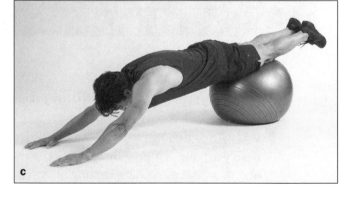

Best Core Exercises in the Lateral Strength Zone

The exercises in this section help you maximize the strength and development of your core in the lateral strength zone.

It's important to note the dynamic side elbow plank with hip abduction, dynamic bent-knee side elbow plank with hip abduction, and the bent-knee Copenhagen hip adduction exercises featured in chapter 11 also work your core in the lateral strength zone.

Dumbbell Unilateral Farmers Walk

Setup

Stand tall at one end of the room while holding a heavy dumbbell on the right side of your body and your palm facing your body by your hip (or at your shoulder) (see figure a).

Action and Coaching Tips

Walk to the other end of the room (see figures b-d), then return to your starting point and complete one full lap, covering 40 to 50 total yards (37-46 m). Switch hands and do another lap. Take normal strides and move as fast as you can without losing control. Maintain a tall, upright posture as you carry the weight.

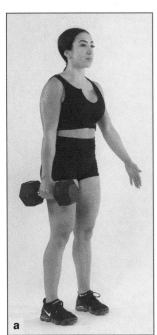 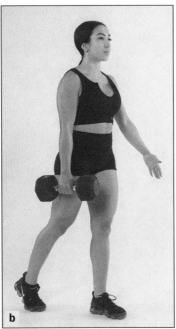 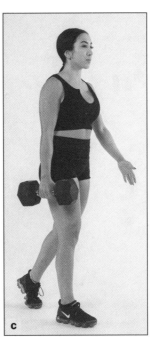 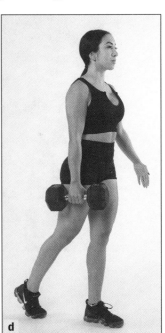

Angled-Barbell Tight Rainbow

This is often mistakenly thought to be a rotational exercise because it can involve twisting of the shoulders. However, true rotational exercises require a line of force that goes horizontally or diagonally across your torso. In this exercise, the line of force is vertical because of gravity. Therefore, your core musculature is mainly resisting side bending while the barbell is out to your side.

Setup

Place one end of a barbell in a corner or into a landmine device. Hold the other end with both hands while standing tall, your feet roughly shoulder-width apart (see figure a).

Action and Coaching Tips

Move the barbell from side to side in a rainbow-like arc from one shoulder to the other while maintaining a straight spine and keeping a slight bend in your elbows throughout (see figures b and c). One rep is completed by moving from one side to the other and back to the start. The movement of the barbell should come from your shoulders, not your elbows. Avoid rotation at your torso; as you move the barbell from side to side, your torso should face the barbell's anchored end.

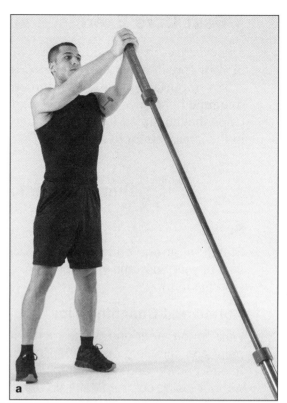

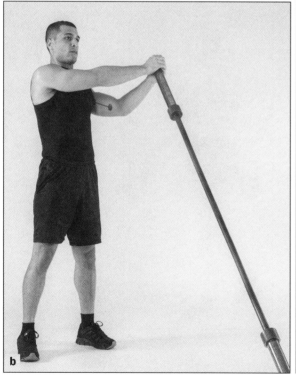

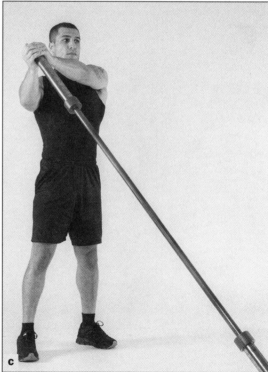

Off-Bench Lateral Hold

Setup

Sit in the center of a weight bench, with one leg on each side. Turn your body to the left so your torso is now in line with the bench. With your knee bent to roughly 90 degrees, lean slightly to your left side while hooking your left heel and right toes under the padded part the bench (see figure a). Your right leg will be your top leg.

Action and Coaching Tips

Once both feet are securely and comfortably hooked under the padded platform of the bench, lower your torso as far as you can without resting the weight of your torso on the bench. Once you've gone as low as you're able while keeping your spine straight, hold this position for 10 to 30 seconds depending on your ability (see figure b). Then perform the same action for the same amount of time on the other side by turning your torso to the right—your left leg will be your top leg—while hooking your left toes and right heel under the padded platform of the bench.

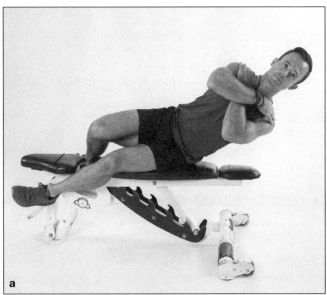
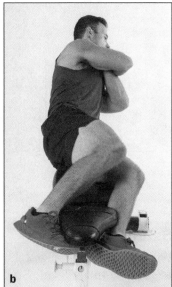

Medicine Ball Side Lean

Setup

With your feet roughly hip-width apart, hold a medicine ball or weight plate directly above your head, with your elbows slightly bent (see figure a).

Action and Coaching Tips

While keeping the medicine ball or weight plate directly above your head, lean your body laterally to one side and shift your hips to the opposite side until you feel a mild stretch (see figure b). Reverse the motion and repeat, leaning your torso and hips in the opposite direction. Alternate sides on each rep.

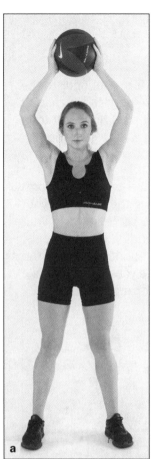
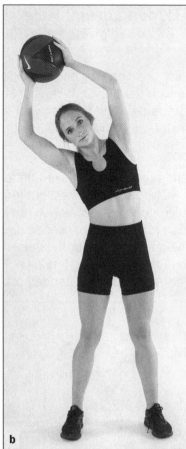
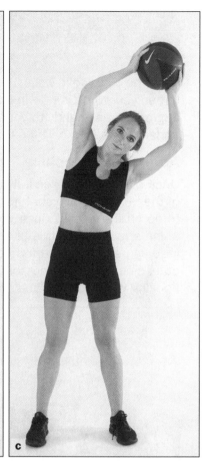

Cable One-Arm Side Bend

Setup

With your right hand, grab the handle of a cable (or resistance band) that's attached at roughly ankle level. Stand tall, with your feet about shoulder-width apart and the cable at your right side (see figure *a*). Stand far enough away from the cable or band that it's at a roughly 45-degree angle to the floor.

Action and Coaching Tips

Without rotating your body, bend your torso sideways to the left until you feel a mild stretch in the right side of your torso (see figure *b*). Reverse the action and finish the rep by slightly flexing your torso to the right against the resistance. Perform all reps on the same side before switching sides.

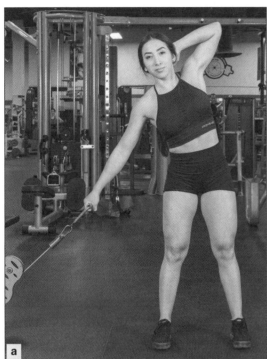
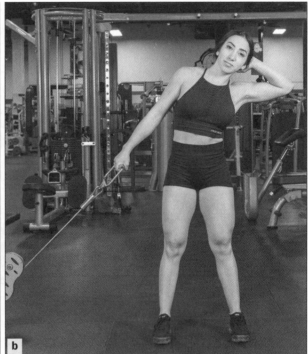

Stability Ball Side Crunch

Setup

Lie on your side over a 22- to 26-inch (55-65 cm) stability ball so your belly button is roughly above the apex of the ball. Anchor your feet against a wall, with your top leg behind your bottom leg. Cross your arms in front of your chest while holding a weight plate. You can also perform this exercise without a weight plate by crossing your arms against your chest (see figure a).

Action and Coaching Tips

Without rotating your body, bend your torso sideways toward the floor until you feel a mild stretch in the opposite side of your torso (see figure b). Reverse the action and finish the rep by slightly flexing your torso laterally away from the floor. Perform all reps on the same side before switching sides.

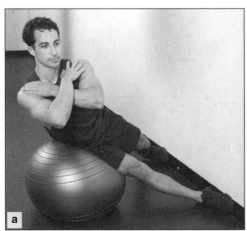
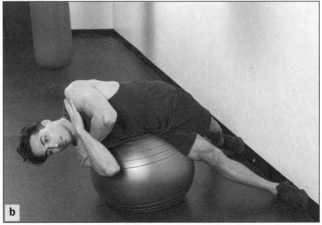

Weight Plate Around the World

Setup

Stand in a wide stance, with your feet about 12 inches (about 30 cm) wider than your shoulders. Hold the weight plate or medicine ball directly above your head, with your elbows slightly bent (see figure a).

Action and Coaching Tips

Keeping your elbows bent, use your entire body to make the biggest circles (more like horizontal ovals) that you can make (see figures b-d). Be sure to bend your knees at the bottom aspects of the movement and shift your weight to the same side the plate or ball is on. Also, reach high at the top parts of this exercise. Perform all reps in the same direction before switching directions.

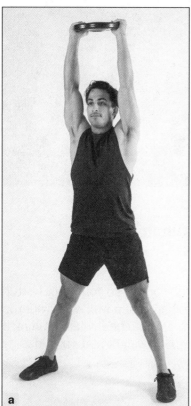
a

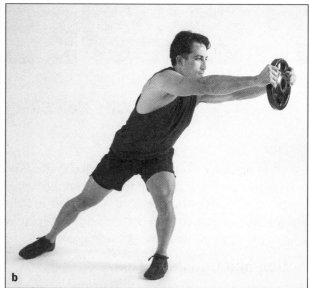
b

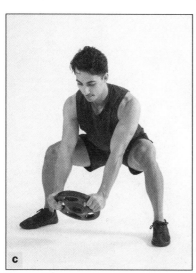
c

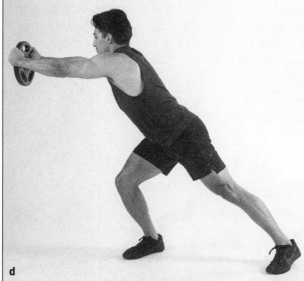
d

Best Core Exercises in the Rotational Strength Zone

The exercises in this section help you maximize the strength and development of the core in the rotational strength zone.

Dumbbell Plank Row

Setup

Begin in a push-up position with each of your hands gripping a dumbbell placed on the floor and palms facing in (see figure a). Your feet are roughly shoulder-width apart, and your wrists are directly below your shoulders. To ensure that the dumbbells do not roll, place your hands directly under your shoulders.

Action and Coaching Tips

From the push-up position, pick up the dumbbell in your left hand and row it into your body (see figure b). Slowly lower it to the floor and repeat the action with your right hand. Continue to alternate hands.

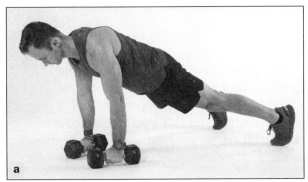
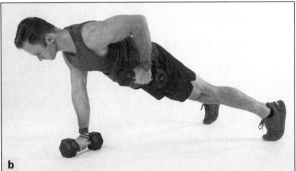

One-Arm Plank

Setup

Begin in a push-up position, with your hands shoulder-width apart and your feet a few inches (about 5 cm) farther than shoulder-width apart (see figure a).

Action and Coaching Tips

Lift one arm off the ground without allowing your shoulders or hips to rotate or your head or belly to sag toward the floor (see figure b). Pause for several seconds before switching hands (see figure c). To make this exercise more difficult, you can perform it from your elbows; if you do so, place a pad, pillow, or folded towel under your elbow for protection. You can also increase the challenge of both the straight-arm and elbow-supported

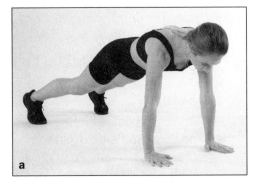

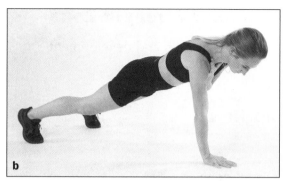

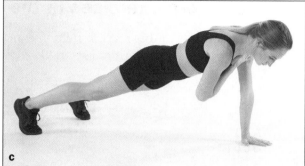

version of this exercise by extending your free arm out to your side, so your arm is parallel with the floor.

Cross-Body Plank

Setup

Begin in a push-up position, your wrists under your shoulders and your feet shoulder-width apart (see figure *a*).

Action and Coaching Tips

Without allowing your head or hips to sag, simultaneously raise your left foot and right hand off the ground. Bring your left knee to your right elbow together while keeping your right hand directly below your chin (see figure *b*). Pause for 2 or 3 seconds, then reverse this motion on the opposite side, touching your right knee to your left elbow. Do not allow your hips or shoulders to rotate at any time.

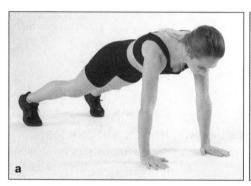

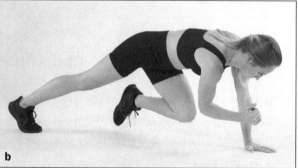

Cable Tight Rotation With Hip Shift

Setup

Attach the cable to the highest position and stand perpendicular to a cable column on your right side. Hold the handle with both hands and extend your arms toward the cable's origin. Position your feet slightly farther than shoulder-width apart and shift your weight toward your right leg, with your shoulders directly over your hips (see figure *a*).

Action and Coaching Tips

Keeping your hips moving with your shoulders, shift your weight to your left leg as you move your arms horizontally, pulling the handle across your body to the right until both arms are just outside your left shoulder (see figure *b*). Stop rotating your hips and shoulders when the cable or band gently touches your forearm. Slowly reverse the motion to return to the starting position and complete the rep. Perform all reps on one side before switching to the other side.

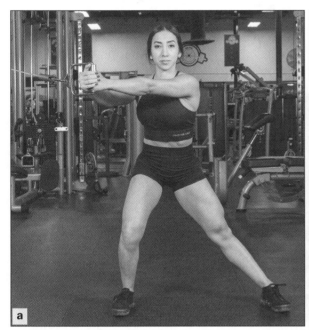 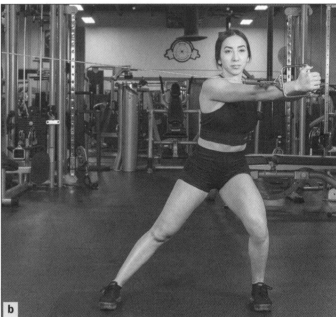

Cable Three-Point Horizontal Chop

This exercise is segmented into three body positions relative to the cable. The exercise sequence fills in the gaps in rotational ranges of motion left by the standard rotational movement where the cable is to your side, which does a great job of strengthening rotation when your arms are in front of your torso, but doesn't create much load at the aspects of rotation when your arms are turning the corner on the side of your torso. Therefore, doing these in all three positions creates complete rotational core strength.

Setup

Attach the cable handle at shoulder level and stand perpendicular to a cable column on your right side. Hold the handle with both hands and extend your arms toward the cable's origin. Position your feet slightly farther than shoulder-width apart and shift your weight toward your right leg, with your shoulders directly over your hips (see figure *a*).

Action and Coaching Tips

Point 1: Keeping your hips moving with your shoulders, shift your weight to your left leg as you move your arms horizontally, pulling the handle across your body to the left until both arms are just outside your left shoulder (see figure *b*). Stop rotating your hips and shoulders when the cable or band gently touches your forearm. Slowly reverse the motion to return to the starting position and complete the rep. Perform all reps on one side before switching to the other side.

Point 2: Stand facing the cable, grabbing the handle first with your left hand, then place your right hand over your left. Rotate your torso to the left while pivoting on the ball of your right foot (see figure c-d). Perform all reps on one side before switching to the other side.

Point 3: To maximally load the muscles that create left-side torso rotation in the lengthened range, stand facing away from the cable so it's roughly behind your right shoulder. Hold the cable handle in the same manner as described in point 2 while pivoting on the ball of your right foot (see figure e). Rotate your torso to the left until the cable touches your right arm (see figure f). Perform all reps on one side before switching to the other side.

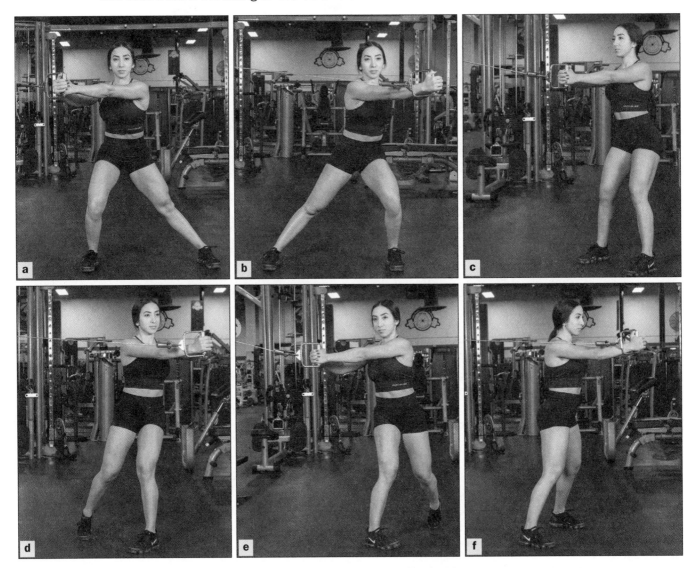

Cable Three-Point High-to-Low Chop

This exercise is segmented into three body positions relative to the cable. The sequence fills in the gaps in rotational ranges of motion left by the standard rotational movement where the cable is to your side, which does a great job of strengthening rotation when your arms are in front of your torso, but doesn't create much load at the aspects of rotation when your arms are turning the corner on the side of your torso. Therefore, doing these in all three positions creates complete rotational core strength.

Setup

Stand perpendicular to a cable column on your right side with the cable attached above your head. Hold the handle with both hands and extend your arms toward the cable's origin (see figure *a*). Position your feet slightly farther than shoulder-width apart.

Action and Coaching Tips

Point 1: With your arms above your head on your right side and most of your weight shifted onto your right leg, drive the cable diagonally downward across your body as you set your hips back slightly and shift your weight to your left leg (see figure *b*). Once the cable touches your arm, slowly reverse the motion to complete the rep. Perform all reps on the same side before switching sides. Throughout this exercise, keep your spine in a neutral position and keep your torso nearly perpendicular to the cable column; do not rotate your torso away from the cable column more than a few degrees as you reach the bottom of the range of motion (doing so greatly reduces the rotational tension on your torso muscles).

Point 2: Stand facing the cable, grabbing the handle first with your left hand, then place your right hand over your left (see figure *c*). Rotate your torso to the left while pivoting on the ball of your right foot (see figure *d*). Perform all reps on one side before switching to the other side.

Point 3: To maximally load the muscles that create left-side torso rotation in the lengthened range, stand facing away from the cable so it's roughly behind your right shoulder. Hold the cable handle in the same manner as described in point 2 while pivoting on the ball of your left foot (see figure *e*). Rotate your torso to the left until the cable touches your right arm (see figure *f*). Perform all reps on one side before switching to the other side.

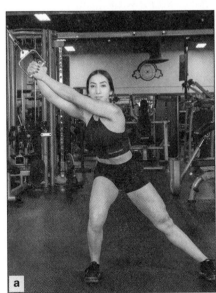
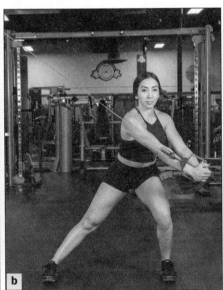
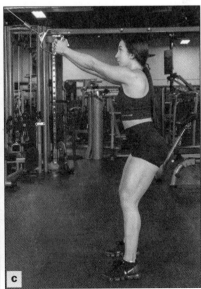

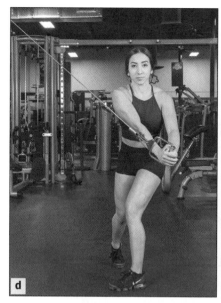 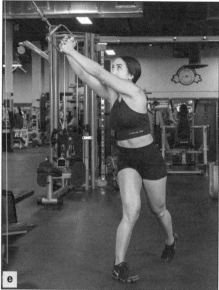 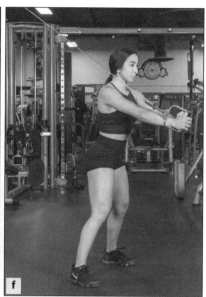

Cable Three-Point Low-to-High Chop

This exercise is segmented into three body positions relative to the cable. This exercise sequence fills in the gaps in rotational ranges of motion left by the standard rotational movement where the cable is to your side, which does a great job of strengthening rotation when your arms are in front of your torso, but doesn't create much load at the aspects of rotation when your arms are turning the corner on the side of your torso. Therefore, doing this in all three positions creates complete rotational core strength.

Setup

Stand perpendicular to a cable column (or resistance band) on your right side. With both hands on the handle, which is attached at ankle level, extend your arms toward the cable's origin. Position your feet slightly farther than shoulder-width apart. Squat and shift most of your weight to your right leg while your arms reach at a downward angle toward the origin of the cable (see figure a).

Action and Coaching Tips

Point 1: Stand up while shifting your weight toward your left leg and driving the cable diagonally, upward across your body. Finish at the top, with your arms above your head on your left side when the rope gently touches your forearm (see figure b). Reverse the motion to return to the starting position, then repeat. Perform all reps on the same side before switching sides.

Point 2: Stand facing the cable, grabbing the handle first with your left hand, then place your right hand over your left (see figure c). Rotate your torso to the left while pivoting on the ball of your right foot (see figure d). Perform all reps on one side before switching to the other side.

Point 3: To maximally load the muscles that create left-side torso rotation in the lengthened range, stand facing away from the cable so it's roughly behind your right shoulder. Hold the cable handle in the same manner as described in point 2 while pivoting on the ball of your left foot (see figure e). Rotate your torso to the left until the cable touches your right arm (see figure f). Perform all reps on one side before switching to the other side.

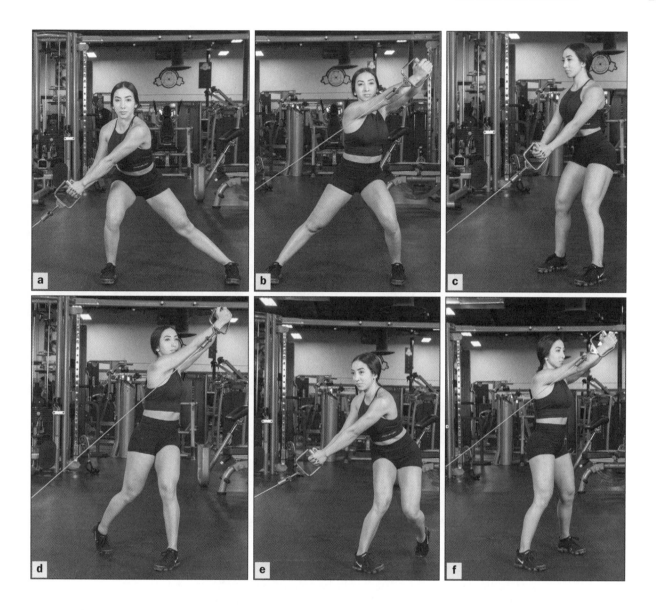

Cable One-Arm Press

This is one of the most underrated exercises. You likely don't see it used in your gym or promoted online nearly as much as Pallof presses are. The one-arm cable press places just as much, if not more, of an antirotation demand on your hips and torso musculature. For one thing, you can use heavier loads because of the split stance. And it gets more done than the Pallof press because it also involves the upper-body pushing musculature, plus the calves and hamstrings of the back leg, which prevent you from being pulled backward.

Setup

Stand facing away from an adjustable cable column while holding the handle at about shoulder height. With the cable handle in your left hand and your elbow at a roughly 45-degree angle from your body, split your stance by putting your left leg behind your right leg (see figure a). Keep your rear foot straight and your back heel off the ground.

Action and Coaching Tips

Press the cable straight out in front of you (see figure *b*). Slowly reverse the motion and bring the handle back into your body as you bring your left arm back toward you in a rowing motion. Don't allow your shoulders or hips to rotate more than a few degrees. Lean slightly forward to be able to move heavier loads.

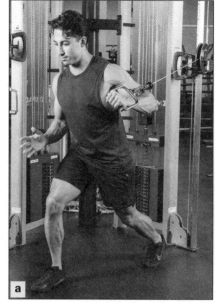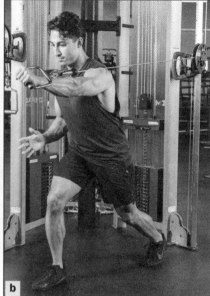

To prevent the cable attachment from digging into your arm, use an extender strap (which can be purchased at a store that sells rock-climbing gear) between the handle and the cable attachment.

Cable Same-Side One-Arm Press

You can also do this exercise with your lead leg on the same side as your pressing arm. This increases the demand on your torso muscles because the cable will try to turn you in the opposite direction of your foot. Therefore, it can't help you as much as when the cable is pulling you toward your back leg.

Setup

Stand facing away from an adjustable cable column while holding a handle at roughly shoulder height. With the cable handle in your right hand and your elbow at a roughly 45-degree angle from your body, split your stance by putting your left leg behind your right leg (see figure *a*). Keep your rear foot straight and your back heel off the ground.

Action and Coaching Tips

Press the cable straight out in front of you (see figure *b*). Slowly reverse the motion and bring the handle back into your body as you bring your right arm back toward you in a rowing motion. Don't allow your shoulders or hips to rotate more than a few degrees. Lean slightly forward to be able to move heavier loads.

To prevent the cable attachment from digging into your arm, use an extender strap (which can be purchased at a store that sells rock-climbing gear) between the handle and the cable attachment.

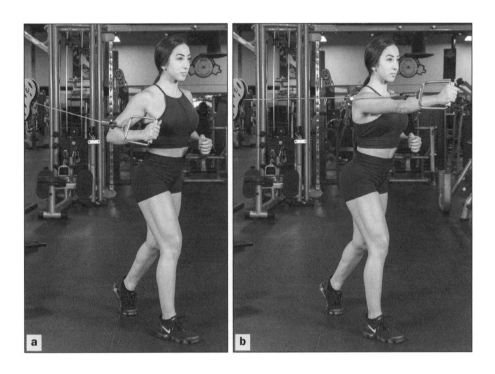

Weight Plate Chop

Setup

Squat and rotate your hips and torso while holding a weight plate weighing 10 to 45 pounds (4.5-20 kg) outside your right knee (see figure a).

Action and Coaching Tips

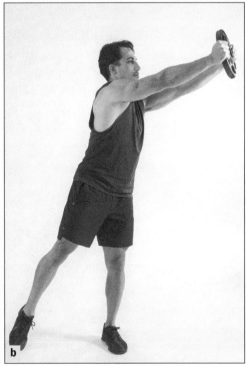

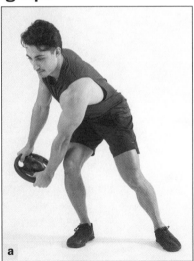

Stand up as you quickly rotate to your left side and drive the plate across your body in a diagonal pattern, finishing with it just above your head (see figure b). Without pausing, quickly reverse the motion by driving the plate back down across your body on the same diagonal path you used to lift it. Perform all reps to one side, then repeat the exercise to the other side. Do this exercise fast, but smoothly and with a consistent rhythm, coordinating your upper body and lower body during both the lifting and the lowering phase of each repetition.

Now let's start putting all these great exercises into workouts, starting with the beginner strength zone training programs.

CHAPTER 14

Beginner Workout Program

This chapter provides a workout program for those who are just starting out or for those who haven't done regular strength training in a while. The workout program in this chapter lays the foundation so you can move on to the more demanding programs in the chapters that follow. The programs in chapters 15, 16, and 17 are designed to be used after first building a solid training foundation. Training smart means using a smart progression of gradually increasing the intensity of your workouts to ensure that you continually improve (i.e., progress) with much less risk of injury or overtraining.

That's where the workout program in this chapter comes in. The phases of the beginner workout program help you build a training foundation to ensure that your body is ready to safely perform the more intense workouts to come. So, regardless of which of the three following chapters you use, it is smartest and safest to start with the progressive, beginner program in this chapter.

Program Overview

Each phase of the beginner workout program progresses from the preceding phase. For example, phase 2 requires you to perform more overall exercises and more overall sets of each exercise than was required in phase 1. Phase 3 involves more exercises and more sets than were asked of you in phase 2. The three workout phases in this chapter gradually increase in intensity. Each training phase builds the foundation needed to more safely and effectively perform the next phase.

Program Guidelines

Each of the three phases of the beginner workout program consists of its own set of unique workouts. Here are a few key points regarding these workouts:

Rest

- Perform the exercises designated with *a* or *b* as paired sets, and perform exercises with *a*, *b*, and *c* as tri-sets. Perform all reps in each set before moving to the next set. Completing 1 round of the exercises in a paired or tri-set is considered 1 set.

- Rest 60 seconds between exercises in a given paired set and tri-set.
- Rest 1 to 3 minutes between each round of a given paired set and tri-set.

Reps

- Focus on the technique of each exercise and use deliberate control on each rep.
- Maintain strict form without cheating by using additional movements or momentum.
- Mentally focus on the working muscles in each exercise.
- Do the concentric (lifting) portion of each rep at a normal tempo and maintain control during the eccentric (lowering) portion.

Weight

- The main goal of the workouts in this chapter is to familiarize your body with the demands of performing basic exercises. Your primary focus when using these workouts, especially in phases 1 and 2, is not to reach full exercise fatigue, but to improve your exercise technique and your muscle awareness when performing the exercises.
- Use a weight load that allows you to maintain proper control and technique while leaving you able to perform 2 to 4 more reps according to what is indicated in each phase of the beginner program.

Work Around—Not Through—Injuries and Limitations

- If an exercise causes pain or discomfort beyond the sensation associated with muscle fatigue, use an alternative exercise that doesn't hurt and targets the same muscle group in the same strength zone. Not every exercise movement is for everybody. There are plenty of movements in the exercise chapters of this book to choose from.

Use Soreness as a Guide, Not as a Goal

As much as we may love to hate feeling sore after a workout and may wish to gauge a workout based on how sore we are afterward, it's crucial to understand that soreness is not needed for muscle and strength development (1). Delayed onset muscle soreness (DOMS) can be the result of performing an unfamiliar exercise. So it's normal and expected to experience some muscle soreness when you're starting these beginner programs.

That said, if you're very sore after your first workout in any phase of the beginner workout program, use that as a guide to go a little easier on your next workout. Mild soreness is okay and an indicator that you are still familiarizing your body with the new workouts and didn't overdo it. However, if you're so sore that it interferes with your daily activities and lasts more than three days, you did too much for your current tolerance. Therefore, you need to dial back the amount of weight you use or the number of reps you perform. These workouts simply provide a guideline to start from, and you must listen to and honor your own body and adapt accordingly. This applies to any workout program you do, regardless of your fitness level.

Beginner Program: Phase 1

The first phase of the beginner program consists of a single workout, which you'll repeat four times, either two, three, or four times a week on nonconsecutive days (see table 14.1 on page 221). If you're exercising four times per week, you'll complete phase 1 of the beginner program in one week's time.

Do not take any sets to muscular failure. In phase 1, (-1) indicates to stop the set 1 rep before muscle failure, (-2) indicates to stop the set 2 reps before muscle failure, (-3) indicates to stop the set 3 reps before muscle failure, and (-4) indicates to stop the set 4 reps before muscle failure.

Beginner Program: Phase 2

The primary goal of this phase is to increase your work volume and movement vocabulary by adding more exercises than in the previous program. Phase 2 of the beginner program consists of two workouts: day A (see table 14.2 on page 222) and day B (see table 14.3 on page 223). You alternate workouts and perform them two, three, or four times per week—but no more than two days in a row to allow for sufficient recovery because these are total-body workouts. Once you've performed each workout six times with the indicated set-and-rep progression, you're ready to move on to phase 3 of the beginner program.

Beginner Program: Phase 3

The primary goal of this phase is to gradually add a muscular fatigue element to your training. Doing so familiarizes your body with reaching muscular failure and achieving a muscle pump in order to focus on adding muscle tissue and increasing connective tissue strength.

So, unlike in phase 1 and phase 2, at the end of phase 3, the workouts call for you to use a weight load that allows you to achieve the indicated number of reps in each set—but no more. In other words, at the end of each set, you should not be able to perform any more reps than indicated while maintaining proper control and technique. This approach is referred to as taking each set to technical failure because your muscle fatigue prevents you from maintaining proper technique. Be sure to maintain control in the eccentric (lowering) portion of each rep.

Like in phase 2, this phase consists of two workouts: day A (see table 14.4 on page 224) and day B (see table 14.5 on page 225). You alternate between day A and day B workouts and perform them two, three, or four times per week—but no more than two days in a row to allow for sufficient recovery because these are total-body workouts. Once you've performed each workout six times with the indicated set-and-rep progression, you're ready to move on to the next stage of training.

Weekly Workout Schedule for Phase 2 and Phase 3

Following are weekly training schedule options for performing both phase 2 and phase 3 of the beginner workout program.

Schedule or Training Twice per Week

Week 1

Monday: Day A–workout 1

Tuesday: Rest

Wednesday: Rest

Thursday: Day B–workout 1

Friday: Rest

Saturday: Rest

Sunday: Rest

Week 2

Monday: Day A–workout 2   Friday: Rest

Tuesday: Rest   Saturday: Rest

Wednesday: Rest   Sunday: Rest

Thursday: Day B–workout 2

Continue the sequence on week 3, starting with day A workout 3 on Monday and so on.

Schedule or Training Three Times per Week

Week 1

Monday: Day A–workout 1   Friday: Day A–workout 2

Tuesday: Rest   Saturday: Rest

Wednesday: Day B–workout 1   Sunday: Rest

Thursday: Rest

Week 2

Monday: Day B–workout 2   Friday: Day B–workout 3

Tuesday: Rest   Saturday: Rest

Wednesday: Day A–workout 3   Sunday: Rest

Thursday: Rest

Continue the sequence on week 3, starting with day A workout 4 on Monday and so on.

Schedule or Training Four Times per Week

Option 1

Monday: Day A–workout 1   Friday: Day B–workout 2

Tuesday: Day B–workout 1   Saturday: Rest

Wednesday: Rest   Sunday: Rest

Thursday: Day A–workout 2

Option 2

Monday: Day A–workout 1   Friday: Rest

Tuesday: Day B–workout 1   Saturday: Day B–workout 2

Wednesday: Rest   Sunday: Rest

Thursday: Day A–workout 2

Continue the sequence on week 2, starting with day A workout 3 and so on.

Regardless of how many days per week you prefer to perform phase 2 and phase 3 of this beginner program, you can change the days of the week that you perform each workout to better fit your schedule. Just make sure to perform the workouts in alternating fashion between workout A and workout B. And try to distribute your workouts and rest days throughout the week in a sequence similar to the samples to maximize recovery.

TABLE 14.1   Beginner Workout Program Phase 1

Strength zone	Exercise name	Page number	Workout 1 (sets × reps)	Workout 2 (sets × reps)	Workout 3 (sets × reps)	Workout 4 (sets × reps)	Workout 5 (sets × reps)	Workout 6 (sets × reps)
Glutes: hip hinging for the lengthened to midrange	1a. Dumbbell hybrid deadlift	157	1 × 10-12 (-4)	1 × 10-12 (-3)	1 × 10-12 (-2)	1 × 10-12 (-2)	1 × 10-12 (-1)	1 × 10-12 (-1)
Chest: horizontal or decline pressing for the lengthened to midrange	1b. Push-up*	30	1 × 10-12 (-4)	1 × 10-12 (-3)	1 × 10-12 (-2)	1 × 10-12 (-2)	1 × 10-12 (-1)	1 × 10-12 (-1)
**Quads and glutes: knee bending for the lengthened to midrange	2a. Dumbbell stability ball wall squat	143	1 × 10-12 (-4)	1 × 10-12 (-3)	1 × 10-12 (-2)	1 × 10-12 (-2)	1 × 10-12 (-1)	1 × 10-12 (-1)
Lats: horizontal pulling for the shortened to midrange	2b. Dumbbell two-arm bent-over row	60	1 × 12-15 (-4)	1 × 12-15 (-3)	1 × 12-15 (-2)	1 × 12-15 (-2)	1 × 12-15 (-1)	1 × 12-15 (-1)
Lats: vertical or diagonal pulling with arms inside for the lengthened to midrange	3a. Neutral-grip lat pull-down	54	1 × 12-15 (-4)	1 × 12-15 (-3)	1 × 12-15 (-2)	1 × 12-15 (-2)	1 × 12-15 (-1)	1 × 12-15 (-1)
Middle delts: shortened to midrange	3b. Dumbbell one-arm overhead press	74	1 × 10-12 (-4) each side	1 × 10-12 (-3) each side	1 × 10-12 (-2) each side	1 × 10-12 (-2) each side	1 × 10-12 (-1) each side	1 × 10-12 (-1) each side
Biceps: shortened to midrange	4a. Dumbbell standing biceps curl	103	1 × 12-15 (-4)	1 × 12-15 (-3)	1 × 12-15 (-2)	1 × 12-15 (-2)	1 × 12-15 (-1)	1 × 12-15 (-1)
Triceps: shortened to midrange	4b. Dumbbell triceps skull crusher	112	1 × 12-15 (-4)	1 × 12-15 (-3)	1 × 12-15 (-2)	1 × 12-15 (-2)	1 × 12-15 (-1)	1 × 12-15 (-1)
Core: rotational	4c. Cable one-arm press	213	1 × 14 each side	1 × 14 each	1 × 16 each side	1 × 16 each side	1 × 18-20 each side	1 × 18-20 each side

(-1) indicates to stop the set 1 rep before muscle failure. (-2) indicates to stop the set 2 reps before muscle failure. (-3) indicates to stop the set 3 reps before muscle failure. And (-4) indicates to stop the set 4 reps before muscle failure.

*If push-ups from the floor are too difficult, perform Hands-Elevated Push-Ups (p. 33). If push-ups from the floor are too easy, perform Feet-Elevated Push-Ups (p. 32).

**As mentioned in chapter 11, due to their multijoint nature, all exercises such as squats, Romanian deadlifts, lunges, and many variations of those exercises provided in chapters 9 and 10 also load your glutes when they're closer to a lengthened (stretched) range.

TABLE 14.2   Beginner Workout Program Phase 2: Day A

Strength zone	Exercise name	Page number	Workout 1 (sets × reps)	Workout 2 (sets × reps)	Workout 3 (sets × reps)	Workout 4 (sets × reps)	Workout 5 (sets × reps)	Workout 6 (sets × reps)
Glutes: hip hinging for the lengthened to midrange	1a. Barbell hybrid deadlift	156	2 × 10-12 (-3)	2 × 10-12 (-3)	2 × 10-12 (-2)	2 × 10-12 (-2)	2 × 10-12 (-1)	2 × 10-12 (-1)
Middle delts: shortened to midrange	1b. Dumbbell rotational overhead press	73	2 × 10-12 (-3) each side	2 × 10-12 (-3) each side	2 × 10-12 (-2) each side	2 × 10-12 (-2) each side	2 × 10-12 (-1) each side	2 × 10-12 (-1) each side
Lats: horizontal pulling for the shortened to midrange	2a. Suspension trainer row	65	2 × 12-15 (-3)	2 × 12-15 (-3)	2 × 12-15 (-2)	2 × 12-15 (-2)	2 × 12-15 (-1)	2 × 12-15 (-1)
*Quads and glutes: knee bending for the lengthened to midrange	2b. Dumbbell goblet squat with NT Loop knee resistance**	138	2 × 10-12 (-3) each side	2 × 10-12 (-3) each side	2 × 10-12 (-2) each side	2 × 10-12 (-2) each side	2 × 10-12 (-1) each side	2 × 10-12 (-1) each side
Biceps: lengthened to midrange	3a. EZ-bar preacher curl	100	2 × 10-12 (-3)	2 × 10-12 (-3)	2 × 10-12 (-2)	2 × 10-12 (-2)	2 × 10-12 (-1)	2 × 10-12 (-1)
Triceps: lengthened to midrange	3b. Dumbbell behind-the-head triceps extension	110	2 × 12-15 (-3)	2 × 12-15 (-3)	2 × 12-15 (-2)	2 × 12-15 (-2)	2 × 12-15 (-1)	2 × 12-15 (-1)
Core: linear	4a. Stability ball rollout	194	2 × 10-12	2 × 10-12	2 × 13-15	2 × 13-15	2 × 15-20	2 × 15-20
Hamstrings: knee flexion for the shortened to midrange	4b. Stability ball leg curl	129	2 × 10-12	2 × 10-12	2 × 13-15	2 × 13-15	2 × 15-20	2 × 15-20

(-1) indicates to stop the set 1 rep before muscle failure. (-2) indicates to stop the set 2 reps before muscle failure. (-3) indicates to stop the set 3 reps before muscle failure. And (-4) indicates to stop the set 4 reps before muscle failure.

*As mentioned in chapter 11, due to their multijoint nature, all exercises such as squats, Romanian deadlifts, lunges, and many variations of those exercises provided in chapters 9 and 10 also load your glutes when they're closer to a lengthened (stretched) range.

**Use body weight or hold dumbbell depending on your strength level.

TABLE 14.3 Beginner Workout Program Phase 2: Day B

Strength zone	Exercise name	Page number	Workout 1 (sets × reps)	Workout 2 (sets × reps)	Workout 3 (sets × reps)	Workout 4 (sets × reps)	Workout 5 (sets × reps)	Workout 6 (sets × reps)
Lats: vertical or diagonal pulling with arms inside for the lengthened to midrange	1a. Neutral-grip lat pull-down	54	2 × 12-15 (-3)	2 × 12-15 (-3)	2 × 12-15 (-2)	2 × 12-15 (-2)	2 × 12-15 (-1)	2 × 12-15 (-1)
*Quads and glutes: knee bending for the lengthened to midrange	1b. Dumbbell elevated split squat**	141	2 × 8 each side	2 × 8 each side	2 × 10 each side	2 × 10 each side	2 × 12 each side	2 × 12 each side
Chest: horizontal or decline pressing for the lengthened to midrange	2a. Dumbbell bench press	26	2 × 10-12 (-3)	2 × 10-12 (-3)	2 × 10-12 (-2)	2 × 10-12 (-2)	2 × 10-12 (-1)	2 × 10-12 (-1)
Glutes: hip extension for the shortened to midrange	2b. One-leg hip thrust**	164	2 × 12-15 (-3) each side	2 × 12-15 (-3) each side	2 × 12-15 (-2) each side	2 × 12-15 (-2) each side	2 × 12-15 (-1) each side	2 × 12-15 (-1) each side
Triceps: lengthened to midrange	3a. Cable rope overhead triceps extension	108	2 × 12-15 (-3)	2 × 12-15 (-3)	2 × 12-15 (-2)	2 × 12-15 (-2)	2 × 12-15 (-1)	2 × 12-15 (-1)
Biceps: shortened to midrange	3b. Dumbbell standing biceps curl	103	2 × 12-15 (-3)	2 × 12-15 (-3)	2 × 12-15 (-2)	2 × 12-15 (-2)	2 × 12-15 (-1)	2 × 12-15 (-1)
Core: rotational	4a. Cable tight rotation with hip shift	208	2 × 10-12 (-3) each side	2 × 10-12 (-3) each side	2 × 10-12 (-2) each side	2 × 10-12 (-2) each side	2 × 10-12 (-1) each side	2 × 10-12 (-1) each side
Middle delts: lengthened to midrange	4b. Cable side shoulder raise	75	2 × 10-12 (-3) each side	2 × 10-12 (-3) each side	2 × 10-12 (-2) each side	2 × 10-12 (-2) each side	2 × 10-12 (-1) each side	2 × 10-12 (-1) each side

(-1) indicates to stop the set 1 rep before muscle failure. (-2) indicates to stop the set 2 reps before muscle failure. (-3) indicates to stop the set 3 reps before muscle failure. And (-4) indicates to stop the set 4 reps before muscle failure.

*As mentioned in chapter 11, due to their multijoint nature, all exercises such as squats, Romanian deadlifts, lunges, and many variations of those exercises provided in chapters 9 and 10 also load your glutes when they're closer to a lengthened (stretched) range.

**Use body weight or hold dumbbell depending on your strength level.

TABLE 14.4 Beginner Workout Program Phase 3: Day A

Strength zone	Exercise name	Page number	Workout 1 (sets × reps)	Workout 2 (sets × reps)	Workout 3 (sets × reps)	Workout 4 (sets × reps)	Workout 5 (sets × reps)	Workout 6 (sets × reps)
Lats: vertical or diagonal pulling with arms outside in the lengthened-to-midrange	1a. Assisted pull-up	48	3 × 12-15 (-2)	3 × 12-15 (-2)	3 × 12-15 (-1)	3 × 12-15 (-1)	3 × 12-15	3 × 12-15
**Quads and glutes: knee bending for the lengthened to midrange	1b. Dumbbell traveling lunge*	139	3 × 8-10 (-2) each side	3 × 8-10 (-2) each side	3 × 8-10 (-1) each side	3 × 8-10 (-1) each side	3 × 8-10 each side	3 × 8-10 each side
Chest: horizontal or decline pressing for the lengthened to midrange	2a. Machine chest press	28	3 × 10-12 (-2)	3 × 10-12 (-2)	3 × 10-12 (-1)	3 × 10-12 (-1)	3 × 10-12	3 × 10-12
Glutes: hip extension for the shortened to midrange	2b. Weight plate one-leg hip lift	166	3 × 12-15 (-2) each side	3 × 12-15 (-2) each side	3 × 12-15 (-1) each side	3 × 12-15 (-1) each side	3 × 12-15 each side	3 × 12-15 each side
Quads: knee extension for the shortened to midrange	3a. Machine leg extension	147	3 × 10-12 (-2)	3 × 10-12 (-2)	3 × 10-12 (-1)	3 × 10-12 (-1)	3 × 10-12	3 × 10-12
Biceps: shortened to midrange	3b. Dumbbell standing biceps curl	103	3 × 12-15 (-2)	3 × 12-15 (-2)	3 × 12-15 (-1)	3 × 12-15 (-1)	3 × 12-15	3 × 12-15
Core: linear	3c. Arm walkout	194	3 × 4-5	3 × 4-5	3 × 6-7	3 × 6-7	3 × 8-10	3 × 8-10
Core: rotational	4a. Cable same-side one-arm press	214	3 × 12-15 (-2) each side	3 × 12-15 (-2) each side	3 × 12-15 (-1) each side	3 × 12-15 (-1) each side	3 × 12-15 each side	3 × 12-15 each side
Middle delts: lengthened to midrange	4b. Cable side shoulder raise	75	3 × 12-15 (-2) each side	3 × 12-15 (-2) each side	3 × 12-15 (-1) each side	3 × 12-15 (-1) each side	3 × 12-15 each side	3 × 12-15 each side
Hip adduction	4c. Side-lying hip adduction	174	3 × 12-14 each side	3 × 12-14 each side	3 × 15-18 each side	3 × 15-18 each side	3 × 20 each side	3 × 20 each side

(-1) indicates to stop the set 1 rep before muscle failure. (-2) indicates to stop the set 2 reps before muscle failure. (-3) indicates to stop the set 3 reps before muscle failure. And (-4) indicates to stop the set 4 reps before muscle failure.

*Use body weight or hold dumbbell depending on your strength level.

**As mentioned in chapter 11, due to their multijoint nature, all exercises such as squats, Romanian deadlifts, lunges, and many variations of those exercises provided in chapters 9 and 10 also load your glutes when they're closer to a lengthened (stretched) range.

TABLE 14.5   Beginner Workout Program Phase 3: Day B

Strength zone	Exercise name	Page number	Workout 1 (sets × reps)	Workout 2 (sets × reps)	Workout 3 (sets × reps)	Workout 4 (sets × reps)	Workout 5 (sets × reps)	Workout 6 (sets × reps)
Hamstrings: hip hinging for the lengthened to midrange **(Glutes: lengthened to midrange)	1a. Dumbbell Romanian deadlift	121	3 × 10-12 (-2)	3 × 10-12 (-2)	3 × 10-12 (-1)	3 × 10-12 (-1)	3 × 10-12	3 × 10-12
Middle delts: shortened to midrange	1b. Kettlebell shoulder-to-shoulder press	73	3 × 10 each side	3 × 10 each side	3 × 12 each side	3 × 12 each side	3 × 13-15 each side	3 × 13-15 each side
Lats: horizontal pulling for the shortened to midrange	2a. Cable one-arm row	62	3 × 12-15 (-2) each side	3 × 12-15 (-2) each side	3 × 12-15 (-1) each side	3 × 12-15 (-1) each side	3 × 12-15 each side	3 × 12-15 each side
*Quads and glutes: knee bending for the lengthened to midrange	2b. Dumbbell step-up*	139	3 × 10-12 (-2) each side	3 × 10-12 (-2) each side	3 × 10-12 (-1) each side	3 × 10-12 (-1) each side	3 × 10-12 each side	3 × 10-12 each side
Hamstrings: knee flexion for the shortened to midrange	3a. Machine lying leg curl	127	3 × 12-15 (-2)	3 × 12-15 (-2)	3 × 12-15 (-1)	3 × 12-15 (-1)	3 × 12-15	3 × 12-15
Triceps: lengthened to midrange	3b. Dumbbell behind-the-head triceps extension	110	3 × 10-12 (-2)	3 × 10-12 (-2)	3 × 10-12 (-1)	3 × 10-12 (-1)	3 × 10-12	3 × 10-12
Core: rotational	3c. One-arm plank	207	3 × 10 sec each side	3 × 10 sec each side	3 × 12 sec each side	3 × 12 sec each side	3 × 15 sec each side	3 × 15 sec each side
Core: linear	4a. Reverse crunch	198	3 × 10-12 (-2)	3 × 10-12 (-2)	3 × 10-12 (-1)	3 × 10-12 (-1)	3 × 10-12	3 × 10-12
Rear delts: lengthened to midrange	4b. Dumbbell side-lying rear-delt fly	81	3 × 10-12 (-2) each side	3 × 10-12 (-2) each side	3 × 10-12 (-1) each side	3 × 10-12 (-1) each side	3 × 10-12 each side	3 × 10-12 each side
Hip abduction	4c. Weight plate side-lying hip abduction	171	3 × 12-14 each side	3 × 12-14 each side	3 × 15-18 each side	3 × 15-18 each side	3 × 20 each side	3 × 20 each side

(-1) indicates to stop the set 1 rep before muscle failure. (-2) indicates to stop the set 2 reps before muscle failure. (-3) indicates to stop the set 3 reps before muscle failure. And (-4) indicates to stop the set 4 reps before muscle failure.

*Use body weight or hold dumbbell depending on your strength level.

**As mentioned in chapter 11, due to their multijoint nature, all exercises such as squats, Romanian deadlifts, lunges, and many variations of those exercises provided in chapters 9 and 10 also load your glutes when they're closer to a lengthened (stretched) range.

CHAPTER 15

Programs for Two or Three Workouts per Week

The workout programs in this chapter are designed for people who want to workout two or three times per week. Three times per week is preferred over twice per week if your schedule allows. If you're dedicated to strength training more frequently than that, you may be interested in trying the workout programs in chapters 16 and 17.

Program Guidelines

The following is a list of key points to remember and follow in order to strength train smart and get the most of out the workout programs in this chapter.

Rest

- Perform the exercises designated with *a* or *b* as paired sets, and perform exercises with *a*, *b*, and *c* as tri-sets. Perform all reps in each set before moving to the next set. Completing 1 round of the exercises in a paired or tri-set is considered 1 set.
- Rest 30 seconds between exercises in a given paired set and tri-set.
- Rest 1 to 2 minutes between each round of a given paired set and tri-set.

Reps

- The rep range (e.g., 10-15 reps) is next to each exercise in the workout. If you're using the same weight for each set, you may be able to do 15 reps on the first set, 12 reps on the next set, and 10 reps on the third set because of accumulated fatigue. Or you can reduce the weight you're using with each consecutive set to achieve the higher end or given rep range on each consecutive set. Both methods are effective at helping you to progress.
- Maintain strict form without cheating by using additional movements or momentum.
- Mentally focus on the working muscles in each exercise.

- Do the concentric (lifting) portion of each rep at a normal tempo and maintain strict control during the eccentric (lowering) portion. Take roughly 3 seconds on the eccentric portion of each rep.

Weight
- Use a weight load that's light enough to allow you to achieve the minimum number of reps indicated for each exercise.
- Use a weight load heavy enough that you're unable to perform any more reps than the maximum number indicated for each exercise while maintaining proper control and technique.

Work Around—Not Through—Injuries and Limitations
- If an exercise causes pain or discomfort beyond the sensation associated with muscle fatigue, use an alternative exercise that doesn't hurt and targets the same muscle group in the same strength zone.
- Not every exercise movement is for everybody. There are plenty of movements in the exercise chapters of this book to choose from.

Program Setup

The following programs consist of two total-body workouts: workout A and workout B (see tables 15.1.-15.10). This section has five programs with two different total-body workouts each. You'll alternate between workout A and workout B on each program. You'll train two or three days per week, allowing at least one rest day between workouts to maximize recovery and minimize the risk of overtraining. The sample weekly workout schedules show how a weekly setup could be used for working out two or three times per week.

Each time you complete day A and day B, it equals one time through the workouts. You'll perform each of the two total-body workouts for seven times through each workout before switching to the next program and repeating those workouts for another seven times. So, if you're training twice per week, it will take you seven weeks to complete each program.

Weekly Workout Schedule for Two or Three Times per Week

Following are weekly training schedule options for training two or three times per week.

Schedule or Training Twice per Week
Sample Option 1
Monday: Day A—total-body workout
Tuesday: Rest
Wednesday: Rest
Thursday: Day B—total-body workout
Friday: Rest
Saturday: Rest
Sunday: Rest

Sample Option 2

Monday: Rest

Tuesday: Day A—total-body workout

Wednesday: Rest

Thursday: Rest

Friday: Day B—total-body workout

Saturday: Rest

Sunday: Rest

You can change the days of the week that you perform each workout to better fit your schedule. Just make sure to alternate total-body workout A and total-body workout B. And to maximize your recovery, allow at least one rest day between workouts.

Schedule or Training Three Time per Week

Sample Option 1

`WEEK 1`

Monday: Day A—total-body workout 1

Tuesday: Rest

Wednesday: Day B—total-body workout 1

Thursday: Rest

Friday: Day A—total-body workout 2

Saturday: Rest

Sunday: Rest

`WEEK 2`

Monday: Day B—total-body workout 2

Tuesday: Rest

Wednesday: Day A—total-body workout 3

Thursday: Rest

Friday: Day B—total-body workout 3

Saturday: Rest

Sunday: Rest

Continue the sequence on week 3, starting with Day A—total-body workout 4 on Monday and so on.

Sample Option 2

`WEEK 1`

Monday: Day A—total-body workout 1

Tuesday: Rest

Wednesday: Rest

Thursday: Day B—total-body workout 1

Friday: Rest

Saturday: Day A—total-body workout 2

Sunday: Rest

WEEK 2

Monday: Day B—total-body workout 2

Tuesday: Rest

Wednesday: Rest

Thursday: Day A—total-body workout 3

Friday: Rest

Saturday: Day B—total-body workout 3

Sunday: Rest

Continue the sequence on week 3, starting with Day A—total-body workout 4 on Monday and so on.

Sample Option 3

WEEK 1

Monday: Day A—total-body workout 1

Tuesday: Rest

Wednesday: Day B—total-body workout 1

Thursday: Rest

Friday: Rest

Saturday: Day A—total-body workout 2

Sunday: Rest

WEEK 2

Monday: Day B—total-body workout 2

Tuesday: Rest

Wednesday: Day A—total-body workout 3

Thursday: Rest

Friday: Rest

Saturday: Day B—total-body workout 3

Sunday: Rest

Continue the sequence on week 3, starting with Day A—total-body workout 4 on Monday and so on.

You can change the days of the week that you perform each workout to better fit your schedule. Just make sure to alternate total-body workout A and total-body workout B. And to maximize your recovery, allow at least one rest day between workouts.

Rest Days

Non-strength-training days, which are indicated as rest days in the sample weekly training schedules, don't mean you have to do nothing. During your days off from using the strength zone training workouts, you can do low-impact activities, such as going for long walks, hikes, bike rides, or swims. Yoga can also be a great option for your active rest days.

Reload Workouts

The first time you do each workout in a program, it's considered a reload workout. A reload workout is simply a lower-intensity version of the workout, which helps you to stay active while recovering between programs. It also acclimates you to the movements and gives you an idea of the appropriate weight loads (based on your strength level) you'll use for the new program you're starting.

Mixed Sets and Reps for Maximal Results

The training system and workout programs provided in this book enable you to incorporate the right blend of exercises to achieve strength through the true full range of motion. They also include a full spectrum of set and repetition ranges. This variety is the reason they can be so effective in helping you get stronger.

Research has shown that daily variations in intensity and volume (sets and reps) are more effective than weekly volume variations for increases in maximal strength; they may also lead to greater gains in muscle size (1, 2, 3, 4). In short, it's best to think about the types of strength training exercises—and the sets and reps you use—in the same way that you think about your nutrition: Make sure to get enough variety, because each type offers unique training or nutritional value.

Warm Up and Build Up

Before you begin a workout from one of the following programs, be sure to perform a general warm-up. Also make sure to perform some build-up sets, which are simply lighter, less intense versions of whatever exercises you're getting ready to perform with heavier loads. Build-up sets are used to gradually build up to your working intensity. For example, if you're going to perform a heavy lift, you first do a few lighter sets of that lift in order to build up to your working weight. As a rule of thumb, if the workout program calls for 4 sets of an exercises, you'll do 2 build-up sets. If the workout program calls for 3 sets of a given exercise, you'll perform 1 build-up set because it involves using lighter loads than when you're performing 4 sets of fewer reps. And because the times you'll be performing only 2 sets of a given exercise involve using lighter loads (because of the higher reps), there's no need to perform a build-up set to get into your working weight.

Why No Exercises for Front Delts?

In each of the following programs, even though there is no strength zone exercise category listed for the front delts, there are multiple exercises included to strengthen your front delts through the true full range of motion.

As mentioned in chapter 3, the front delts are worked during decline, horizontal, and diagonal pressing exercises. More specifically, these pressing exercises strengthen your front delts in the lengthened-to-midrange strength zone. While many of the exercises in chapter 5 are for the shortened-to-midrange strength zone for your middle delts, they also strengthen your front delts in the shortened-to-midrange strength zone.

TABLE 15.1   Program 1, Total-Body Workout Day A

Strength zone	Exercise name	Page number	Workout 1: reload (sets × reps or time)	Workouts 2 and 5 (sets × reps or time)	Workouts 3 and 6 (sets × reps or time)	Workouts 4 and 7 (sets × reps or time)
*Glutes and hamstrings: hip hinging for the lengthened to midrange	1a. Barbell elevated Romanian deadlift	120	2 × 10-12	4 × 5-8	2 × 20-25	3 × 10-15
Core: linear	1b. Stability ball plate crunch	196	2 × 8-10	4 × 6-8 (pause 2 sec at the top of each rep)	2 × 20-25	3 × 12-15
Glutes: hip extension for the shortened to midrange	2a. Cable one-leg Romanian deadlift	163	2 × 8-12 each side	4 × 6-8 each side	2 × 20 each side	3 × 12-15 each side
Core: rotational	2b. Cable three-point high-to-low chop	210	2 × 6 in each position, each side	4 × 6-8 in each position, each side	2 × 15 in each position, each side	3 × 10-12 in each position, each side
Lats: vertical or diagonal pulling with arms inside for the lengthened to midrange	3a. Chin-up (assisted if needed with band or machine)	53	2 × 6-8	3 × 10-15	4 × 5-8	2 × 20-30
Chest: incline pressing for the lengthened to midrange	3b. Angled-barbell one-arm press	36	2 × 10-12 each side	3 × 10-12 each side	4 × 6-8 each side	2 × 15-20 each side
Chest: horizontal or diagonal shoulder adduction for the shortened to midrange	4a. Cable crossover pec fly	41	2 × 10-12	3 × 12-15	4 × 10-12	2 × 20-25
Traps: scapular retraction	4b. Cable one-arm horizontal shrug	93	2 × 10-12 each side	3 × 10-15 each side	4 × 6-8 each side	2 × 20-25 each side
Hips: adduction	4c. Side-lying hip adduction leg scissors	173	2 × 10 each side	3 × 12-15 (1 sec hold at top each rep) each side	4 × 6-8 (3 sec hold at top each rep) each side	2 × 20-25 each side
Middle delts: lengthened to midrange	5a. Cable side shoulder raise	75	2 × 10-12 each side	2 × 20-25 each side	3 × 12-15 each side	4 × 6-8 each side
Biceps: lengthened to midrange	5b. Cable one-arm face-away biceps curl	99	2 × 10-12 each side	2 × 20-25 each side	3 × 12-15 each side	4 × 6-8 each side
Calf: straight knee	5c. Dumbbell traveling calf raise	180	2 × 20 sec	4 × 30 sec	4 × 30 sec	2 × 50 sec

Strength zone	Exercise name	Page number	Workout 1: reload (sets × reps or time)	Workouts 2 and 5 (sets × reps or time)	Workouts 3 and 6 (sets × reps or time)	Workouts 4 and 7 (sets × reps or time)
Triceps: shortened to midrange	6a. Dumbbell triceps skull crusher	112	2 × 10-12	2 × 20-25	3 × 12-15	4 × 6-8
Rear delts: length-ened to midrange	6b. Dumbbell side-lying rear-delt fly	81	2 × 10-12 each side	2 × 20-25 each side	3 × 12-15 each side	4 × 6-8 each side
Core: lateral	6c. Dumbbell unilateral farmers walk	201	2 × 20 sec each side	2 × 50 sec each side	3 × 40 sec each side	4 × 30 sec each side

Rest 30 seconds between exercises and 1 to 2 minutes between paired sets or tri-sets.

*As mentioned in chapter 11, due to their multijoint nature, all exercises such as squats, Romanian deadlifts, lunges, and many variations of those exercises provided in chapters 9 and 10 also load your glutes when they're closer to a lengthened (stretched) range.

TABLE 15.2 Program 1, Total-Body Workout Day B

Strength zone	Exercise name	Page number	Workout 1: reload (sets × reps or time)	Workouts 2 and 5 (sets × reps or time)	Workouts 3 and 6 (sets × reps or time)	Workouts 4 and 7 (sets × reps or time)
*Quads and glutes: knee bending for the lengthened to midrange	1a. Dumbbell traveling lunge	139	2 × 8-10 each side	3 × 12-15 each side	4 × 5-8 each side	2 × 20-25 each side
Core: rotational	1b. Cable tight rotation with hip shift	208	2 × 12 each side	3 × 12 each side	4 × 8 each side	2 × 20 each side
Chest: horizontal or decline pressing for the lengthened to midrange	2a. Machine chest press	28	2 × 10-12	3 × 10-15	4 × 6-8	2 × 20-25
Lats: horizontal pull-ing for the short-ened to midrange	2b. Dumbbell two-arm bent-over row	60	2 × 10-12	3 × 12-15	4 × 8-10	2 × 20-25
Lats: vertical or diagonal pulling with arms outside for the lengthened to midrange	3a. Cable one-arm half-kneel-ing lat pull-down	50	2 × 10-12 each side	2 × 20-25 each side	3 × 10-15 each side	4 × 6-8 each side
Traps: scapular ele-vation	3b. Cable one-arm shrug	90	2 × 10-12 each side	2 × 20-25 each side	3 × 10-15 each side	4 × 6-8 each side
Quads: knee exten-sion for the short-ened to midrange	4a. Machine leg extension	147	2 × 10-12	2 × 20-25	3 × 12-15	4 × 6-8
Calves: bent-knee	4b. Dumbbell half-kneeling calf raise	183	2 × 20 each side	2 × 30 each side	3 × 20 each side	4 × 12-15 each side

> *continued*

Table 15.2 > *continued*

Strength zone	Exercise name	Page number	Workout 1: reload (sets × reps or time)	Workouts 2 and 5 (sets × reps or time)	Workouts 3 and 6 (sets × reps or time)	Workouts 4 and 7 (sets × reps or time)
Biceps: shortened to midrange	4c. Dumbbell biceps curl	103	2 × 10-12	2 × 20-25	3 × 12-15	4 × 6-8
Hamstrings: knee flexion for the shortened to midrange	5a. Machine seated leg curl	125	2 × 10-12	2 × 20-30	3 × 10-15	4 × 6-8
Core: lateral	5b. Medicine ball side lean	203	2 × 8-10 each side	2 × 20 each side	3 × 12-15 each side	4 × 8-10 each side
Hips: abduction	6a. Machine seated hip abduction	169	2 × 10-12	4 × 6-8	2 × 20-30	3 × 10-15
Core: linear	6b. Core exercise indicated	192	Stability ball rollout 2 × 10-12	Ab wheel rollout 4 × 6-8	Stability ball rollout 2 × 20	Arm walkout 3 × 8-10
Triceps: shortened to midrange	7a. Cable rope overhead triceps extension	108	2 × 10-12	4 × 6-8	2 × 20-25	3 × 12-15
Middle and rear delts: shortened to midrange	7b. Barbell 45-degree row	71	2 × 10-12	4 × 8-10	2 × 20-25	3 × 12-15

Rest 30 seconds between exercises and 1 to 2 minutes between paired sets or tri-sets.

*As mentioned in chapter 11, due to their multijoint nature, all exercises such as squats, Romanian deadlifts, lunges, and many variations of those exercises provided in chapters 9 and 10 also load your glutes when they're closer to a lengthened (stretched) range.

TABLE 15.3 Program 2, Total-Body Workout Day A

Strength zone	Exercise name	Page number	Workout 1: reload (sets × reps or time)	Workouts 2 and 5 (sets × reps or time)	Workouts 3 and 6 (sets × reps or time)	Workouts 4 and 7 (sets × reps or time)
*Glutes and hamstrings: hip hinging for the lengthened to midrange	1a. Dumbbell traveling Romanian deadlift lunge	122	2 × 10-12 each side	4 × 5-8 each side	2 × 17-20 each side	3 × 10-15 each side
Core: linear	1b. Band leg lowering	192	2 × 8-10	4 × 6-8	2 × 15-20	3 × 10-12
Chest: incline pressing for the lengthened to midrange	2a. Dumbbell incline bench press	34	2 × 10-12	4 × 5-8	2 × 20-25	3 × 10-15
Lats: horizontal pulling for the shortened to midrange	2b. One-arm anti-rotation suspension row	66	2 × 8-10 each side	4 × 6-8 each side	2 × 15-20 each side	3 × 10-12 each side

Strength zone	Exercise name	Page number	Workout 1: reload (sets × reps or time)	Workouts 2 and 5 (sets × reps or time)	Workouts 3 and 6 (sets × reps or time)	Workouts 4 and 7 (sets × reps or time)
Core: lateral	2c. Cable one-arm side bend	204	2 × 10 each side	4 × 8-10 each side	2 × 20 each side	3 × 15 each side
Quads: knee extension for the shortened to midrange	3a. Reverse sled drag	148	2 × 40 yards (36 m)	3 × 60-70 yards (55-64 m)	4 × 40 yards (36 m)	2 × 100 yards (91 m)
Calves: straight knee	3b. Dumbbell one-leg leaning calf raise	180	2 × 12-15 each side	3 × 12-15 each side	4 × 8-10 each side	2 × 25-30 each side
Middle delts: shortened to midrange	3c. Kettlebell shoulder-to-shoulder press	73	2 × 5-6 each side	3 × 10-12 each side	4 × 6-8 each side	2 × 16-20 each side
Chest: horizontal or diagonal shoulder adduction for the shortened to midrange	4a. Machine one-arm rotated chest press	40	2 × 10-12 each side	3 × 12-15 each side	4 × 8-10 each side	2 × 20-25 each side
Traps: scapular retraction	4b. Dumbbell off-bench one-arm horizontal shrug	92	2 × 10-12 each side	3 × 12-15 each side	4 × 8-10 each side	2 × 20-25 each side
Hips: abduction	4c. Band lateral hip shuffle	170	2 × 10 each side	3 × 12-15 each side	4 × 8-10 each side	2 × 20-25 each side
Biceps: lengthened to midrange	5a. EZ-bar preacher curl	100	2 × 10-12	2 × 20-25	3 × 12-15	4 × 6-8
Triceps: lengthened to midrange	5b. Kettlebell behind-the-head triceps extension	109	2 × 10-12	2 × 20-25	3 × 12-15	4 × 6-8
Middle delts: lengthened to midrange	5c. Dumbbell side-lying side shoulder raise	76	2 × 10-12 each side	2 × 20-25 each side	3 × 12-15 each side	4 × 6-8 each side
Core: rotational	6a. Cable three-point low-to-high chop	212	2 × 6 in each position, each side	2 × 15 in each position, each side	3 × 10-12 in each position, each side	4 × 6-8 in each position, each side
Calves: bent knee	6b. Machine seated calf raise	185	2 × 15	2 × 25-30	3 × 12-15	4 × 6-8

Rest 30 seconds between exercises and 1 to 2 minutes between paired sets or tri-sets.

*As mentioned in chapter 11, due to their multijoint nature, all exercises such as squats, Romanian deadlifts, lunges, step-ups, and many variations of those exercises provided in chapters 9 and 10 also load your glutes when they're closer to a lengthened (stretched) range.

TABLE 15.4   Program 2, Total-Body Workout Day B

Strength zone	Exercise name	Page number	Workout 1: reload (sets × reps or time)	Workouts 2 and 5 (sets × reps or time)	Workouts 3 and 6 (sets × reps or time)	Workouts 4 and 7 (sets × reps or time)
*Quads and glutes: knee bending for the lengthened to midrange	1a. Trap bar squat	136	2 × 8-10	3 × 12-15	4 × 5-8	2 × 20-25
Core: linear	1b. Core exercise indicated	192	Reverse crunch 2 × 8-10	Reverse crunch 3 × 10-15	Incline bench reverse crunch 4 × 6-8	Stability ball knee tuck 2 × 20-30
Chest: horizontal or decline pressing for the lengthened to midrange	2a. Push-up exercise indicated	26	Push-up 2 × 10-15	Box crossover push-up 3 × max reps	NT Loop resisted push-up 4 × max reps	Push-up 2 × max reps
Lats: vertical or diagonal pulling with arms outside for the lengthened to midrange	2b. Overhand-grip lat pull-down	49	2 × 10-12	3 × 10-15	4 × 6-8	2 × 20-25
Lats: vertical or diagonal pulling with arms inside for the lengthened to midrange	3a. Band one-arm neutral-grip lat pull-down	59	2 × 10-12 each side	2 × 20-25 each side	3 × 12-15 each side	4 × 5-8 each side
Traps: scapular elevation	3b. Dumbbell one-arm leaning shrug	90	2 × 10-12 each side	2 × 20-25 each side	3 × 12-15 each side	4 × 8-10 each side
Glutes: hip extension for the shortened to midrange	4a. 45-degree hip extension	166	2 × 8-12	2 × 20-25	3 × 12-15	4 × 6-10
Core: lateral	4b. Angled-barbell tight rainbow	201	2 × 15 sec	2 × 30 sec	3 × 20 sec	4 × 15 sec
Hamstrings: knee flexion for the shortened to midrange	5a. Machine lying one-leg curl	127	2 × 10-12 each side	2 × 20-30 each side	3 × 10-15 each side	4 × 6-8 each side
Core: rotational	5b. Weight plate chop	215	2 × 10-12 each side	2 × 20 each side	3 × 10-15 each side	4 × 6-8 each side
Hips: adduction	6a. Bent-knee Copenhagen hip adduction	174	2 × 8-10 each side	4 × 5-8 each side (pause 3 sec at top of each rep)	2 × 15 each side	3 × 10-12 each side (pause 2 sec at top of each rep)
Triceps: shortened to midrange	6b. Cable rope triceps extension	114	2 × 10-12	4 × 6-8	2 × 20-25	3 × 12-15

Strength zone	Exercise name	Page number	Workout 1: reload (sets × reps or time)	Workouts 2 and 5 (sets × reps or time)	Workouts 3 and 6 (sets × reps or time)	Workouts 4 and 7 (sets × reps or time)
Rear delts: shortened to midrange	6c. Cable rope face pull	79	2 × 10-12	4 × 6-8	2 × 20-25	3 × 12-15
Biceps: shortened to midrange	7a. Cable EZ-bar biceps curl	105	2 × 10-12	4 × 6-8	2 × 20-25	3 × 12-15
Rear delts: lengthened to midrange	7b. Cable one-arm rear-delt fly	82	2 × 10-12 each side	4 × 6-8 each side	2 × 20-25 each side	3 × 12-15 each side

Rest 30 seconds between exercises and 1 to 2 minutes between paired sets or tri-sets.

*As mentioned in chapter 11, due to their multijoint nature, all exercises such as squats, Romanian deadlifts, lunges, step-ups and many variations of those exercises provided in chapters 9 and 10 also load your glutes when they're closer to a lengthened (stretched) range.

TABLE 15.5   Program 3, Total-Body Workout Day A

Strength zone	Exercise name	Page number	Workout 1: reload (sets × reps or time)	Workouts 2 and 5 (sets × reps or time)	Workouts 3 and 6 (sets × reps or time)	Workouts 4 and 7 (sets × reps or time)
*Glutes and hamstrings: hip hinging for the lengthened to midrange	1a. Angled-barbell leaning Romanian deadlift	124	2 × 10-12	4 × 6-8	2 × 17-20	3 × 10-15
Core: linear	1b. Stability ball arc	193	2 × 8-10 each side	4 × 6-8 each side	2 × 14-15 each side	3 × 10-12 each side
Chest: horizontal or decline pressing for the lengthened to midrange	2a. Dumbbell bench press	26	2 × 10-12	4 × 5-8	2 × 20-25	3 × 10-15
Lats: horizontal pulling for the shortened to midrange	2b. Dumbbell one-arm bench row	61	2 × 10-12 each side	4 × 6-8 each side	2 × 20-25 each side	3 × 10-12 each side
Quads: knee extension for the shortened to midrange	3a. Machine unilateral leg extension	148	2 × 10-12 each side	4 × 6-8 each side	2 × 20-25 each side	3 × 12-15 each side
Core: rotational	3b. Dumbbell plank row	207	2 × 8 each side	4 × 6-8 each side	2 × 12-15 each side	3 × 8-10 each side
Chest: horizontal or diagonal shoulder adduction for the shortened to midrange	4a. Machine pec fly	43	2 × 10-12	3 × 12-15	4 × 8-10	2 × 20-25
Traps: scapular retraction	4b. Dumbbell bent-over horizontal shrug	91	2 × 10-12	3 × 15	4 × 10	2 × 25
Hamstrings: knee flexion for the shortened to midrange	4c. Hamstring exercise indicated	125	Stability ball leg curl 2 × 10-15	Stability ball one-leg curl 3 × 12-20 each side	Nordic hamstring curl 4 × 4-8	Stability ball leg curl 2 × 25-30

> continued

Table 15.5   > *continued*

Strength zone	Exercise name	Page number	Workout 1: reload (sets × reps or time)	Workouts 2 and 5 (sets × reps or time)	Workouts 3 and 6 (sets × reps or time)	Workouts 4 and 7 (sets × reps or time)
Triceps: lengthened to midrange	5a. Cable rope overhead triceps extension	108	2 × 10-12	3 × 12-15	4 × 6-8	2 × 20-25
Middle delts: lengthened to midrange	5b. NT Loop side shoulder raise	77	2 × 10-12 each side	3 × 12-15 each side	4 × 6-8 each side	2 × 20-25 each side
Core: lateral	5c. Stability ball side crunch	205	2 × 10 each side	3 × 12-15 each side	4 × 6-10	2 × 20-30
Biceps: lengthened to midrange	6a. Cable one-arm face-away biceps curl	99	2 × 10-12 each side	2 × 20 each side	3 × 12-15 each side	4 × 6-8 each side
Rear delts: lengthened to midrange	6b. Low-cable rear-delt fly	82	2 × 10-12 each side	2 × 20 each side	3 × 12-15 each side	4 × 6-8 each side
Hips: abduction	7a. Machine seated hip abduction	169	2 × 10-12	2 × 20-25	3 × 10-15	4 × 6-8
Calves: bent knee	7b. Dumbbell half-kneeling calf raise	183	2 × 10-12 each side	2 × 25-30 each side	3 × 15-20 each side	4 × 8-12 each side

Rest 30 seconds between exercises and 1 to 2 minutes between paired sets or tri-sets.

*As mentioned in chapter 11; due to their multijoint nature, all exercises such as squats, Romanian deadlifts, lunges, step-ups and many variations of those exercises provided in chapters 9 and 10 also load your glutes when they're closer to a lengthened (stretched) range.

TABLE 15.6   Program 3, Total-Body Workout Day B

Strength zone	Exercise name	Page number	Workout 1: reload (sets × reps or time)	Workouts 2 and 5 (sets × reps or time)	Workouts 3 and 6 (sets × reps or time)	Workouts 4 and 7 (sets × reps or time)
*Quads and glutes: knee bending for the lengthened to midrange	1a. Dumbbell step-up	139	2 × 8-10 each side	3 × 12-15 each side	4 × 5-8 each side	2 × 20 each side
Core: lateral	1b. Bench lateral hold	203	2 × 12-15 sec each side	3 × 25-30 sec each side	4 × 15-20 sec each side	2 × 35-40 sec each side
Glutes: hip extension for the shortened to midrange	2a. Weight plate one-leg hip lift	166	2 × 10-12 each side	3 × 12-15 each side	4 × 8-10 each side	2 × 25-30 each side
Hips: adduction	2b. NT Loop quadruped hip adduction	176	2 × 10-12 each side	3 × 12-15 each side	4 × 8-10 each side	2 × 20-25 each side

Strength zone	Exercise name	Page number	Workout 1: reload (sets × reps or time)	Workouts 2 and 5 (sets × reps or time)	Workouts 3 and 6 (sets × reps or time)	Workouts 4 and 7 (sets × reps or time)
Chest: incline pressing for the lengthened to midrange	3a. Angled-barbell shoulder-to-shoulder press	35	2 × 10 each side	3 × 12-15 each side	4 × 6-8 each side	2 × 20 each side
Lats: vertical or diagonal pulling with arms outside for the lengthened to midrange	3b. Cable fighters lat pulldown	51	2 × 10-12 each side	3 × 12-15 each side	4 × 8-10 each side	2 × 20-25 each side
Lats: vertical or diagonal pulling with arms inside for the lengthened to midrange	4a. Cable straight-arm compound pull-down	57	2 × 10-12	2 × 20-25	3 × 12-15	4 × 8-10
Traps: scapular elevation	4b. Cable wide-grip angled upright row	88	2 × 10-12	2 × 30	3 × 15-20	4 × 10-12
Calves: straight knee	5a. Machine ankles-together calf raise	182	2 × 15	2 × 25-30	3 × 12-15	4 × 8-10
Core: linear	5b. Band leg lowering	192	2 × 20-30 sec	2 × 50 sec	3 × 40 sec	4 × 40 sec
Core: rotational	6a. Cable three-point horizontal chop	209	2 × 6-8 each position, each side	4 × 6-8 each position, each side	2 × 12-15 each position, each side	3 × 10 each position, each side
Triceps: shortened to midrange	6b. Suspension trainer skull crusher	114	2 × 10-12	4 × 8-10	2 × 20-25	3 × 15
Rear delts: shortened to midrange	6c. Suspension trainer wide-grip row	80	2 × 10-12	4 × 8-10	2 × 20-25	3 × 15
Middle delts: shortened to midrange	7a. Machine overhead press	75	2 × 10-12	4 × 6-8	2 × 20-25	3 × 10-15
Biceps: shortened to midrange	7b. EZ-bar biceps curl	102	2 × 10-12	4 × 6-8	2 × 20-25	3 × 10-15

Rest 30 seconds between exercises and 1 to 2 minutes between paired sets or tri-sets.

*As mentioned in chapter 11; due to their multijoint nature, all exercises such as squats, Romanian deadlifts, lunges, step-ups and many variations of those exercises provided in chapters 9 and 10 also load your glutes when they're closer to a lengthened (stretched) range.

TABLE 15.7 Program 4, Total-Body Workout Day A

Strength zone	Exercise name	Page number	Workout 1: Reload (sets × reps or time)	Workouts 2 and 5 (sets × reps or time)	Workouts 3 and 6 (sets × reps or time)	Workouts 4 and 7 (sets × reps or time)
*Glutes and hamstrings: hip hinging for the lengthened to midrange	1a. Dumbbell one-leg one-arm Romanian deadlift	123	2 × 10-12 each side	4 × 6-8 each side	2 × 20 each side	3 × 12-15 each side
Core: linear	1b. Suspension trainer arm fallout	195	2 × 8-10	4 × 6-8	2 × 20	3 × 12-15
Lats: horizontal pulling for the shortened to midrange	2a. Machine row	64	2 × 10-12	4 × 5-8	2 × 20-25	3 × 10-15
Traps: scapular retraction	2b. Machine row horizontal shrug	65	2 × 10-12	4 × 5-8	2 × 20-25	3 × 10-15
Chest: horizontal or decline pressing for the lengthened to midrange	2c. Push-up exercise indicated	26	Push-up 2 × 12-15	Lock-off push-up 4 × 6-8 each side	Push-up 2 × max reps	Box crossover push-up 3 × max reps
Lats: vertical or diagonal pulling with arms outside for the lengthened to midrange	3a. Cable one-arm half-kneeling lat pull-down	50	2 × 10-12 each side	3 × 10-15 each side	4 × 6-8 each side	2 × 20 each side
Chest: horizontal or diagonal shoulder adduction for the shortened to midrange	3b. Cable one-arm diagonal pec fly	39	2 × 10-12 each side	3 × 10-15 each side	4 × 6-8 each side	2 × 20 each side
Hamstrings: knee flexion for the shortened to midrange	4a. Machine seated one-leg curl	126	2 × 8-10 each side	3 × 10-15 each side	4 × 6-8 each side	2 × 20-25 each side
Core: rotational	4b. Cross-body plank	208	2 × 15 sec	3 × 30 sec	4 × 20 sec	2 × 40 sec
Rear delts: shortened to midrange	4c. Dumbbell rear-delt fly	78	2 × 10-12	3 × 12-15	4 × 8-10	2 × 20-25
Biceps: lengthened to midrange	5a. EZ-bar preacher curl	100	2 × 10-12	2 × 20-25	3 × 10-15	4 × 6-8
Glutes: hip extension for the shortened to midrange	5b. NT Loop glute walk	168	2 × 30 sec	2 × 50 sec	3 × 40 sec	4 × 30 sec
Hips adduction	5c. Hip adduction exercise indicated	173	Side-lying hip adduction 2 × 8 each side	Side-lying hip adduction 2 × 20-25 each side	Side-lying hip adduction leg scissor 3 × 12-15 each side	Bent-knee Copenhagen hip adduction 4 × 8-10

Strength zone	Exercise name	Page number	Workout 1: Reload (sets × reps or time)	Workouts 2 and 5 (sets × reps or time)	Workouts 3 and 6 (sets × reps or time)	Workouts 4 and 7 (sets × reps or time)
Calves: bent knee	6a. Machine seated calf raise	185	2 × 10-12	2 × 25-30	3 × 15-20	4 × 8-12
Core: lateral	6b. Weight plate around the world	206	2 × 6 each side	2 × 12 each side	3 × 8 each side	4 × 6 each side
Triceps: lengthened to midrange	6c. Dumbbell one-arm behind-the-head triceps extension	110	2 × 10-12 each side	2 × 20-25 each side	3 × 12-15 each side	4 × 8-10 each side
Rear delts: lengthened to midrange	7. Cable one-arm rear-delt fly	82	2 × 10-12 each side	4 × 6-8 each side	2 × 20-25 each side	3 × 12-15 each side

Rest 30 seconds between exercises and 1 to 2 minutes between paired sets or tri-sets.

*As mentioned in chapter 11; due to their multijoint nature, all exercises such as squats, Romanian deadlifts, lunges, step-ups and many variations of those exercises provided in chapters 9 and 10 also load your glutes when they're closer to a lengthened (stretched) range.

TABLE 15.8 Program 4, Total-Body Workout Day B

Strength zone	Exercise name	Page number	Workout 1: reload (sets × reps or time)	Workouts 2 and 5 (sets × reps or time)	Workouts 3 and 6 (sets × reps or time)	Workouts 4 and 7 (sets × reps or time)
*Quads and glutes: knee bending for the lengthened to midrange	1a. Dumbbell reverse lunge with NT Loop knee resistance	140	2 × 8-10 each side	3 × 12-15 each side	4 × 6-8 each side	2 × 20 each side
Core: rotational	1b. Cable one-arm press	213	2 × 8-10 each side	3 × 15 each side	4 × 8-10 each side	2 × 20-25 each side
Lats: vertical or diagonal pulling with arms inside for the lengthened to midrange	2a. Underhand-grip lat pull-down	55	2 × 10-12	3 × 12-15	4 × 8-10	2 × 20-25
Traps: scapular elevation	2b. Dumbbell one-arm leaning shrug	90	2 × 10-12 each side	3 × 12-15 each side	4 × 8-10 each side	2 × 20-25 each side
Middle delts: lengthened to midrange	2c. NT Loop Mini side shoulder raise	77	2 × 10-12 each side	3 × 12-15 each side	4 × 6-8 each side	2 × 20-25 each side
Quads: knee extension for the shortened to midrange	3a. Unilateral reverse sled drag	149	2 × 30 yards (27 m) each leg	3 × 50-60 yards (46-55 m) each let	4 × 20-30 yards (18-27 m) each leg	2 × 80 yards (73 m) each leg
Core: linear	3b. Core exercise indicated	192	Stability ball rollout 2 × 10-12	Arm walkout 3 × 8	Ab wheel rollout 4 × 5-6	Stability ball rollout 2 × 20

> continued

Table 15.8 *> continued*

Strength zone	Exercise name	Page number	Workout 1: reload (sets × reps or time)	Workouts 2 and 5 (sets × reps or time)	Workouts 3 and 6 (sets × reps or time)	Workouts 4 and 7 (sets × reps or time)
Hips: abduction	4a. Machine seated hip abduction	169	2 × 10-12	2 × 25	3 × 12-15	4 × 8-10
Calves: straight knee	4b. Dumbbell one-leg leaning calf raise	180	2 × 10-12 each side	2 × 25-30 each side	3 × 12-15 each side	4 × 8-12 each side
Core: lateral	5a. Dumbbell unilateral farmers walk	201	2 × 30 sec each side	2 × 50-60 sec each side	3 × 40 sec each side	4 × 20-30 sec each side
Chest: incline pressing for the lengthened to midrange	5b. Machine incline chest press	37	2 × 10-12	2 × 20-25	3 × 12-15	4 × 8-10
Middle delts: shortened to midrange	6a. Dumbbell side shoulder raise	72	2 × 10-12	4 × 6-8	2 × 20-25	3 × 12-15
Triceps: shortened to midrange	6b. Cable one-arm triceps kickback	115	2 × 10-12 each side	4 × 8-10 each side	2 × 20-25 each side	3 × 12-15 each side
Biceps: shortened to midrange	7a. Dumbbell concentration biceps curl	103	2 × 10-12 each side	4 × 6-8 each side	2 × 20 each side	3 × 12-15 each side
Rear delts: lengthened to midrange	7b. Dumbbell side-lying rear-delt fly	81	2 × 10-12 each side	4 × 6-8 each side	2 × 20-25 each side	3 × 12-15 each side

Rest 30 seconds between exercises and 1 to 2 minutes between paired sets or tri-sets.

*As mentioned in chapter 11; due to their multijoint nature, all exercises such as squats, Romanian deadlifts, lunges, step-ups and many variations of those exercises provided in chapters 9 and 10 also load your glutes when they're closer to a lengthened (stretched) range.

TABLE 15.9 Program 5, Total-Body Workout Day A

Strength zone	Exercise name	Page number	Workout 1: reload (sets × reps or time)	Workouts 2 and 5 (sets × reps or time)	Workouts 3 and 6 (sets × reps or time)	Workouts 4 and 7 (sets × reps or time)
*Glutes and hamstrings: hip hinging for the lengthened to midrange	1a. Dumbbell lateral Romanian deadlift lunge	122	2 × 10-12 each side	4 × 6-8 each side	2 × 18-20 each side	3 × 10-12 each side
Core: linear	1b. Core exercise indicated	192	Reverse crunch 2 × 8	Incline bench reverse crunch 4 × 6-8	Reverse crunch 2 × 15-20	Stability ball pike rollout 3 × 8-12
Lats: vertical or diagonal pulling with arms outside for the lengthened to midrange	2a. Pull-up (assisted if needed with band or machine)	48	2 × 8-10	4 × 5-8	2 × 20-25	3 × 10-12

Strength zone	Exercise name	Page number	Workout 1: reload (sets × reps or time)	Workouts 2 and 5 (sets × reps or time)	Workouts 3 and 6 (sets × reps or time)	Workouts 4 and 7 (sets × reps or time)
Traps: scapular elevation	2b. Barbell wide-grip shrug	89	2 × 8-10	4 × 8-10	2 × 20-25	3 × 12-15
Lats: horizontal pulling for the shortened to midrange	3a. Barbell bent-over row	59	2 × 10-12	3 × 10-15	4 × 6-8	2 × 20-25
Chest: incline pressing for the lengthened to midrange	3b. Dumbbell incline bench press	34	2 × 10-12	3 × 10-15	4 × 6-8	2 × 20-25
Hamstrings: knee flexion for the shortened to midrange	4a. Hamstring exercise indicated	125	Stability ball leg curl 2 × 10-15	Stability ball one-leg curl 3 × 12-15 each side	Nordic hamstring curl 4 × 5-8	Stability ball leg curl 2 × 25-30
Core: lateral	4b. Cable one-arm side bend	204	2 × 8-10 each side	3 × 12-15 each side	4 × 8-10 each side	2 × 20-25 each side
Core: rotational	4c. Cable same-side one-arm press	214	2 × 10-12 each side	3 × 12-15 each side	4 × 8-10 each side	2 × 20-25 each side
Biceps: lengthened to midrange	5a. Dumbbell incline bench one-arm preacher curl	101	2 × 10-12 each side	2 × 20-25 each side	3 × 12-15 each side	4 × 8-10 each side
Middle and rear delts: shortened to midrange	5b. Dumbbell incline bench 45-degree row	70	2 × 10-12	2 × 20-25	3 × 12-15	4 × 8-10
Calves: straight knee	5c. Dumbbell foot-elevated calf raise	181	2 × 12-15 each side	2 × 25-30 each side	3 × 15 each side	4 × 8-12 each side
Triceps: shortened to midrange	6a. Machine triceps extension	117	2 × 10-12	2 × 20-25	3 × 12-15	4 × 8-10
Hips: abduction	6b. Hip abduction exercise indicated	169	Weight plate side-lying hip abduction 2 × 10-12 each side	Weight plate side-lying hip abduction 2 × 20-30 each side	Dynamic bent-knee side elbow plank with hip abduction 3 × 15 each side	Dynamic side elbow plank with hip abduction 4 × 6-10 each side
Quads: knee extension for the shortened to midrange	6c. NT Loop inverted leg extension exercise indicated	151	NT Loop inverted leg extension 2 × 10-12	NT Loop inverted leg extension 2 × 20-25	NT Loop inverted leg extension 3 × 12-15	NT Loop feet-elevated inverted leg extension 4 × 6-10

Rest 30 seconds between exercises and 1 to 2 minutes between paired sets or tri-sets.

*As mentioned in chapter 11; due to their multijoint nature, all exercises such as squats, Romanian deadlifts, lunges, step-ups and many variations of those exercises provided in chapters 9 and 10 also load your glutes when they're closer to a lengthened (stretched) range.

TABLE 15.10 Program 5, Total-Body Workout Day B

Strength zone	Exercise name	Page number	Workout 1: reload (sets × reps or time)	Workouts 2 and 5 (sets × reps or time)	Workouts 3 and 6 (sets × reps or time)	Workouts 4 and 7 (sets × reps or time)
*Quads and glutes: knee bending for the lengthened to midrange	1a. Barbell squat	134	2 × 8-10	3 × 10-15	4 × 6-8	2 × 20-25
Core: linear	1b. Core exercise indicated	192	Stability ball rollout 2 × 8-10	Ab wheel rollout 3 × 12-15	Arm walkout 4 × 5-8	Stability ball rollout 2 × 20-25
Lats: vertical or diagonal pulling with arms inside for the lengthened to midrange	2a. Cable one-arm half-kneeling neutral-grip lat pull-down	56	2 × 10-12 each side	3 × 12-15 each side	4 × 8-10 each side	2 × 20-25 each side
Chest: horizontal or diagonal shoulder adduction for the shortened to mid-range	2b. Cable one-arm horizontal pec fly	39	2 × 10-12 each side	3 × 12-15 each side	4 × 8-10 each side	2 × 20-25 each side
Chest: horizontal or decline pressing for the lengthened to midrange	3a. Dumbbell decline hip bridge press	27	2 × 10-12	3 × 12-15	4 × 6-8	2 × 20-25
Traps: scapular retraction	3b. Dumbbell bench one-arm horizontal shrug	92	2 × 10-12 each side	3 × 12-15 each side	4 × 8-10 each side	2 × 20-25 each side
Glutes: hip extension for the shortened to midrange	4a. 45-degree hip extension	166	2 × 10-12	2 × 20-30	3 × 12-15	4 × 6-10
Hips: adduction	4b. NT Loop quadruped hip adduction	176	2 × 10-12 each side	2 × 20 each side	3 × 12-15 each side	4 × 8-10 each side
Triceps: lengthened to midrange	4c. NT Loop overhead triceps press	111	2 × 10-12	2 × 20-25	3 × 12-15	4 × 6-8
Biceps: shortened to midrange	5a. Dumbbell incline bench biceps curl	104	2 × 10-12	2 × 20-25	3 × 12-15	4 × 6-8
Rear delts: lengthened to midrange	5b. NT Loop Mini rear-delt fly	84	2 × 10-12 each side	2 × 20-25 each side	3 × 12-15 each side	4 × 8-10 each side
Middle delts: lengthened to midrange	6a. NT Loop side shoulder raise	77	2 × 10-12 each side	4 × 6-10 each side	2 × 20-25 each side	3 × 12-15 each side

Strength zone	Exercise name	Page number	Workout 1: reload (sets × reps or time)	Workouts 2 and 5 (sets × reps or time)	Workouts 3 and 6 (sets × reps or time)	Workouts 4 and 7 (sets × reps or time)
Calves: bent knee	6b. Dumbbell one-leg seated calf raise	184	2 × 10-12 each side	4 × 8-12 each side	2 × 25-30 each side	3 × 15 each side
Core: lateral	6c. Off-bench lateral hold	203	2 × 10-15 sec each side	4 × 10-15 sec each side	2 × 30 sec each side	3 × 20 sec each side
Core: rotational	7. Cable three-point horizontal chop	209	2 × 6-8 each position, each side	4 × 6-8 each position, each side	2 × 12-15 each position, each side	3 × 10 each position, each side

Rest 30 seconds between exercises and 1 to 2 minutes between paired sets or tri-sets.

*As mentioned in chapter 11; due to their multijoint nature, all exercises such as squats, Romanian deadlifts, lunges, step-ups and many variations of those exercises provided in chapters 9 and 10 also load your glutes when they're closer to a lengthened (stretched) range.

CHAPTER 16

Programs for Four Workouts per Week

The workout programs featured in the chapter are designed for people who prefer to work out four times per week. If you're dedicated to strength training more frequently than that, you'll want to try the workouts in chapter 17.

Program Guidelines

The following is a list of key points to remember and follow in order to strength train smart and get the most of out the workout programs in the chapter.

Rest

- Perform the exercises designated with *a* or *b* as paired sets, and perform exercises with *a*, *b*, and *c* as tri-sets. Perform all reps in each set before moving to the next set. Completing 1 round of the exercises in a paired or tri-set is considered 1 set.
- Rest 30 seconds between exercise in a given paired set and tri-set.
- Rest 1 to 2 minutes between each round of a given paired set and tri-set.

Reps

- The rep range (e.g., 10-15 reps) is next to each exercise in the workout. If you're using the same weight for each set, you may be able to do 15 reps on the first set, 12 reps on the next set, and 10 reps on the third set because of accumulated fatigue. Or you can reduce the weight you're using with each consecutive set to achieve the higher end or given rep range on each consecutive set. Both methods are effective in helping you to progress.
- Maintain strict form without cheating by using additional movements or momentum.
- Mentally focus on the working muscles in each exercise.
- Do the concentric (lifting) portion of each rep at a normal tempo and maintain strict control during the eccentric (lowering) portion. Take roughly 3 seconds on the eccentric portion of each rep.

Weight

- Use a weight load that's light enough to allow you to achieve the minimum number of reps indicated for each exercise.
- Use a weight load heavy enough that you're unable to perform any more reps than the maximum number indicated for each exercise while maintaining proper control and technique.

Work Around—Not Through—Injuries and Limitations

- If an exercise causes pain or discomfort beyond the sensation associated with muscle fatigue, use an alternative exercise that doesn't hurt that targets the same muscle group in the same strength zone.
- Not every exercise movement is for everybody. There are plenty of movements in the exercise chapters of this book to choose from.

Program Setup

The five workout programs in this chapter each consist of four different workouts: two lower-body and core workouts and two upper-body workouts (see tables 16.1-16.5). You'll alternate between lower-body and core workouts and upper-body workouts, performing the workouts in order: A, B, C, and D. And there are no more than two consecutive training days so you have time for recovery.

Completing workouts A, B, C, and D equals one time through. You'll perform each of the five total programs for seven times through, which is seven weeks total before switching to the next program and repeating those workouts for another seven times through for seven weeks total.

Weekly Workout Schedule for Four Times per Week

Following are weekly training schedule options for training four times per week using the workout programs in the chapter.

Sample Option 1

Monday: Day A—lower body and core

Tuesday: Day B—upper body

Wednesday: Rest

Thursday: Day C—lower body and core

Friday: Rest

Saturday: Day D—upper body

Sunday: Rest

Sample Option 2

Monday: Day A—lower body and core

Tuesday: Rest

Wednesday: Day B—upper body

Thursday: Day C—lower body and core

Friday: Rest

Saturday: Day D—upper body

Sunday: Rest

Sample Option 3

    Monday: Day A—lower body and core

    Tuesday: Day B—upper body

    Wednesday: Rest

    Thursday: Day C—lower body and core

    Friday: Day D—upper body

    Saturday: Rest

    Sunday: Rest

You can change the days of the week that you perform each workout to better fit your schedule. Just make sure to perform the workouts in the same order: A, B, C, and D. And to maximize your recovery, make sure to follow the same pattern shown in these samples by training no more than two consecutive days before taking a rest day.

Rest Days

The non-strength-training days, which are indicated as rest days in the sample weekly training setups, don't mean you have to do nothing. During your days off from using the smarter strength training workouts, you can do low-impact activities, such as going for long walks, hikes, bike rides, or swims. Yoga can also be a great option for your active rest days.

Reload Workouts

The first time you do each workout in a program, it's considered a reload workout. A reload workout is simply a lower-intensity version of the workout, which helps you to stay active while recovering between programs. It also acclimates you to the movements and gives you an idea of the appropriate weight loads (based on your strength level) to use for the new program you're starting.

Mixed Sets and Reps for Maximal Results

The training system and workout programs provided in this book enable you to incorporate the right blend of exercises to achieve strength in the true full range of motion. They also include a full spectrum of set and repetition ranges. This variety is the reason they can be so effective in helping you get stronger.

Research has shown that daily variations in intensity and volume (sets and reps) are more effective than weekly volume variations for increases in maximal strength; they may also lead to greater gains in muscle size (1, 2, 3, 4).

In short, it's best to think about the types of strength training exercise—and the sets and reps you use—in the same way that you think about your nutrition: Make sure to get enough variety, because each type offers unique training or nutritional value.

Warm Up and Build Up

Before you begin a workout in the following programs, be sure to perform a general warm-up. Also make sure to perform some build-up sets, which are simply lighter, less intense versions of whatever exercises you're getting ready to perform with heavier loads. Build-up sets are used to gradually build up to your working intensity. For example, if you're going to perform a heavy lift, first do a few lighter sets of that lift in order to build up to your working weight. As a rule of thumb, if the workout program calls for 4 sets of an exercises, you'll do 2 build-up sets. If the workout program calls for 3 sets of a given exercise, you'll perform 1 build-up set because it involves using lighter loads than when you're performing 4 sets for fewer reps. And because the times you'll be performing only 2 sets of a given exercise involve using lighter loads (because of the higher reps), there's no need to perform a build-up set to get into your working weight.

Why No Exercises for Front Delts?

In each of the following programs, even though there is no strength zone exercise category listed for the front delts, there are multiple exercises included to strengthen your front delts through the true full range of motion.

As mentioned in chapter 3, the front delts are worked during decline, horizontal, and diagonal pressing exercises. More specifically, these pressing exercises strengthen your front delts in the lengthened-to-midrange strength zone. While many of the exercises in chapter 5 are for the shortened-to-midrange strength zone for your middle delts, they also strengthen your front delts in the shortened-to-midrange strength zone.

TABLE 16.1   Program 1

DAY A: LOWER BODY AND CORE

Strength zone	Exercise name	Page number	Workout 1: reload (sets × reps or time)	Workouts 2 and 5 (sets × reps or time)	Workouts 3 and 6 (sets × reps or time)	Workouts 4 and 7 (sets × reps or time)
*Glutes and hamstrings: hip hinging for the lengthened to midrange	1a. Barbell elevated Romanian deadlift	120	2 × 10-12	4 × 5-8	2 × 20-25	3 × 10-15
Core: linear	1b. Stability ball plate crunch	196	2 × 8-10	4 × 6-8 (pause 2 sec at the top of each rep)	2 × 20-25	3 × 12-15
Glutes: hip extension for the shortened to midrange	2a. Cable one-leg Romanian deadlift	163	2 × 8-12 each side	4 × 6-8 each side	2 × 20 each side	3 × 12-15 each side
Core: rotational	2b. Cable three-point high-to-low chop	210	2 × 6 in each position, each side	4 × 6-8 in each position, each side	2 × 15 in each position, each side	3 × 10-12 in each position, each side
Hips: adduction	3a. Side-lying hip adduction leg scissors	173	2 × 10 each side	3 × 12-15 (1 sec hold at top of each rep) each side	4 × 6-8 (3 sec hold at top of each rep) each side	2 × 20-25 each side
Calves: straight knee	3b. Dumbbell traveling calf raise	180	2 × 20 sec	3 × 40 sec	4 × 30 sec	2 × 50 sec
Core: lateral	Dumbbell unilateral farmers walk	201	2 × 20 sec each side	2 × 50 sec each side	3 × 40 sec each side	4 × 30 sec each side

DAY B: UPPER BODY

Strength zone	Exercise name	Page number	Workout 1: reload (sets × reps or time)	Workouts 2 and 5 (sets × reps or time)	Workouts 3 and 6 (sets × reps or time)	Workouts 4 and 7 (sets × reps or time)
Lats: vertical or diagonal pulling with arms inside for the lengthened to midrange	1a. Chin-up (assisted if needed)	53	2 × 6-8	2 × 20-30	3 × 10-15	4 × 5-8
Chest: incline pressing for the lengthened to midrange	1b. Angled-barbell one-arm press	36	2 × 10-12 each side	2 × 15-20 each side	3 × 10-12 each side	4 × 6-8 each side
Middle delts: lengthened to midrange	2a. Cable side shoulder raise	75	2 × 10-12 each side	2 × 20-25 each side	3 × 12-15 each side	4 × 6-8 each side
Biceps: lengthened to midrange	2b. Cable one-arm face-away biceps curl	99	2 × 10-12 each side	2 × 20-25 each side	3 × 12-15 each side	4 × 6-8 each side

> continued

Table 16.1 > *continued*

DAY B: UPPER BODY *(continued)*

Strength zone	Exercise name	Page number	Workout 1: reload (sets × reps or time)	Workouts 2 and 5 (sets × reps or time)	Workouts 3 and 6 (sets × reps or time)	Workouts 4 and 7 (sets × reps or time)
Triceps: shortened to midrange	3a. Dumbbell triceps skull crusher	112	2 × 10-12	4 × 6-8	2 × 20-25	3 × 12-15
Rear delts: lengthened to midrange	3b. Dumbbell side-lying rear-delt fly	81	2 × 10-12 each side	4 × 6-8 each side	2 × 20-25 each side	3 × 12-15 each side
Chest: horizontal or diagonal shoulder adduction for the shortened to midrange	4a. Cable crossover pec fly	41	2 × 10-12	3 × 12-15	4 × 10-12	2 × 20-25
Traps: scapular retraction	4b. Cable one-arm horizontal shrug	93	2 × 10-12 each side	3 × 10-15 each side	4 × 6-8 each side	2 × 20-25 each side

DAY C: LOWER BODY AND CORE

Strength zone	Exercise name	Page number	Workout 1: reload (sets × reps or time)	Workouts 2 and 5 (sets × reps or time)	Workouts 3 and 6 (sets × reps or time)	Workouts 4 and 7 (sets × reps or time)
*Quads and glutes: knee bending for the lengthened to midrange	1a. Dumbbell traveling lunge	139	2 × 8-10 each side	3 × 12-15 each side	4 × 5-8 each side	2 × 20-25 each side
Core: rotational	1b. Cable tight rotation with hip shift	208	2 × 12 each side	3 × 12 each side	4 × 8 each side	2 × 20 each side
Quads: knee extension for the shortened to midrange	2a. Machine leg extension	147	2 × 10-12	3 × 12-15	4 × 6-8	2 × 20-25
Calves: bent knee	2b. Dumbbell half-kneeling calf raise	183	2 × 20 each side	3 × 20 each side	4 × 12-15 each side	2 × 30 each side
Hamstrings: knee flexion for the shortened to midrange	3a. Machine seated leg curl	125	2 × 10-12	2 × 20-30	3 × 10-15	4 × 6-8
Core: lateral	3b. Medicine ball side lean	203	2 × 8-10 each side	2 × 20 each side	3 × 12-15 each side	4 × 8-10 each side
Hips: abduction	4a. Machine seated hip abduction	169	2 × 10-12	4 × 6-8	2 × 20-30	3 × 10-15
Core: linear	4b. Core exercise indicated	192	Stability ball rollout 2 × 10-12	Ab wheel rollout 4 × 6-8	Stability ball rollout 2 × 20	Arm walkout 3 × 8-10

DAY D: UPPER BODY

Strength zone	Exercise name	Page number	Workout 1: reload (sets × reps or time)	Workouts 2 and 5 (sets × reps or time)	Workouts 3 and 6 (sets × reps or time)	Workouts 4 and 7 (sets × reps or time)
Chest: horizontal or decline pressing for the lengthened to midrange	1a. Machine chest press	28	2 × 10-12	3 × 10-15	4 × 6-8	2 × 20-25
Lats: horizontal pulling for the shortened to midrange	1b. Dumbbell two-arm bent-over row	60	2 × 10-12	3 × 12-15	4 × 8-10	2 × 20-25
Lats: vertical or diagonal pulling with arms outside for the lengthened to midrange	2a. Cable one-arm half-kneeling lat pull-down	50	2 × 10-12 each side	3 × 10-15 each side	4 × 6-8 each side	2 × 20-25 each side
Traps: scapular elevation	2b. Cable one-arm shrug	90	2 × 10-12 each side	3 × 10-15 each side	4 × 6-8 each side	2 × 20-25 each side
Biceps: shortened to midrange	3a. Dumbbell biceps curl	103	2 × 10-12	2 × 20-25	3 × 12-15	4 × 6-8
Triceps: lengthened to midrange	3b. Cable rope overhead triceps extension	108	2 × 10-12	2 × 20-25	3 × 12-15	4 × 6-8
Middle and rear delts: shortened to midrange	4. Barbell 45-degree row	71	2 × 10-12	4 × 8-10	2 × 20-25	3 × 12-15

Rest 30 seconds between exercises and 1 to 2 minutes between paired sets or tri-sets.

*As mentioned in chapter 11, due to their multijoint nature, all exercises such as squats, Romanian deadlifts, lunges, step-ups and many variations of those exercises provided in chapters 9 and 10 also load your glutes when they're closer to a lengthened (stretched) range.

TABLE 16.2   Program 2

DAY A: LOWER BODY AND CORE

Strength zone	Exercise name	Page number	Workout 1: reload (sets × reps or time)	Workouts 2 and 5 (sets × reps or time)	Workouts 3 and 6 (sets × reps or time)	Workouts 4 and 7 (sets × reps or time)
*Glutes and hamstrings: hip hinging for the lengthened to midrange	1a. Dumbbell traveling Romanian deadlift lunge	122	2 × 10-12 each side	4 × 5-8 each side	2 × 17-20 each side	3 × 10-15 each side
Core: linear	1b. Band leg lowering	192	2 × 8-10	4 × 6-8	2 × 15-20	3 × 10-12
Quads: knee extension for the shortened to midrange	2a. Reverse sled drag	148	2 × 40 yards (36 m)	4 × 40 yards (36 m)	2 × 100 yards (91 m)	3 × 60-70 yards (55-64 m)
Calves: straight knee	2b. Dumbbell one-leg leaning calf raise	180	2 × 12-15 each side	4 × 8-10 each side	2 × 25-30 each side	3 × 12-15 each side

> continued

Table 16.2 > *continued*

DAY A: LOWER BODY AND CORE *(continued)*

Strength zone	Exercise name	Page number	Workout 1: reload (sets × reps or time)	Workouts 2 and 5 (sets × reps or time)	Workouts 3 and 6 (sets × reps or time)	Workouts 4 and 7 (sets × reps or time)
Hips: abduction	3a. Band lateral hip shuffle	170	2 × 10 each side	3 × 20-25 each side	4 × 15 each side	2 × 30-35 each side
Core: lateral	3b. Cable one-arm side bend	204	2 × 10 each side	3 × 15 each side	4 × 8-10 each side	2 × 20 each side
Core: rotational	4a. Cable three-point low-to-high chop	212	2 × 6 in each position, each side	2 × 15 in each position, each side	3 × 10-12 in each position, each side	4 × 6-8 in each position, each side
Calves: bent knee	4b. Machine seated calf raise	185	2 × 15	2 × 25-30	3 × 12-15	4 × 6-8

DAY B: UPPER BODY

Strength zone	Exercise name	Page number	Workout 1: reload (sets × reps or time)	Workouts 2 and 5 (sets × reps or time)	Workouts 3 and 6 (sets × reps or time)	Workouts 4 and 7 (sets × reps or time)
Chest: incline pressing for the lengthened to midrange	1a. Dumbbell incline bench press	34	2 × 10-12	2 × 20-25	3 × 10-15	4 × 5-8
Lats: horizontal pulling for the shortened to midrange	1b. One-arm anti-rotation suspension row	66	2 × 8-10 each side	2 × 15-20 each side	3 × 10-12 each side	4 × 6-8 each side
Chest: horizontal or diagonal shoulder adduction for the shortened to midrange	2a. Machine one-arm rotated chest press	40	2 × 10-12 each side	2 × 20-25 each side	3 × 12-15 each side	4 × 8-10 each side
Traps: scapular retraction	2b. Dumbbell off-bench one-arm horizontal shrug	92	2 × 10-12 each side	2 × 20-25 each side	3 × 12-15 each side	4 × 8-10 each side
Middle delts: shortened to midrange	3a. Kettlebell shoulder-to-shoulder press	73	2 × 5-6 each side	4 × 6-8 each side	2 × 16-20 each side	3 × 10-14 each side
Biceps: lengthened to midrange	3b. EZ-bar preacher curl	100	2 × 10-12	4 × 6-8	2 × 20-25	3 × 12-15
Triceps: lengthened to midrange	4a. Kettlebell behind-the-head triceps extension	109	2 × 10-12	3 × 12-15	4 × 6-8	2 × 20-25
Middle delts: lengthened to midrange	4b. Dumbbell side-lying side shoulder raise	76	2 × 10-12 each side	3 × 12-15 each side	4 × 6-8 each side	2 × 20-25 each side

DAY C: LOWER BODY AND CORE

Strength zone	Exercise name	Page number	Workout 1: reload (sets × reps or time)	Workouts 2 and 5 (sets × reps or time)	Workouts 3 and 6 (sets × reps or time)	Workouts 4 and 7 (sets × reps or time)
*Quads and glutes: knee bending for the lengthened to midrange	1a. Trap bar squat	136	2 × 8-10	3 × 12-15	4 × 5-8	2 × 20-25
Core: linear	1b. Core exercise indicated	192	Reverse crunch 2 × 8-10	Reverse crunch 3 × 10-15	Incline bench reverse crunch 4 × 6-8	Stability ball knee tuck 2 × 20-30
Glutes: hip extension for the shortened to midrange	2a. 45-degree hip extension	166	2 × 8-12	3 × 12-15	4 × 6-10	2 × 20-25
Core: lateral	2b. Angled-barbell tight rainbow	201	2 × 15 sec	3 × 20 sec	4 × 15 sec	2 × 30 sec
Hamstrings: knee flexion for the shortened to midrange	3a. Machine lying one-leg curl	127	2 × 10-12 each side	2 × 20-30 each side	3 × 10-15 each side	4 × 6-8 each side
Core: rotational	3b. Weight plate chop	215	2 × 10-12 each side	2 × 20 each side	3 × 10-15 each side	4 × 6-8 each side
Hips: adduction	4. Bent-knee Copenhagen hip adduction	174	2 × 8-10 each side	4 × 5-8 (pause 2 sec at top of each rep) each side	2 × 15 each side	3 × 10-12 each side

DAY D: UPPER BODY

Strength zone	Exercise name	Page number	Workout 1: reload (sets × reps or time)	Workouts 2 and 5 (sets × reps or time)	Workouts 3 and 6 (sets × reps or time)	Workouts 4 and 7 (sets × reps or time)
Chest: horizontal or decline pressing for the lengthened to midrange	1a. Push-up exercise indicated	29	Push-up 2 × 10-15	Box crossover push-up 3 × max reps	NT Loop resisted push-up 4 × max reps	Push-up 2 × max reps
Lats: vertical or diagonal pulling with arms outside for the lengthened to midrange	1b. Overhand-grip lat pull-down	49	2 × 10-12	3 × 10-15	4 × 6-8	2 × 20-25
Lats: vertical or diagonal pulling with arms inside for the lengthened to midrange	2a. Neutral-grip one-arm lat pull-down	56	2 × 10-12 each side	3 × 12-15 each side	4 × 5-8 each side	2 × 20-25 each side
Traps: scapular elevation	2b. Dumbbell one-arm leaning shrug	90	2 × 10-12 each side	3 × 12-15 each side	4 × 8-10 each side	2 × 20-25 each side

> continued

Table 16.2 *> continued*

DAY D: UPPER BODY *(continued)*

Strength zone	Exercise name	Page number	Workout 1: reload (sets × reps or time)	Workouts 2 and 5 (sets × reps or time)	Workouts 3 and 6 (sets × reps or time)	Workouts 4 and 7 (sets × reps or time)
Biceps: shortened to midrange	3a. Cable EZ-bar biceps curl	105	2 × 10-12	2 × 20-25	3 × 12-15	4 × 6-8
Rear delts: lengthened to midrange	3b. Cable one-arm rear-delt fly	82	2 × 10-12 each side	2 × 20-25 each side	3 × 12-15 each side	4 × 6-8 each side
Triceps: shortened to midrange	4a. Cable rope triceps extension	114	2 × 10-12	4 × 6-8	2 × 20-25	3 × 12-15
Rear delts: shortened to midrange	4b. Cable rope face pull	79	2 × 10-12	4 × 6-8	2 × 20-25	3 × 12-15

Rest 30 seconds between exercises and 1 to 2 minutes between paired sets or tri-sets.

*As mentioned in chapter 11, due to their multijoint nature, all exercises such as squats, Romanian deadlifts, lunges, step-ups and many variations of those exercises provided in chapters 9 and 10 also load your glutes when they're closer to a lengthened (stretched) range.

TABLE 16.3   Program 3

DAY A: LOWER BODY AND CORE

Strength zone	Exercise name	Page number	Workout 1: reload (sets × reps or time)	Workouts 2 and 5 (sets × reps or time)	Workouts 3 and 6 (sets reps or time)	Workouts 4 and 7 (sets × reps or time)
*Glutes and hamstrings: hip hinging for the lengthened to midrange	1a. Angled-barbell leaning Romanian deadlift	124	2 × 10-12	4 × 6-8	2 × 17-20	3 × 10-15
Core: linear	1b. Stability ball arc	193	2 × 8-10 each side	4 × 6-8 each side	2 × 14-15 each side	3 × 10-12 each side
Quads: knee extension for the shortened to midrange	2a. Machine unilateral leg extension	148	2 × 10-12 each side	4 × 6-8 each side	2 × 20-25 each side	3 × 12-15 each side
Core: rotational	2b. Dumbbell plank row	207	2 × 8 each side	4 × 6-8 each side	2 × 12-15 each side	3 × 8-10 each side
Hamstrings: knee flexion for the shortened to midrange	3a. Hamstring exercise indicated	125	Stability ball leg curl 2 × 10-15	Stability ball one-leg curl 3 × 12-20 each side	Nordic hamstring curl 4 × 4-8	Stability ball leg curl 2 × 25-30
Core: lateral	3b. Stability ball side crunch	205	2 × 10 each side	3 × 12-15 each side	4 × 6-10 each side	2 × 20-30 each side
Hips: abduction	4a. Machine seated hip abduction	169	2 × 10-12	2 × 20-25	3 × 10-15	4 × 6-8
Calves: bent knee	4b. Dumbbell half-kneeling calf raise	183	2 × 10-12 each side	2 × 25-30 each side	3 × 15-20 each side	4 × 8-12 each side

DAY B: UPPER BODY

Strength zone	Exercise name	Page number	Workout 1: reload (sets × reps or time)	Workouts 2 and 5 (sets × reps or time)	Workouts 3 and 6 (sets × reps or time)	Workouts 4 and 7 (sets × reps or time)
Chest: horizontal or decline pressing for the lengthened to midrange	1a. Dumbbell bench press	26	2 × 10-12	2 × 20-25	3 × 10-15	4 × 5-8
Lats: horizontal pulling for the shortened to midrange	1b. Dumbbell one-arm bench row	61	2 × 10-12 each side	2 × 20-25 each side	3 × 10-12 each side	4 × 6-8 each side
Chest: horizontal or diagonal shoulder adduction for the shortened to midrange	2a. Machine pec fly	43	2 × 10-12	2 × 20-25	3 × 12-15	4 × 8-10
Traps: scapular retraction	2b. Dumbbell bent-over horizontal shrug	91	2 × 10-12	2 × 25	3 × 15	4 × 10
Triceps: lengthened to midrange	3a. Cable rope overhead triceps extension	108	2 × 10-12	4 × 6-8	2 × 20-25	3 × 12-15
Middle delts: lengthened to midrange	3b. NT Loop side shoulder raise	77	2 × 10-12 each side	4 × 6-8 each side	2 × 20-25 each side	3 × 12-15 each side
Biceps: lengthened to midrange	4a. Cable one-arm face-away biceps curl	99	2 × 10-12 each side	3 × 12-15 each side	4 × 6-8 each side	2 × 20 each side
Rear delts: lengthened to midrange	4b. Low-cable rear-delt fly	82	2 × 10-12 each side	3 × 12-15 each side	4 × 6-8 each side	2 × 20-25 each side

DAY C: LOWER BODY AND CORE

Strength zone	Exercise name	Page number	Workout 1: reload (sets × reps or time)	Workouts 2 and 5 (sets × reps or time)	Workouts 3 and 6 (sets × reps or time)	Workouts 4 and 7 (sets × reps or time)
*Quads and glutes: knee bending for the lengthened to midrange	1a. Dumbbell step-up	139	2 × 8-10 each side	3 × 12-15 each side	4 × 5-8 each side	2 × 20 each side
Core: lateral	1b. Off-bench lateral hold	203	2 × 12-15 sec each side	3 × 25-30 sec each side	4 × 15-20 sec each side	2 × 35-40 sec each side
Glutes: hip extension for the shortened to midrange	2a. Weight plate one-leg hip lift	166	2 × 10-12 each side	3 × 12-15 each side	4 × 8-10 each side	2 × 25-30 each side
Hips: adduction	2b. NT Loop quadruped hip adduction	176	2 × 10-12 each side	3 × 12-15 each side	4 × 8-10 each side	2 × 20-25 each side

> *continued*

Table 16.3 > *continued*

DAY C: LOWER BODY AND CORE *(continued)*

Strength zone	Exercise name	Page number	Workout 1: reload (sets × reps or time)	Workouts 2 and 5 (sets × reps or time)	Workouts 3 and 6 (sets × reps or time)	Workouts 4 and 7 (sets × reps or time)
Calves: straight knee	3a. Machine ankles-to-gether calf raise	182	2 × 15	2 × 25-30	3 × 12-15	4 × 8-10
Core: linear	3b. Band leg lowering	192	2 × 20-30 sec	2 × 50 sec	3 × 40 sec	4 × 40 sec
Core: rotational	4. Cable three-point horizontal chop	209	2 × 6-8 each position, each side	4 × 6-8 each position, each side	2 × 12-15 each position, each side	3 × 10 each position, each side

DAY D: UPPER BODY

Strength zone	Exercise name	Page number	Workout 1: reload (sets × reps or time)	Workouts 2 and 5 (sets × reps or time)	Workouts 3 and 6 (sets × reps or time)	Workouts 4 and 7 (sets × reps or time)
Chest: incline pressing for the lengthened to midrange	1a. Angled-barbell shoulder-to-shoulder press	35	2 × 20 total	3 × 24-30 total	4 × 12-16 total	2 × 40 total
Lats: vertical or diagonal pulling with arms outside for the lengthened to midrange	1b. Cable fighters lat pull-down	51	2 × 10-12 each side	3 × 12-15 each side	4 × 8-10 each side	2 × 20-25 each side
Lats: vertical or diagonal pulling with arms inside for the lengthened to midrange	2a. Cable straight-arm compound pull-down	57	2 × 10-12	3 × 12-15	4 × 8-10	2 × 20-25
Traps: scapular elevation	2b. Cable wide-grip angled upright row	88	2 × 10-12	3 × 15-20	4 × 10-12	2 × 30
Middle delts: shortened to midrange	3a. Machine overhead press	75	2 × 10-12	2 × 20-25	3 × 10-15	4 × 6-8
Biceps: shortened to midrange	3b. EZ-bar biceps curl	102	2 × 10-12	2 × 20-25	3 × 10-15	4 × 6-8
Triceps: shortened to midrange	4a. Suspension trainer skull crusher	114	2 × 10-12	4 × 8-10	2 × 20-25	3 × 15
Rear delts: shortened to midrange	4b. Suspension trainer wide-grip row	80	2 × 10-12	4 × 8-10	2 × 20-25	3 × 15

Rest 30 seconds between exercises and 1 to 2 minutes between paired sets or tri-sets.

*As mentioned in chapter 11, due to their multijoint nature, all exercises such as squats, Romanian deadlifts, lunges, step-ups and many variations of those exercises provided in chapters 9 and 10 also load your glutes when they're closer to a lengthened (stretched) range.

TABLE 16.4   Program 4

DAY A: LOWER BODY AND CORE

Strength zone	Exercise name	Page number	Workout 1: reload (sets × reps or time)	Workouts 2 and 5 (sets × reps or time)	Workouts 3 and 6 (sets × reps or time)	Workouts 4 and 7 (sets × reps or time)
*Glutes and hamstrings: hip hinging for the lengthened to midrange	1a. Dumbbell one-leg one-arm Romanian deadlift	123	2 × 10-12 each side	4 × 6-8 each side	2 × 20 each side	3 × 12-15 each side
Core: linear	1b. Suspension trainer arm fallout	195	2 × 8-10	4 × 6-8	2 × 20	3 × 12-15
Hamstrings: knee flexion for the shortened to midrange	2a. Machine seated one-leg curl	126	2 × 8-10 each side	4 × 6-8 each side	2 × 20-25 each side	3 × 10-15 each side
Core: rotational	2b. Cross-body plank	208	2 × 15 sec	4 × 20 sec	2 × 40 sec	3 × 30 sec
Glutes: hip extension for the shortened to midrange	3a. NT Loop glute walk	168	2 × 30 sec	3 × 40 sec	4 × 30 sec	2 × 50 sec
Hips: adduction	3b. Hip adduction exercise indicated	173	Side-lying hip adduction 2 × 8 each side	Side-lying hip adduction leg scissors 3 × 12-15 each side	Bent-knee Copenhagen hip adduction 4 × 8-10 each side	Side-lying hip adduction 2 × 20-25 each side
Calves: bent knee	4a. Machine seated calf raise	185	2 × 10-12	2 × 25-30	3 × 15-20	4 × 8-12
Core: lateral	4b. Weight plate around the world	206	2 × 6 each side	2 × 12 each side	3 × 8 each side	4 × 6 each side

DAY B: UPPER BODY

Strength zone	Exercise name	Page number	Workout 1: reload (sets × reps or time)	Workouts 2 and 5 (sets × reps or time)	Workouts 3 and 6 (sets × reps or time)	Workouts 4 and 7 (sets × reps or time)
Lats: horizontal pulling for the shortened to midrange	1a. Machine row	64	2 × 10-12	2 × 20-25	3 × 10-15	4 × 5-8
Traps: scapular retraction	1b. Machine row horizontal shrug	94	2 × 10-12	2 × 20-25	3 × 10-15	4 × 5-8
Chest: horizontal or decline pressing for the lengthened to midrange	1c. Push-up exercise indicated	30	Push-up 2 × 12-15	Push-up 2 × max reps	Box cross-over push-up 3 × max reps	Lock-off push-up 4 × 6-8 each side

> continued

Table 16.4 > *continued*

DAY B: UPPER BODY *(continued)*

Strength zone	Exercise name	Page number	Workout 1: reload (sets × reps or time)	Workouts 2 and 5 (sets × reps or time)	Workouts 3 and 6 (sets × reps or time)	Workouts 4 and 7 (sets × reps or time)
Lats: vertical or diagonal pulling with arms outside for the lengthened to midrange	2a. Cable one-arm half-kneeling lat pull-down	50	2 × 10-12 each side	4 × 6-8 each side	2 × 20 each side	3 × 10-15 each side
Chest: horizontal or diagonal shoulder adduction for the shortened to midrange	2b. Cable one-arm diagonal pec fly	39	2 × 10-12 each side	4 × 6-8 each side	2 × 20 each side	3 × 10-15 each side
Biceps: lengthened to midrange	3a. EZ-bar preacher curl	100	2 × 10-12	3 × 10-15	4 × 6-8	2 × 20-25
Triceps: lengthened to midrange	3b. Dumbbell one-arm behind-the-head triceps extension	110	2 × 10-12 each side	3 × 12-15 each side	4 × 8-10 each side	2 × 20-25 each side
Rear delts: shortened to midrange	3c. Dumbbell rear-delt fly	78	2 × 10-12	3 × 12-15	4 × 8-10	2 × 20-25

DAY C: LOWER BODY AND CORE

Strength zone	Exercise name	Page number	Workout 1: reload (sets × reps or time)	Workouts 2 and 5 (sets × reps or time)	Workouts 3 and 6 (sets × reps or time)	Workouts 4 and 7 (sets × reps or time)
*Quads and glutes: knee bending for the lengthened to midrange	1a. Dumbbell reverse lunge with NT Loop knee resistance	140	2 × 8-10 each side	3 × 12-15 each side	4 × 6-8 each side	2 × 20 each side
Core: rotational	1b. Cable one-arm press	213	2 × 8-10 each side	3 × 15 each side	4 × 8-10 each side	2 × 20-25 each side
Quads: knee extension for the shortened to midrange	2a. Unilateral reverse sled drag	149	2 × 30 yards (27 m) each leg	3 × 50-60 yards (46-55 m) each leg	4 × 20-30 yards (18-27 m) each leg	2 × 80 yards (73 m) each leg
Core: linear	2b. Core exercise indicated	192	Stability ball rollout 2 × 10-12	Arm walkout 3 × 8	Ab wheel rollout 4 × 5-6	Stability ball rollout 2 × 20
Hips: abduction	3a. Machine seated hip abduction	169	2 × 10-12	2 × 25	3 × 12-15	4 × 8-10
Calves: straight knee	3b. Dumbbell one-leg leaning calf raise	180	2 × 10-12 each side	2 × 25-30 each side	3 × 12-15 each side	4 × 8-12 each side
Core: lateral	4. Dumbbell unilateral farmers walk	201	2 × 30 sec each side	4 × 20-30 sec each side	2 × 50-60 sec each side	3 × 40 sec each side

DAY D: UPPER BODY

Strength zone	Exercise name	Page number	Workout 1: reload (sets × reps or time)	Workouts 2 and 5 (sets × reps or time)	Workouts 3 and 6 (sets × reps or time)	Workouts 4 and 7 (sets × reps or time)
Lats: vertical or diagonal pulling with arms inside for the lengthened to midrange	1a. Underhand-grip lat pull-down	55	2 × 10-12	3 × 12-15	4 × 8-10	2 × 20-25
Traps: scapular elevation	1b. Dumbbell one-arm leaning shrug	90	2 × 10-12 each side	3 × 12-15 each side	4 × 8-10 each side	2 × 20-25 each side
Middle delts: lengthened to midrange	1c. NT Loop Mini side shoulder raise	77	2 × 10-12 each side	3 × 12-15 each side	4 × 6-8 each side	2 × 20-25 each side
Middle delts: shortened to midrange	2a. Dumbbell side shoulder raise	72	2 × 10-12	3 × 12-15	4 × 6-8	2 × 20-25
Triceps: shortened to midrange	2b. Cable one-arm triceps kickback	115	2 × 10-12 each side	3 × 12-15 each side	4 × 8-10 each side	2 × 20-25 each side
Biceps: shortened to midrange	3a. Dumbbell concentration biceps curl	103	2 × 10-12 each side	2 × 20 each side	3 × 12-15 each side	4 × 6-8 each side
Rear delts: lengthened to midrange	3b. Dumbbell side-lying rear-delt fly	81	2 × 10-12 each side	2 × 20-25 each side	3 × 12-15 each side	4 × 6-8 each side
Chest: incline pressing for the lengthened to midrange	4. Machine incline chest press	37	2 × 10-12	4 × 8-10	2 × 20-25	3 × 12-15

Rest 30 seconds between exercises and 1 to 2 minutes between paired sets or tri-sets.

*As mentioned in chapter 11, due to their multijoint nature, all exercises such as squats, Romanian deadlifts, lunges, step-ups and many variations of those exercises provided in chapters 9 and 10 also load your glutes when they're closer to a lengthened (stretched) range.

TABLE 16.5   Program 5

DAY A: LOWER BODY AND CORE

Strength zone	Exercise name	Page number	Workout 1: reload (sets × reps or time)	Workouts 2 and 5 (sets × reps or time)	Workouts 3 and 6 (sets × reps or time)	Workouts 4 and 7 (sets × reps or time)
*Glutes and hamstrings: hip hinging for the lengthened to midrange	1a. Dumbbell lateral Romanian deadlift lunge	122	2 × 10-12 each side	4 × 6-8 each side	2 × 20 each side	3 × 10-15 each side
Core: linear	1b. Core exercise indicated	192	Reverse crunch 2 × 8	Incline bench reverse crunch 4 × 6-8	Reverse crunch 2 × 15-20	Stability ball pike rollout 3 × 8-12

> *continued*

Table 16.5   *> continued*

DAY A: LOWER BODY AND CORE *(continued)*

Strength zone	Exercise name	Page number	Workout 1: reload (sets × reps or time)	Workouts 2 and 5 (sets × reps or time)	Workouts 3 and 6 (sets × reps or time)	Workouts 4 and 7 (sets × reps or time)
Hamstrings: knee flexion for the shortened to mid-range	2a. Hamstring exercise indicated	128	Stability ball leg curl 2 × 10-15	Nordic hamstring curl 4 × 5-8	Stability ball leg curl 2 × 25-30	Stability ball one-leg curl 3 × 12-15 each side
Core: lateral	2b. Cable one-arm side bend	204	2 × 8-10 each side	4 × 8-10 each side	2 × 20-25 each side	3 × 12-15 each side
Quads: knee extension for the shortened to midrange	3a. NT Loop inverted leg extension exercise indicated	151	NT Loop inverted leg extension 2 × 10-12	NT Loop inverted leg extension 3 × 12-15	NT Loop feet-elevated inverted leg extension 4 × 6-10	NT Loop inverted leg extension 2 × 20-25
Core: rotational	3b. Cable same-side one-arm press	214	2 × 10-12 each side	3 × 12-15 each side	4 × 8-10 each side	2 × 20-25 each side
Calves: straight knee	4a. Dumbbell foot-elevated calf raise	181	2 × 12-15 each side	2 × 25-30 each side	3 × 15 each side	4 × 8-12 each side
Hips: abduction	4b. Hip abduction exercise indicated	171	Weight plate side-lying hip abduction 2 × 10-12 each side	Weight plate side-lying hip abduction 2 × 20-30 each side	Dynamic bent-knee side elbow plank with hip adduction 3 × 12-15 each side	Dynamic side elbow plank with hip abduction 4 × 6-10 each side

DAY B: UPPER BODY

Strength zone	Exercise name	Page number	Workout 1: reload (sets × reps or time)	Workouts 2 and 5 (sets × reps or time)	Workouts 3 and 6 (sets × reps or time)	Workouts 4 and 7 (sets × reps or time)
Lats: vertical or diagonal pulling with arms outside for the lengthened to midrange	1a. Pull-up (assisted if needed with band or machine)	48	2 × 8-10	2 × 20-25	3 × 10-12	4 × 5-8
Traps: scapular elevation	1b. Barbell wide-grip shrug	89	2 × 8-10	2 × 20-25	3 × 12-15	4 × 8-10
Lats: horizontal pulling for the shortened to midrange	2a. Barbell bent-over row	59	2 × 10-12	2 × 20-25	3 × 10-15	4 × 6-8
Chest: incline pressing for the lengthened to midrange	2b. Dumbbell incline bench press	34	2 × 10-12	2 × 20-25	3 × 10-15	4 × 6-8

DAY B: UPPER BODY *(continued)*

Strength zone	Exercise name	Page number	Workout 1: reload (sets × reps or time)	Workouts 2 and 5 (sets × reps or time)	Workouts 3 and 6 (sets × reps or time)	Workouts 4 and 7 (sets × reps or time)
Biceps: lengthened to midrange	3a. Dumbbell incline bench one-arm preacher curl	101	2 × 10-12 each side	4 × 8-10 each side	2 × 20-25 each side	3 × 12-15 each side
Middle and rear delts: shortened to midrange	3b. Dumbbell incline bench 45-degree row	70	2 × 10-12	4 × 8-10	2 × 20-25	3 × 12-15
Triceps: shortened to midrange	4. Machine triceps extension	117	2 × 10-12	3 × 12-15	4 × 8-10	2 × 20-25

DAY C: LOWER BODY AND CORE

Strength zone	Exercise name	Page number	Workout 1: reload (sets × reps or time)	Workouts 2 and 5 (sets × reps or time)	Workouts 3 and 6 (sets × reps or time)	Workouts 4 and 7 (sets × reps or time)
*Quads and glutes: knee bending for the lengthened to midrange	1a. Barbell squat	134	2 × 8-10	3 × 10-15	4 × 6-8	2 × 20-25
Core: linear	1b. Core exercise indicated	192	Stability ball rollout 2 × 8-10	Ab wheel rollout 3 × 12-15	Arm walkout 4 × 5-8	Stability ball rollout 2 × 20-25
Glutes: hip extension for the shortened to midrange	2a. 45-degree hip extension	166	2 × 10-12	3 × 12-15	4 × 6-10	2 × 20-30
Hips: adduction	2b. NT Loop quadruped hip adduction	176	2 × 10-12 each side	3 × 12-15 each side	4 × 8-10 each side	2 × 20 each side
Calves: bent knee	3a. Dumbbell one-leg seated calf raise	184	2 × 10-12 each side	2 × 25-30 each side	3 × 15 each side	4 × 8-12 each side
Core: lateral	3b. Off-bench lateral hold	203	2 × 10-15 sec each side	2 × 30 sec each side	3 × 20 sec each side	4 × 10-15 sec each side
Core: rotational	4. Cable three-point horizontal chop	209	2 × 6-8 each position, each side	4 × 6-8 each position, each side	2 × 12-15 each position, each side	3 × 10 each position, each side

DAY D: UPPER BODY

Strength zone	Exercise name	Page number	Workout 1: reload (sets × reps or time)	Workouts 2 and 5 (sets × reps or time)	Workouts 3 and 6 (sets × reps or time)	Workouts 4 and 7 (sets × reps or time)
Lats: vertical or diagonal pulling with arms inside for the lengthened to midrange	1a. Cable one-arm half-kneeling neutral-grip lat pull-down	56	2 × 10-12 each side	3 × 12-15 each side	4 × 8-10 each side	2 × 20-25 each side

> *continued*

Table 16.5 *> continued*

			DAY D: UPPER BODY *(continued)*			
Strength zone	**Exercise name**	**Page number**	**Workout 1: reload (sets × reps or time)**	**Workouts 2 and 5 (sets × reps or time)**	**Workouts 3 and 6 (sets × reps or time)**	**Workouts 4 and 7 (sets × reps or time)**
Chest: horizontal or diagonal shoulder adduction for the shortened to mid-range	1b. Cable one-arm horizontal pec fly	39	2 × 10-12 each side	3 × 12-15 each side	4 × 8-10 each side	2 × 20-25 each side
Chest: horizontal or decline pressing for the lengthened to midrange	2a. Dumbbell decline hip bridge press	27	2 × 10-12	3 × 12-15	4 × 6-8	2 × 20-25
Traps: scapular retraction	2b. Dumbbell bench one-arm horizontal shrug	92	2 × 10-12 each side	3 × 12-15 each side	4 × 8-10 each side	2 × 20-25 each side
Middle delts: length-ened to midrange	3a. NT Loop side shoulder raise	77	2 × 10-12 each side	2 × 20-25 each side	3 × 12-15 each side	4 × 6-10 each side
Triceps: lengthened to midrange	3b. NT Loop overhead tri-ceps press	111	2 × 10-12	2 × 20-25	3 × 12-15	4 × 6-8
Biceps: shortened to midrange	4a. Dumbbell incline bench biceps curl	104	2 × 10-12	4 × 6-8	2 × 20-25	3 × 12-15
Rear delts: length-ened to midrange	4b. NT Loop Mini rear-delt fly	84	2 × 10-12 each side	4 × 8-10 each side	2 × 20-25 each side	3 × 12-15 each side

Rest 30 seconds between exercises and 1 to 2 minutes between paired sets or tri-sets.

*As mentioned in chapter 11, due to their multijoint nature, all exercises such as squats, Romanian deadlifts, lunges, step-ups and many varia-tions of those exercises provided in chapters 9 and 10 also load your glutes when they're closer to a lengthened (stretched) range.

CHAPTER 17

Programs for Five or Six Workouts per Week

The workout programs featured in the chapter are designed for people who prefer to work out five or six times per week. If you enjoy bodybuilding-style workouts that involve body-part split training, this workout programming chapter has your name on it! These programs differ from the earlier programs because they create more overall training volume (i.e., number of exercises, total sets and reps) per muscle group per week.

Program Guidelines

The following is a list of key points to remember and follow in order to strength train smart and get the most of out the workout programs in the chapter.

Rest

- Perform the exercises designated with *a* or *b* as paired sets, and perform exercises with *a*, *b*, and *c* as tri-sets. Perform all reps in each set before moving to the next set. Completing 1 round of the exercises in a paired or tri-set is considered 1 set.
- Rest 30 seconds between exercise in a given paired set and tri-set.
- Rest 1 to 2 minutes between each round of a given paired set and tri-set.

Reps

- The rep range (e.g., 10-15 reps) is next to each exercise in the workout. If you're using the same weight for each set, you may be able to do 15 reps on the first set, 12 reps on the next set, and 10 reps on the third because of accumulated fatigue. Or you can reduce the weight you're using with each consecutive set to achieve the higher end or given rep range on each consecutive set. Both methods are effective in helping you to progress.
- Maintain strict form without cheating by using additional movements or momentum.
- Mentally focus on the working muscles in each exercise.

- Do the concentric (lifting) portion of each rep at a normal tempo and maintain strict control during the eccentric (lowering) portion. Take roughly 3 seconds on the eccentric portion of each rep.

Weight

- Use a weight load that's light enough to allow you to achieve the minimum number of reps indicated for each exercise.
- Use a weight load heavy enough that you're unable to perform any more reps than the maximum number indicated for each exercise while maintaining proper control and technique.

Work Around—Not Through—Injuries and Limitations

- If an exercise causes pain or discomfort beyond the sensation associated with muscle fatigue, use an alternative exercise that doesn't hurt that targets the same muscle group in the same strength zone.
- Not every exercise movement is for everybody. There are plenty of movements in the exercise chapters of this book to choose from.

Program Setup

Two types of programs appear in this chapter: a three-day split (training three days in a row with the fourth day off; see tables 17.1-17.5) and a four-day split (training four days in a row with the fifth day off; see tables 17.6-17.10). There are five programs for each type.

The three-day split rotates through workouts focusing on the following:

1. Lower body and core (day A)
2. Back, triceps, middle delts, and traps (day B)
3. Chest, biceps, rear delts (day C)
4. Rest day

Repeat sequence starting again with day A.

You'll always perform the workouts in order: A, B, and C. There are five programs in all.

The four-day split rotates through workouts focusing on the following:

1. Glute and hamstring focus for lower body and core (day A)
2. Pressing, pulling, and traps (day B)
3. Quad and calf focus for lower body and core (day C)
4. Biceps, triceps, and shoulders (day D)
5. Rest day

Repeat sequence starting again with day A.

You'll always perform the workouts in order: A, B, C, and D. There are five programs for the four-day split.

A three-day split or four-day split doesn't mean you're only training three or four days per week. In both the three- and four-day splits, you're using strength training workouts five or six times per week. Here's the weekly setup for using the three-day and four-day split programs in this chapter.

Weekly Setup for Three-Day Split

Week 1

Monday: Day A – Workout 1	Friday: Day A – Workout 2
Tuesday: Day B – Workout 1	Saturday: Day B – Workout 2
Wednesday: Day C – Workout 1	Sunday: Day C – Workout 2
Thursday: Rest	

Week 2

Monday: Rest	Friday: Rest
Tuesday: Day A – Workout 3	Saturday: Day A – Workout 4
Wednesday: Day B – Workout 3	Sunday: Day B – Workout 4
Thursday: Day C – Workout 3	

Week 3

Monday: Day C – Workout 4	Friday: Day C – Workout 5
Tuesday: Rest	Saturday: Rest
Wednesday: Day A – Workout 5	Sunday: Day A – Workout 6
Thursday: Day B – Workout 5	

Continue the sequence on week 4, starting with day B, workout 6 on Monday and so on.

Weekly Setup for Four-Day Split

Week 1

Monday: Day A – Workout 1	Friday: Rest
Tuesday: Day B – Workout 1	Saturday: Day A – Workout 2
Wednesday: Day C – Workout 1	Sunday: Day B – Workout 2
Thursday: Day D – Workout 1	

Week 2

Monday: Day C – Workout 2	Friday: Day B – Workout 3
Tuesday: Day D – Workout 2	Saturday: Day C – Workout 3
Wednesday: Rest	Sunday: Day D – Workout 3
Thursday: Day A – Workout 3	

Week 3

Monday: Day A – Workout 4	Friday: Rest
Tuesday: Day B – Workout 4	Saturday: Day A – Workout 5
Wednesday: Day C – Workout 4	Sunday: Day B – Workout 5
Thursday: Day D – Workout 4	

Continue the sequence on week 4, starting with day C, workout 5 on Monday and so on.

Each time you complete day A through day C, or day A through day D, it equals one time through the workouts. You'll perform each of the five total three-day split programs, or the five total four-day split programs for seven times through each workout before switching to the next program and repeating those workouts for another seven times.

Rest Days

Your non-strength-training days, which are indicated as rest days in the sample weekly training setups, don't mean you have to do nothing. During your days off from using the smarter strength training workouts, you can do low-impact activities, such as going for long walks, hikes, bike rides, or swims. Yoga can also be a great option for your active rest days.

Reload Workouts

The first time you do each workout in a program, it's considered a reload workout. A reload workout is simply a lower-intensity version of the workout, which helps you to stay active while recovering between programs. It also acclimates you to the movements and gives you an idea of the appropriate weight loads (based on your strength level) to use for the new program you're starting.

Mixed Sets and Reps for Maximal Results

The training system and workout programs in this book enable you to incorporate the right blend of exercises to achieve strength through the true full range of motion. They also include a full spectrum of set and repetition ranges. This variety is the reason that they can be so effective in helping you get stronger.

Research has shown that daily variations in intensity and volume (sets and reps) are more effective than weekly volume variations for increases in maximal strength; they may also lead to greater gains in muscle size (1, 2, 3, 4).

In short, it's best to think about the types of strength training exercise—and the sets and reps you use—in the same way that you think about your nutrition: Make sure to get enough variety, because each type offers unique training or nutritional value.

Warm Up and Build Up

Before you begin a workout in the following programs, be sure to perform a general warm-up. Also make sure to perform build-up sets, which are simply lighter, less intense versions of whatever exercises you're getting ready to perform with heavier loads. Build-up sets are used to gradually build up to your working intensity. For example, if you're going to perform a heavy lift, you first do a few lighter sets of that lift in order to build up to your working weight. As a rule of thumb, if the workout program calls for four sets of an exercise, you'll do two build-up sets. If the workout program calls for 3 sets of a given exercise, you'll perform 1 build-up set because it involves using lighter loads than when you're performing 4 sets for fewer reps. And because the times you'll be performing only 2 sets of a given exercise involve using lighter loads (because of the higher reps), there's no need to perform a build-up set to get into your working weight.

Why No Exercises for Front Delts?

In each of the following programs, even though there is no strength zone exercise category listed for the front delts, there are multiple exercises included to strengthen your front delts through the true full range of motion.

As mentioned in chapter 3, the front delts are worked during decline, horizontal, and diagonal pressing exercises. More specifically, these pressing exercises strengthen your front delts in the lengthened-to-midrange strength zone. While many of the exercises in chapter 5 are for the shortened-to-midrange strength zone for your middle delts, they also strengthen your front delts in the shortened-to-midrange strength zone.

TABLE 17.1   Program 1, Three-Day Split

DAY A: LOWER BODY AND CORE

Strength zone	Exercise name	Page number	Workout 1: reload (sets × reps or time)	Workouts 2 and 5 (sets × reps or time)	Workouts 3 and 6 (sets × reps or time)	Workouts 4 and 7 (sets × reps or time)
*Glutes and hamstrings: hip hinging for the lengthened to midrange	1a. Barbell elevated Romanian deadlift	120	2 × 10-12	4 × 5-8	2 × 20-30	3 × 10-15
Core: linear	1b. Stability ball plate crunch	196	2 × 8-10	4 × 6-8	2 × 15-20	3 × 10-12
*Quads and glutes: knee bending for the lengthened to midrange	2a. Dumbbell traveling lunge	139	2 × 8-10 each side	4 × 5-8 each side	2 × 20-25 each side	3 × 12-15 each side
Calves: bent knee	2b. Dumbbell half-kneeling calf raise	183	2 × 8-10 each side	4 × 8-10 each side	2 × 25-30 each side	3 × 15-20 each side
Glutes: hip extension for the shortened to midrange	3a. Cable one-leg Romanian deadlift	163	2 × 8-12 each side	3 × 10-15 each side	4 × 6-8 each side	2 × 20-25 each side
Core: rotational	3b. Cable three-point high-to-low chop	210	2 × 6 in each position, each side	3 × 10-12 in each position, each side	4 × 6-8 in each position, each side	2 × 15 in each position, each side
Hamstrings: knee flexion for the shortened to midrange	4a. Machine seated leg curl	125	2 × 10-12	3 × 10-15	4 × 6-8	2 × 20-30
Hips: abduction Core: lateral	4b. Hip and core exercise indicated	172	Dynamic bent-knee side elbow plank with hip abduction 2 × 8-10 each side	Dynamic bent-knee side elbow plank with hip abduction 3 × 10-15	Dynamic side elbow plank with hip abduction 4 × 6-8 each side	Dynamic bent-knee side elbow plank with hip abduction 2 × 20-30

> continued

Table 17.1 > *continued*

DAY A: LOWER BODY AND CORE *(continued)*

Strength zone	Exercise name	Page number	Workout 1: reload (sets × reps or time)	Workouts 2 and 5 (sets × reps or time)	Workouts 3 and 6 (sets × reps or time)	Workouts 4 and 7 (sets × reps or time)
Quads: knee extension for the shortened to midrange	5a. Machine leg extension	147	2 × 10-12	2 × 20-25	3 × 12-15	4 × 6-8
Calves: straight knee	5b. Dumbbell traveling calf raise	180	2 × 20 sec	2 × 50 sec	3 × 40 sec	4 × 30 sec
Hips: adduction	5c. Side-lying hip adduction	174	2 × 10 each side	2 × 20-25 each side	3 × 12-15 (1 sec hold at top each rep) each side	4 × 6-8 (3 sec hold at top each rep) each side

DAY B: BACK, TRICEPS, MIDDLE DELTS, TRAPS

Strength zone	Exercise name	Page number	Workout 1: reload (sets × reps or time)	Workouts 2 and 5 (sets × reps or time)	Workouts 3 and 6 (sets × reps or time)	Workouts 4 and 7 (sets × reps or time)
Lats: vertical or diagonal pulling with arms inside for the lengthened to midrange	1a. Chin-up (assisted if needed)	53	2 × 6-8	2 × 20	3 × 10-15	4 × 5-8
Triceps: shortened to midrange	1b. Dumbbell triceps skull crusher	112	2 × 10-12	2 × 20-25	3 × 12-15	4 × 6-8
Lats: horizontal pulling for the shortened to midrange	2a. Cable one-arm row	62	2 × 10-12 each side	2 × 20-25 each side	3 × 10-15 each side	4 × 6-8 each side
Middle delts: lengthened to midrange	2b. Cable side shoulder raise	75	2 × 10-12 each side	2 × 20-25 each side	3 × 12-15 each side	4 × 6-8 each side
Traps: scapular elevation	3a. Cable wide-grip angled upright row	88	2 × 10-12	4 × 6-8	3 × 12-15	2 × 20-25
Triceps: lengthened to midrange	3b. Cable rope overhead triceps extension	108	2 × 10-12	4 × 6-8	3 × 12-15	2 × 20-25
Middle delts: shortened to midrange	4a. Dumbbell rotational overhead press	73	2 × 10-12 each side	4 × 6-8 each side	2 × 16-20 each side	3 × 10-12 each side
Traps: scapular retraction	4b. Machine row horizontal shrug	94	2 × 8-10	4 × 8-10	2 × 25-30	3 × 15-20

DAY B: BACK, TRICEPS, MIDDLE DELTS, TRAPS *(continued)*

Strength zone	Exercise name	Page number	Workout 1: reload (sets × reps or time)	Workouts 2 and 5 (sets × reps or time)	Workouts 3 and 6 (sets × reps or time)	Workouts 4 and 7 (sets × reps or time)
Lats: vertical or diagonal pulling with arms outside for the lengthened to midrange	5. One-arm lat pull-down	50	2 × 10-12 each side	4 × 6-8 each side	2 × 16-20 each side	3 × 10-12 each side

DAY C: CHEST, BICEPS, REAR DELTS

Strength zone	Exercise name	Page number	Workout 1: reload (sets × reps or time)	Workouts 2 and 5 (sets × reps or time)	Workouts 3 and 6 (sets × reps or time)	Workouts 4 and 7 (sets × reps or time)
Chest: horizontal or decline pressing for the lengthened to midrange	1a. Machine chest press	28	2 × 10-12	3 × 10-15	4 × 6-8	2 × 20-25
Rear delts: lengthened to midrange	1b. NT Loop Mini rear-delt fly	84	2 × 10-12 each side	3 × 10-15 each side	4 × 6-8 each side	2 × 20 each side
Chest: incline pressing for the lengthened to midrange	2a. Dumbbell incline bench press	34	2 × 10-12	2 × 20-25	3 × 12-15	4 × 8-10
Rear delts: shortened to midrange	2b. Dumbbell face pull	79	2 × 10-12	2 × 20-25	3 × 12-15	4 × 6-8
Biceps: lengthened to midrange	3a. Cable one-arm face-away biceps curl	99	2 × 10-12 each side	3 × 12-15 each side	4 × 6-8 each side	2 × 20-25 each side
Chest: horizontal or diagonal shoulder adduction for the shortened to midrange	3b. NT Loop one-arm pec deck fly	41	2 × 10-12 each side	3 × 10-15 each side	4 × 6-8 each side	2 × 20-25 each side
Biceps: shortened to midrange	4a. Cable EZ-bar biceps curl	105	2 × 10-12	4 × 6-8	3 × 10-12	2 × 15-20
**Lats: vertical or diagonal pulling with arms outside for the lengthened to midrange	4b. Cable one-arm half-kneeling lat pull-down	50	2 × 10-12 each side	4 × 6-8 each side	3 × 12-15 each side	2 × 20-25 each side

Rest 30 seconds between exercises and 1 to 2 minutes between paired sets or tri-sets.

*As mentioned in chapter 11, due to their multijoint nature, all exercises such as squats, Romanian deadlifts, lunges, step-ups and many variations of those exercises provided in chapters 9 and 10 also load your glutes when they're closer to a lengthened (stretched) range.

**This exercise is included in this workout to balance out the total workout time of each workout.

TABLE 17.2   Program 2, Three-Day Split

			DAY A: LOWER BODY AND CORE			
Strength zone	**Exercise name**	**Page number**	**Workout 1: reload (sets × reps or time)**	**Workouts 2 and 5 (sets × reps or time)**	**Workouts 3 and 6 (sets × reps or time)**	**Workouts 4 and 7 (sets × reps or time)**
*Quads and glutes: knee bending for the lengthened to midrange	1a. Dumbbell reverse lunge with NT Loop knee resistance	140	2 × 6-8 each side	4 × 5-8 each side	2 × 20-25 each side	3 × 12-15 each side
Calves: bent knee	1b. Machine seated calf raise	185	2 × 10-12	4 × 6-8	2 × 25-30	3 × 12-15
*Glutes and hamstrings: hip hinging for the lengthened to midrange	2a. Dumbbell traveling Romanian deadlift lunge	122	2 × 10-12 each side	4 × 5-8 each side	2 × 17-20 each side	3 × 10-12 each side
Core: linear	2b. Core exercise indicated	192	Reverse crunch 2 × 8-10	Incline bench reverse crunch 4 × 6-8	Stability ball knee tuck 2 × 20-30	Reverse crunch 3 × 10-15
Quads: knee extension for the shortened to midrange	3a. Reverse sled drag	148	2 × 40 yards (36 m)	3 × 60-70 yards (55-64 m)	4 × 40 yards (36 m)	2 × 100 yards (91 m)
Core: lateral	3b. Angled-barbell tight rainbow	201	2 × 10 each side	3 × 12-15 each side	4 × 8-10 each side	2 × 20 each side
Glutes: hip extension for the shortened to midrange	4a. 45-degree hip extension	166	2 × 8-10	3 × 12-15	4 × 6-10	2 × 20-25
Core: rotational	4b. Dumbbell plank row	207	2 × 5-6 each side	3 × 9-10 each side	4 × 5-7 each side	2 × 12-15 each side
Hamstrings: knee flexion for the shortened to midrange	5a. Machine lying leg curl	127	2 × 10-12	2 × 20-30	3 × 10-15	4 × 6-8
Hips: abduction	5b. Band lateral hip shuffle	170	2 × 15 each side	2 × 30 each side	3 × 20 each side	4 × 15 each side
Calves: straight knee	6a. Dumbbell one-leg leaning calf raise	180	2 × 10-12 each side	2 × 25-30 each side	3 × 15-20 each side	4 × 10-12 each side
Hips: adduction	6b. Bent-knee Copenhagen hip adduction	174	2 × 6-8 each side	2 × 15 each side	3 × 10 (pause 1 sec at top of each rep) each side	4 × 5-8 (pause 2 sec at top of each rep) each side

DAY B: BACK, TRICEPS, MIDDLE DELTS, TRAPS

Strength zone	Exercise name	Page number	Workout 1: reload (sets × reps or time)	Workouts 2 and 5 (sets × reps or time)	Workouts 3 and 6 (sets × reps or time)	Workouts 4 and 7 (sets × reps or time)
Lats: horizontal pulling for the shortened to midrange	1a. Dumbbell one-arm bench row	61	2 × 10-12 each side	2 × 15-20 each side	3 × 10-12 each side	4 × 6-8 each side
Middle delts: lengthened to midrange	1b. Dumbbell side-lying side shoulder raise	76	2 × 10-12 each side	2 × 20-25 each side	3 × 12-15 each side	4 × 6-8 each side
Lats: vertical or diagonal pulling with arms outside for the lengthened to midrange	2a. Lat pull-down	49	2 × 10-12	4 × 5-8	2 × 20-25	3 × 12-15
Triceps: shortened to midrange	2b. NT Loop one-arm triceps kickback	116	2 × 10-12 each side	4 × 6-8 each side	2 × 20-25 each side	3 × 12-15 each side
Lats: vertical or diagonal pulling with arms inside for the lengthened to midrange	3a. Cable straight-arm compound pull-down	57	2 × 10-12	4 × 8-10	2 × 20	3 × 12-15
Traps: scapular retraction	3b. Cable one-arm horizontal shrug	93	2 × 20 each side	4 × 8-10 each side	2 × 20 each side	3 × 12-15 each side
Triceps: lengthened to midrange	4a. Kettlebell behind-the-head triceps extension	109	2 × 10-12	2 × 20-25	3 × 12-15	4 × 6-8
Middle delts: shortened to midrange	4b. Kettlebell shoulder-to-shoulder press	73	2 × 5-6 each side	2 × 16-20 each side	3 × 10-12 each side	4 × 6-8 each side
Traps: scapular elevation	5. Barbell wide-grip shrug	89	2 × 10-12	3 × 15	4 × 6-8	2 × 25-30

DAY C: CHEST, BICEPS, REAR DELTS

Strength zone	Exercise name	Page number	Workout 1: reload (sets × reps or time)	Workouts 2 and 5 (sets × reps or time)	Workouts 3 and 6 (sets × reps or time)	Workouts 4 and 7 (sets × reps or time)
Chest: incline pressing for the lengthened to midrange	1a. Angled-barbell one-arm press	36	2 × 8-10 each side	3 × 12-15 each side	4 × 5-8 each side	2 × 20-25 each side
Biceps: shortened to midrange	1b. Dumbbell standing biceps curl	103	2 × 8-10	3 × 12-15	4 × 6-8 each side	2 × 20-25

> continued

Table 17.2   > *continued*

			DAY C: CHEST, BICEPS, REAR DELTS *(continued)*			
Strength zone	**Exercise name**	**Page number**	**Workout 1: reload (sets × reps or time)**	**Workouts 2 and 5 (sets × reps or time)**	**Workouts 3 and 6 (sets × reps or time)**	**Workouts 4 and 7 (sets × reps or time)**
Chest: horizontal or decline pressing for the lengthened to midrange	2a. Push-up exercise indicated	29	Push-up 2 × 10-15	Box crossover push-up 3 × max reps	NT Loop resisted push-up 4 × max reps	Push-up 2 × max reps
Rear delts: lengthened to midrange	2b. Machine rear-delt fly	84	2 × 10-12	3 × 12-15	4 × 6-8	2 × 20-25
Chest: horizontal or diagonal shoulder adduction for the shortened to midrange	3a. Dumbbell squeeze press	38	2 × 10-12	2 × 20-25	3 × 12-15	4 × 8-10
Rear delts: shortened to midrange	3b. Dumbbell rear-delt fly	78	2 × 10-12	2 × 20-25	3 × 12-15	4 × 8-10
Biceps: lengthened to midrange	4. EZ-bar preacher curl	100	2 × 10-12	2 × 20-25	3 × 12-15	4 × 6-8

Rest 30 seconds between exercises and 1 to 2 minutes between paired sets or tri-sets.

*As mentioned in chapter 11, due to their multijoint nature, all exercises such as squats, Romanian deadlifts, lunges, step-ups and many variations of those exercises provided in chapters 9 and 10 also load your glutes when they're closer to a lengthened (stretched) range.

TABLE 17.3   Program 3, Three-Day Split

			DAY A: LOWER BODY AND CORE			
Strength zone	**Exercise name**	**Page number**	**Workout 1: reload (sets × reps or time)**	**Workouts 2 and 5 (sets × reps or time)**	**Workouts 3 and 6 (sets × reps or time)**	**Workouts 4 and 7 (sets × reps or time)**
*Glutes and hamstrings: hip hinging for the lengthened to midrange	1a. Angled-barbell leaning Romanian deadlift	124	2 × 8-10 each side	4 × 6-8 each side	2 × 17-20 each side	3 × 10-12 each side
Core: rotational	1b. Cable one-arm press	213	2 × 6-8 each side	4 × 6-8 each side	2 × 17-20 each side	3 × 10-12 each side
*Quads and glutes: knee bending for the lengthened to midrange	2a. Dumbbell step-up	139	2 × 8-10 each side	4 × 6-8 each side	2 × 20-25 each side	3 × 12-15 each side
Calves: bent knee	2b. Dumbbell one-leg seated calf raise	184	2 × 10-12 each side	4 × 8-10 each side	2 × 25-30 each side	3 × 15 each side
Quads: knee extension for the shortened to midrange	3a. Machine unilateral leg extension	148	2 × 10-12 each side	3 × 12-15 each side	4 × 6-8 each side	2 × 20-25 each side
Core: lateral	3b. Weight plate around the world	206	2 × 6-8	3 × 8 each side	4 × 5 each side	2 × 10-12 each side

DAY A: LOWER BODY AND CORE *(continued)*

Strength zone	Exercise name	Page number	Workout 1: reload (sets × reps or time)	Workouts 2 and 5 (sets × reps or time)	Workouts 3 and 6 (sets × reps or time)	Workouts 4 and 7 (sets × reps or time)
Hamstrings: knee flexion for the shortened to midrange	4a. Hamstring exercise indicated	128	Stability ball leg curl 2 × 10-15	Stability ball one-leg curl 3 × 12-15	Nordic hamstring curl 4 × 4-6	Stability ball leg curl 2 × 20-30
Hips: abduction	4b. Machine seated hip abduction	169	2 × 10-12	3 × 12-15	4 × 6-8	2 × 25-30
Calves: straight knee	4c. Dumbbell foot-elevated calf raise	181	2 × 10-12 each side	3 × 12-15 each side	4 × 6-8 each side	2 × 25-30 each side
Core: linear	5a. Core exercise indicated	194	Stability ball knee tuck 2 × 12-15	Stability ball rollout 3 × 12-15	Stability ball pike rollout 4 × 6-8	Stability ball knee tuck 2 × 20-30
Hips: adduction	5b. NT Loop quadruped hip adduction	176	2 × 10 each side	2 × 20 each side	3 × 12 each side	4 × 8 each side
Glutes: hip extension for the shortened to midrange	5c. NT Loop glute walk	168	2 × 30 sec	2 × 60 sec (use light band tension)	3 × 45 sec (use medium band tension)	4 × 30 sec (use heavy band tension)

DAY B: BACK, TRICEPS, MIDDLE DELTS, TRAPS

Strength zone	Exercise name	Page number	Workout 1: reload (sets × reps or time)	Workouts 2 and 5 (sets × reps or time)	Workouts 3 and 6 (sets × reps or time)	Workouts 4 and 7 (sets × reps or time)
Lats: horizontal pulling for the shortened to midrange	1a. Dumbbell one-arm off-bench row	61	2 × 10-12 each side	2 × 20 each side	3 × 12-15 each side	4 × 6-8 each side
Middle delts: shortened to midrange	1b. Machine overhead press	75	2 × 10-12	2 × 20-25	3 × 10-15	4 × 6-8
Lats: vertical or diagonal pulling with arms outside for the lengthened to midrange	2a. Cable fighters lat pull-down	51	2 × 10-12 each side	2 × 20-24 each side	3 × 12-15 each side	4 × 6-8 each side
Middle delts: lengthened to midrange	2b. Cable side shoulder raise	75	2 × 10-12 each side	2 × 20-25 each side	3 × 12-15 each side	4 × 6-8 each side
Triceps: lengthened to midrange	3a. Cable rope overhead triceps extension	108	2 × 10-12	4 × 6-8	2 × 20-25	3 × 12-15
Lats: vertical or diagonal pulling with arms inside for the lengthened to midrange	3b. Cable straight-arm compound pull-down	57	2 × 10-12	4 × 8-10	2 × 20-25	3 × 12-15

> continued

Table 17.3 *> continued*

DAY B: BACK, TRICEPS, MIDDLE DELTS, TRAPS *(continued)*

Strength zone	Exercise name	Page number	Workout 1: reload (sets × reps or time)	Workouts 2 and 5 (sets × reps or time)	Workouts 3 and 6 (sets × reps or time)	Workouts 4 and 7 (sets × reps or time)
Triceps: shortened to midrange	4a. Suspension trainer skull crusher	114	2 × 10-12	4 × 6-8	2 × 20-25	3 × 12-15
Traps: scapular retraction	4b. Suspension trainer horizontal shrug	94	2 × 10-12	4 × 10-12	2 × 30	3 × 20
Traps: scapular elevation	5. Cable wide-grip angled upright row	88	2 × 10	3 × 15-20	4 × 10-12	2 × 25-30

DAY C: CHEST, BICEPS, REAR DELTS

Strength zone	Exercise name	Page number	Workout 1: reload (sets × reps or time)	Workouts 2 and 5 (sets × reps or time)	Workouts 3 and 6 (sets × reps or time)	Workouts 4 and 7 (sets × reps or time)
Chest: horizontal or decline pressing for the lengthened to midrange	1a. Dumbbell bench press	26	2 × 10-12	3 × 12-15	4 × 5-8	2 × 20-25
Rear delts: shortened to midrange	1b. Dumbbell 45-degree row	71	2 × 12-15	3 × 15	4 × 8-10	2 × 20-25
Chest: incline pressing for the lengthened to midrange	2a. Machine incline chest press	37	2 × 10-12	3 × 10-15	4 × 6-8	2 × 20-25
Biceps: shortened to midrange	2b. Cable EZ-bar biceps curl	105	2 × 10-12	3 × 10-15	4 × 6-8	2 × 20-25
Biceps: lengthened to midrange	3a. Cable one-arm face-away biceps curl	99	2 × 10-12 each side	2 × 20-25 each side	3 × 12-15 each side	4 × 6-8 each side
Rear delts: lengthened to midrange	3b. Low-cable rear-delt fly	82	2 × 10-12 each side	2 × 20-25 each side	3 × 12-15 each side	4 × 6-8 each side
Chest: horizontal or diagonal shoulder adduction for the shortened to midrange	4. Cable crossover pec fly	41	2 × 10-12	4 × 8-10	3 × 12-15	2 × 20-25

Rest 30 seconds between exercises and 1 to 2 minutes between paired sets or tri-sets.

*As mentioned in chapter 11, due to their multijoint nature, all exercises such as squats, Romanian deadlifts, lunges, step-ups and many variations of those exercises provided in chapters 9 and 10 also load your glutes when they're closer to a lengthened (stretched) range.

TABLE 17.4   Program 4, Three-Day Split

DAY A: LOWER BODY AND CORE

Strength zone	Exercise name	Page number	Workout 1: reload (sets × reps or time)	Workouts 2 and 5 (sets × reps or time)	Workouts 3 and 6 (sets × reps or time)	Workouts 4 and 7 (sets × reps or time)
*Quads and glutes: knee bending for the lengthened to midrange	1a. Trap bar squat	136	2 × 8-10	4 × 5-8	2 × 20	3 × 12-15
Core: linear	1b. Reverse crunch	198	2 × 8-10 each side	4 × 8-10 each side	2 × 20 each side	3 × 12-15 each side
*Glutes and hamstrings: hip hinging for the lengthened to midrange	2a. Dumbbell one-leg one-arm Romanian deadlift	123	2 × 10-12 each side	4 × 6-8 each side	2 × 20 each side	3 × 10-15 each side
Quads: knee extension for the shortened to midrange	2b. NT Loop inverted leg extension	151	2 × 30 yards (27 m) each leg	4 × 20-30 yards (18-27 m) each leg	2 × 80 yards (73 m) each leg	3 × 50-60 yards (46-55 m) each leg
Hamstrings: knee flexion for the shortened to midrange	3a. Machine seated one-leg curl	126	2 × 8-10 each side	3 × 10-15 each side	4 × 6-8 each side	2 × 20-25 each side
Core: lateral	3b. Angled-barbell tight rainbow	201	2 × 8-10 each side	3 × 12-15 each side	4 × 8-10 each side	2 × 20-25 each side
Calves: straight knee	4a. Machine ankles-together calf raise	182	2 × 10-12	3 × 15-20	4 × 8-12	2 × 25-30
Glutes: hip extension for the shortened to midrange	4b. Hip extension exercise indicated	166	Weight plate one-leg hip lift 2 × 15	Weight plate one-leg hip bridge 3 × 15-20 each side	Weight plate one-leg hip lift 4 × 8-10 each side	Stability ball reverse hip extension 2 × 25-30
Hips: adduction	5a. Machine seated hip adduction	175	2 × 10-12	2 × 25	3 × 15	4 × 8-10
Calves: bent knee	5b. Dumbbell half-kneeling calf raise	183	2 × 10-12 each side	2 × 30 each side	3 × 20 each side	4 × 12-15 each side
Core: rotational	6. Cable three-point horizontal chop	209	2 × 6 in each position, each side	2 × 15 in each position, each side	3 × 10-12 in each position, each side	4 × 6-8 in each position, each side

> continued

Table 17.4 > *continued*

DAY B: BACK, TRICEPS, MIDDLE DELTS, TRAPS

Strength zone	Exercise name	Page number	Workout 1: reload (sets × reps or time)	Workouts 2 and 5 (sets × reps or time)	Workouts 3 and 6 (sets × reps or time)	Workouts 4 and 7 (sets × reps or time)
Lats: horizontal pulling for the shortened to midrange	1a. Machine row	64	2 × 10-12	2 × 20-25	3 × 12-15	4 × 5-8
Triceps: lengthened to midrange	1b. Dumbbell one-arm behind-the-head triceps extension	110	2 × 10-12 each side	2 × 20 each side	3 × 12-15 each side	4 × 8-10 each side
Traps: scapular retraction	2a. Machine row horizontal shrug	94	2 × 15	2 × 25-30	3 × 15-20	4 × 10-12
Middle delts: shortened to midrange	2b. Dumbbell side shoulder raise	72	2 × 8-10	2 × 20	3 × 12-15	4 × 8-10
Lats: vertical or diagonal pulling with arms outside for the lengthened to midrange	3a. Cable one-arm half-kneeling lat pull-down	50	2 × 10-12 each side	2 × 20 each side	3 × 10-15 each side	4 × 6-8 each side
Middle delts: lengthened to midrange	3b. NT Loop Mini side shoulder raise	77	2 × 10-12 each side	2 × 20-25 each side	3 × 12-15 each side	4 × 6-10 each side
Lats: vertical or diagonal pulling with arms inside for the lengthened to midrange	4a. Cable one-arm half-kneeling neutral-grip lat pull-down	56	2 × 10-12 each side	4 × 6-8 each side	2 × 20-25 each side	3 × 12-15 each side
Triceps: shortened to midrange	4b. Cable one-arm triceps kickback	115	2 × 8-10 each side	4 × 6-10 each side	2 × 20-25 each side	3 × 15 each side
Traps: scapular elevation	5. Dumbbell one-arm leaning shrug	90	2 × 10-12 each side	4 × 8-10 each side	2 × 20-30 each side	3 × 12-15 each side

DAY C: CHEST, BICEPS, REAR DELTS

Strength zone	Exercise name	Page number	Workout 1: reload (sets × reps or time)	Workouts 2 and 5 (sets × reps or time)	Workouts 3 and 6 (sets × reps or time)	Workouts 4 and 7 (sets × reps or time)
Chest: horizontal or decline pressing for the lengthened to midrange	1a. Dumbbell decline hip bridge press	27	2 × 10-12	3 × 12-15	4 × 6-8	2 × 20-25

DAY C: CHEST, BICEPS, REAR DELTS (continued)

Strength zone	Exercise name	Page number	Workout 1: reload (sets × reps or time)	Workouts 2 and 5 (sets × reps or time)	Workouts 3 and 6 (sets × reps or time)	Workouts 4 and 7 (sets × reps or time)
Rear delts: lengthened to midrange	1b. Dumbbell side-lying rear-delt fly	81	2 × 10-12 each side	3 × 12-15 each side	4 × 8-10 each side	2 × 20-25 each side
Chest: incline pressing for the lengthened to midrange	2a. Dumbbell incline bench press	34	2 × 10-12	3 × 15	4 × 6-8	2 × 20-25
Biceps: lengthened to midrange	2b. Dumbbell incline bench one-arm preacher curl	101	2 × 8-10 each side	3 × 12-15 each side	4 × 8-10 each side	2 × 20-25 each side
Rear delts: shortened to midrange	3a. Suspension trainer face pull	80	2 × 10-12	3 × 15	4 × 8-10	2 × 20-25
Biceps: shortened to midrange	3b. Dumbbell concentration biceps curl	103	2 × 8-10 each side	3 × 12-15 each side	4 × 8-10 each side	2 × 20-25 each side
Chest: horizontal or diagonal shoulder adduction for the shortened to midrange	4. Wide-cable crossover chest press	42	2 × 10-12	3 × 12-15	4 × 8-10	2 × 20-25

Rest 30 seconds between exercises and 1 to 2 minutes between paired sets or tri-sets.

*As mentioned in chapter 11, due to their multijoint nature, all exercises such as squats, Romanian deadlifts, lunges, step-ups and many variations of those exercises provided in chapters 9 and 10 also load your glutes when they're closer to a lengthened (stretched) range.

TABLE 17.5 Program 5, Three-Day Split

DAY A: LOWER BODY AND CORE

Strength zone	Exercise name	Page number	Workout 1: reload (sets × reps or time)	Workouts 2 and 5 (sets × reps or time)	Workouts 3 and 6 (sets × reps or time)	Workouts 4 and 7 (sets × reps or time)
*Glutes and hamstrings: hip hinging for the lengthened to midrange	1a. Dumbbell lateral Romanian deadlift lunge	122	2 × 8-10 each side	4 × 6-8 each side	2 × 20 each side	3 × 10-12 each side
Core: linear	1b. Band leg lowering	192	2 × 30 sec	4 × 30 sec	2 × 50 sec	3 × 40 sec
*Quads and glutes: knee bending for the lengthened to midrange	2a. Cable front-to-back split squat	142	2 × 8-10 each side	4 × 6-8 each side	2 × 20 each side	3 × 12-15 each side
Calves: straight knee	2b. Dumbbell one-leg leaning calf raise	180	2 × 10-12 each side	4 × 8-12 each side	2 × 25-30 each side	3 × 15 each side

> continued

Table 17.5 > *continued*

DAY A: LOWER BODY AND CORE (*continued*)

Strength zone	Exercise name	Page number	Workout 1: reload (sets × reps or time)	Workouts 2 and 5 (sets × reps or time)	Workouts 3 and 6 (sets × reps or time)	Workouts 4 and 7 (sets × reps or time)
Glutes: hip extension for the shortened to midrange	3a. Dumbbell one-leg hip thrust	165	2 × 10-12 each side	3 × 15 each side	4 × 8-10 each side	2 × 20-25 each side
Calves: bent knee	3b. Dumbbell one-leg seated calf raise	184	2 × 12-15 each side	3 × 20 each side	4 × 12-15 each side	2 × 25-30 each side
Core: lateral	3c. Off-bench lateral hold	203	2 × 15 sec each side	3 × 20 sec each side	4 × 15 sec each side	2 × 30 sec each side
Hamstrings: knee flexion for the shortened to midrange	4a. Hamstring exercise indicated	128	Stability ball leg curl 2 × 10-12	Stability ball one-leg curl 3 × 12-15 each side	Nordic hamstring curl 4 × 6-8	Stability ball leg curl 2 × 20-30
Quads: knee extension for the shortened to midrange	4b. Weight plate push	150	2 × 40 yards (36 m)	3 × 60-70 yards (55-64 m)	4 × 40-50 yards (36-46 m)	2 × 80-100 yards (73-91 m)
Hips: adduction	5a. Machine seated hip adduction	175	2 × 10-12	3 × 12-15	4 × 8-10	2 × 25-30
Hips: abduction	5b. Band low lateral hip shuffle	171	2 × 15 each side	3 × 20-25 each side	4 × 12-15 each side	2 × 30 each side
Core: rotational	6. Weight plate chop	215	2 × 8 each side	2 × 20 each side	3 × 12 each side	4 × 8 each side

DAY B: BACK, TRICEPS, MIDDLE DELTS, TRAPS

Strength zone	Exercise name	Page number	Workout 1: reload (sets × reps or time)	Workouts 2 and 5 (sets × reps or time)	Workouts 3 and 6 (sets × reps or time)	Workouts 4 and 7 (sets × reps or time)
Lats: vertical or diagonal pulling with arms outside for the lengthened to midrange	1a. Pull-up (can be assisted using a band or machine)	48	2 × 8-10	2 × 20-25	3 × 10-12	4 × 4-6
Middle delts: shortened to midrange	1b. Dumbbell one-arm overhead press	74	2 × 8-10 each side	2 × 20 each side	3 × 12-15 each side	4 × 6-8 each side
Lats: horizontal pulling for the shortened to midrange	2a. Seated row	64	2 × 10-12	2 × 20-25	3 × 12-15	4 × 6-8
Triceps: shortened to midrange	2b. Dumbbell triceps skull crusher	112	2 × 10-12	2 × 20-25	3 × 12-15	4 × 8-10
Middle delts: lengthened to midrange	3a. Dumbbell side-lying side shoulder raise	76	2 × 10-12 each side	4 × 8-10 each side	2 × 20 each side	3 × 12-15 each side

DAY B: BACK, TRICEPS, MIDDLE DELTS, TRAPS *(continued)*

Strength zone	Exercise name	Page number	Workout 1: reload (sets × reps or time)	Workouts 2 and 5 (sets × reps or time)	Workouts 3 and 6 (sets × reps or time)	Workouts 4 and 7 (sets × reps or time)
Traps: scapular retraction	3b. Dumbbell bench one-arm horizontal shrug	92	2 × 10-12 each side	4 × 8-10 each side	2 × 20-25 each side	3 × 12-15 each side
Lats: vertical or diagonal pulling with arms inside for the lengthened to midrange	4a. Neutral-grip lat pull-down	54	2 × 10-12	4 × 5-6	2 × 20-25	3 × 10-15
Triceps: lengthened to midrange	4b. NT Loop behind-the-head triceps extension	111	2 × 10-12	4 × 8-10	2 × 20-25	3 × 12-15
Traps: scapular elevation	5. Cable one-arm shrug	90	2 × 10-12 each side	3 × 15 each side	4 × 8-10 each side	2 × 20-25 each side

DAY C: CHEST, BICEPS, REAR DELTS

Strength zone	Exercise name	Page number	Workout 1: reload (sets × reps or time)	Workouts 2 and 5 (sets × reps or time)	Workouts 3 and 6 (sets × reps or time)	Workouts 4 and 7 (sets × reps or time)
Pecs: horizontal or decline pressing for the lengthened to midrange	1a. Push-up exercise indicated	29	Push-up 2 × 10-12	Box crossover push-up 3 × max reps	NT Loop resisted push-up 4 × max reps	Push-up 2 × max reps
Biceps: lengthened to midrange	1b. EZ-bar preacher curl	100	2 × 10-12	3 × 12-15	4 × 8-10	2 × 20-25
Pecs: horizontal or diagonal shoulder adduction for the shortened to midrange	2a. Cable one-arm diagonal pec fly	39	2 × 10-12 each side	3 × 12-15 each side	4 × 8-10 each side	2 × 20-25 each side
Rear delts: lengthened to midrange	2b. Cable one-arm rear-delt fly	82	2 × 10-12 each side	3 × 12-15 each side	4 × 8-10 each side	2 × 20 each side
Biceps: shortened to midrange	3a. Dumbbell incline bench biceps curl	104	2 × 10-12	2 × 20	3 × 12-15	4 × 7-9
Rear delts: shortened to midrange	3b. Suspension trainer wide-grip row	80	2 × 10-12	2 × 25-30	3 × 15	4 × 8-10
Pecs: incline pressing for the lengthened to midrange	4. Angled-barbell shoulder-to-shoulder press	35	2 × 20 total	2 × 30 total	3 × 20 total	4 × 8-12 total

Rest 30 seconds between exercises and 1 to 2 minutes between paired sets or tri-sets.

*As mentioned in chapter 11, due to their multijoint nature, all exercises such as squats, Romanian deadlifts, lunges, step-ups and many variations of those exercises provided in chapters 9 and 10 also load your glutes when they're closer to a lengthened (stretched) range.

TABLE 17.6   Program 1, Four-Day Split

DAY A: GLUTE AND HAMSTRING FOCUS FOR LOWER BODY AND CORE

Strength zone	Exercise name	Page number	Workout 1: reload (sets × reps or time)	Workouts 2 and 5 (sets × reps or time)	Workouts 3 and 6 (sets × reps or time)	Workouts 4 and 7 (sets × reps or time)
*Glutes and hamstrings: hip hinging for the lengthened to midrange	1a. Barbell elevated Romanian deadlift	120	2 × 10-12	4 × 5-8	2 × 20-25	3 × 10-15
Core: linear	1b. Stability ball plate crunch	196	2 × 8-10	4 × 6-8 (pause 2 sec at the top of each rep)	2 × 20-25	3 × 12-15
Glutes: hip extension for the shortened to midrange	2a. Cable one-leg Romanian deadlift	163	2 × 8-12 each side	3 × 12-15 each side	4 × 6-8 each side	2 × 20-25 each side
Core: rotational	2b. Cable three-point high-to-low chop	210	2 × 6 in each position, each side	3 × 10-12 in each position, each side	4 × 6-8 in each position, each side	2 × 15 reps in each position, each side
Hamstrings: knee flexion for the shortened to midrange	3a. Machine seated leg curl	125	2 × 10-12	2 × 20-30	3 × 10-15	4 × 6-8
Core: lateral	3b. Medicine ball side lean	203	2 × 8-10 each side	2 × 20 each side	3 × 12-15 each side	4 × 8-10 each side
Hips: abduction	4. Machine seated hip abduction	169	2 × 10-12	2 × 20-30	3 × 10-15	4 × 6-8

DAY B: PRESSING, PULLING, TRAPS

Strength zone	Exercise name	Page number	Workout 1: reload (sets × reps or time)	Workouts 2 and 5 (sets × reps or time)	Workouts 3 and 6 (sets × reps or time)	Workouts 4 and 7 (sets × reps or time)
Lats: vertical or diagonal pulling with arms inside for the lengthened to midrange	1a. Chin-up (assisted if needed with band or machine)	53	2 × 6-8	4 × 5-8	2 × 20-30	3 × 10-15
Chest: incline pressing for the lengthened to midrange	1b. Angled-barbell one-arm press	36	2 × 10-12 each side	4 × 6-8 each side	2 × 15-20 each side	3 × 10-12 each side
Chest: horizontal or decline pressing for the lengthened to midrange	2a. Machine chest press	28	2 × 10-12	3 × 10-15	4 × 6-8	2 × 20-25
Lats: horizontal pulling for the shortened to midrange	2b. Dumbbell two-arm bent-over row	60	2 × 10-12	3 × 12-15	4 × 8-10	2 × 20-25

DAY B: PRESSING, PULLING, TRAPS *(continued)*

Strength zone	Exercise name	Page number	Workout 1: reload (sets × reps or time)	Workouts 2 and 5 (sets × reps or time)	Workouts 3 and 6 (sets × reps or time)	Workouts 4 and 7 (sets × reps or time)
Lats: vertical or diagonal pulling with arms outside for the lengthened to midrange	3a. Cable one-arm half-kneeling lat pull-down	50	2 × 10-12 each side	2 × 20-25 each side	3 × 10-15 each side	4 × 6-8 each side
Traps: scapular elevation	3b. Cable one-arm shrug	90	2 × 10-12 each side	2 × 20-25 each side	3 × 10-15 each side	4 × 6-8 each side
Chest: horizontal or diagonal shoulder adduction for the shortened to midrange	4a. Cable crossover pec fly	41	2 × 10-12	2 × 20-25	3 × 12-15	4 × 10-12
Traps: scapular retraction	4b. Cable one-arm horizontal shrug	93	2 × 10-12 each side	2 × 20-25 each side	3 × 10-15 each side	4 × 6-8 each side

DAY C: QUAD AND CALF FOCUS FOR LOWER BODY AND CORE

Strength zone	Exercise name	Page number	Workout 1: reload (sets × reps or time)	Workouts 2 and 5 (sets × reps or time)	Workouts 3 and 6 (sets × reps or time)	Workouts 4 and 7 (sets × reps or time)
*Quads and glutes: knee bending for the lengthened to midrange	1a. Dumbbell traveling lunge	139	2 × 8-10 each side	3 × 12-15 each side	4 × 5-8 each side	2 × 20-25 each side
Core: linear	1b. Core exercise indicated	192	Stability ball rollout 2 × 10-12	Arm walkout 3 × 8-10	Ab wheel roll-out 4 × 6-8	Stability ball rollout 2 × 20
Quads: knee extension for the shortened to midrange	2a. Machine leg extension	147	2 × 10-12	2 × 20-25	3 × 12-15	4 × 6-8
Calves: bent knee	2b. Dumbbell half-kneeling calf raise	183	2 × 20 each side	2 × 30 each side	3 × 20 each side	4 × 12-15 each side
Hips: adduction	3a. Side-lying hip adduction leg scissors	173	2 × 10 each side	4 × 6-8 (3 sec hold at top each rep) each side	2 × 20-25 each side	3 × 12-15 (1 sec hold at top each rep) each side
Calves: straight knee	3b. Dumbbell traveling calf raise	180	2 × 20 sec	4 × 30 sec	2 × 50 sec	3 × 40 sec
Core: lateral	4a. Dumbbell unilateral farmers walk	201	2 × 20 sec each side	4 × 30 sec each side	2 × 50 sec each side	3 × 40 sec each side
Core: rotational	4b. Cable tight rotation with hip shift	208	2 × 12 each side	2 × 20 each side	3 × 12 each side	4 × 8 each side

Table 17.6 > *continued*

DAY D: BICEPS, TRICEPS, SHOULDERS

Strength zone	Exercise name	Page number	Workout 1: reload (sets × reps or time)	Workouts 2 and 5 (sets × reps or time)	Workouts 3 and 6 (sets × reps or time)	Workouts 4 and 7 (sets × reps or time)
Middle delts: lengthened to midrange	1a. Cable side shoulder raise	75	2 × 10-12 each side	3 × 12-15 each side	4 × 6-8 each side	2 × 20-25 each side
Biceps: lengthened to midrange	1b. Cable one-arm face-away biceps curl	99	2 × 10-12 each side	3 × 12-15 each side	4 × 6-8 each side	2 × 20-25 each side
Triceps: shortened to midrange	2a. Dumbbell triceps skull crusher	112	2 × 10-12	2 × 20-25	3 × 12-15	4 × 6-8
Rear delts: lengthened to midrange	2b. Dumbbell side-lying rear-delt fly	81	2 × 10-12 each side	2 × 20-25 each side	3 × 12-15 each side	4 × 6-8 each side
Biceps: shortened to midrange	3a. Dumbbell biceps curl	103	2 × 10-12	2 × 20-25	3 × 12-15	4 × 6-8
Triceps: lengthened to midrange	3b. Cable rope overhead triceps extension	108	2 × 10-12	2 × 20-25	3 × 12-15	4 × 6-8
Middle and rear delts: shortened to midrange	4. Barbell 45-degree row	71	2 × 10-12	4 × 8-10	2 × 20-25	3 × 12-15

Rest 30 seconds between exercises and 1 to 2 minutes between paired sets or tri-sets.

*As mentioned in chapter 11, due to their multijoint nature, all exercises such as squats, Romanian deadlifts, lunges, step-ups and many variations of those exercises provided in chapters 9 and 10 also load your glutes when they're closer to a lengthened (stretched) range.

TABLE 17.7   Program 2, Four-Day Split

DAY A: GLUTE AND HAMSTRING FOCUS FOR LOWER BODY AND CORE

Strength zone	Exercise name	Page number	Workout 1: reload (sets × reps or time)	Workouts 2 and 5 (sets × reps or time)	Workouts 3 and 6 (sets × reps or time)	Workouts 4 and 7 (sets × reps or time)
*Glutes and hamstrings: hip hinging for the lengthened to midrange	1a. Dumbbell traveling Romanian deadlift lunge	122	2 × 10-12 each side	4 × 5-8 each side	2 × 17-20 each side	3 × 10-15 each side
Core: linear	1b. Band leg lowering	192	2 × 8-10	4 × 6-8	2 × 15-20	3 × 10-12
Glutes: hip extension for the shortened to midrange	2a. 45-degree hip extension	166	2 × 8-12	3 × 12-15	4 × 6-10	2 × 20-25
Core: lateral	2b. Angled-barbell tight rainbow	201	2 × 15 sec	3 × 20 sec	4 × 15 sec	2 × 30 sec

DAY A: GLUTE AND HAMSTRING FOCUS FOR LOWER BODY AND CORE *(continued)*

Strength zone	Exercise name	Page number	Workout 1: reload (sets × reps or time)	Workouts 2 and 5 (sets × reps or time)	Workouts 3 and 6 (sets × reps or time)	Workouts 4 and 7 (sets × reps or time)
Hamstrings: knee flexion for the shortened to midrange	3a. Machine lying one-leg curl	127	2 × 10-12 each side	2 × 20-30 each side	3 × 10-15 each side	4 × 6-8 each side
Core: rotational	3b. Weight plate chop	215	2 × 10-12 each side	2 × 20 each side	3 × 10-15 each side	4 × 6-8 each side
Hips: adduction	4. Bent-knee Copenhagen hip adduction	174	2 × 8-10 each side	2 × 15 each side	3 × 10-12 each side	4 × 5-8 (pause 2 sec at top of each rep) each side

DAY B: PRESSING, PULLING, TRAPS

Strength zone	Exercise name	Page number	Workout 1: reload (sets × reps or time)	Workouts 2 and 5 (sets × reps or time)	Workouts 3 and 6 (sets × reps or time)	Workouts 4 and 7 (sets × reps or time)
Chest: incline pressing for the lengthened to midrange	1a. Dumbbell incline bench press	34	2 × 10-12	4 × 5-8	2 × 20-25	3 × 10-15
Lats: horizontal pulling for the shortened to midrange	1b. One-arm anti-rotation suspension row	66	2 × 8-10 each side	4 × 6-8 each side	2 × 15-20 each side	3 × 10-12 each side
Chest: horizontal or decline pressing for the lengthened to midrange	2a. Push-up exercise indicated	29	Push-up 2 × 10-15	Box crossover push-up 3 × max reps	NT Loop resisted push-up 4 × max reps	Push-up 2 × max reps
Lats: vertical or diagonal pulling with arms outside for the lengthened to midrange	2b. Overhand-grip lat pull-down	49	2 × 10-12	3 × 10-15	4 × 6-8	2 × 20-25
Chest: horizontal or diagonal shoulder adduction for the shortened to midrange	3a. Machine one-arm rotated chest press	40	2 × 10-12 each side	2 × 20-25 each side	3 × 12-15 each side	4 × 8-10 each side
Traps: scapular retraction	3b. Dumbbell off-bench one-arm horizontal shrug	92	2 × 10-12 each side	2 × 20-25 each side	3 × 12-15 each side	4 × 8-10 each side
Lats: vertical or diagonal pulling with arms inside for the lengthened to midrange	4a. Neutral-grip one-arm lat pull-down	56	2 × 10-12 each side	2 × 20-25 each side	3 × 12-15 each side	4 × 5-8 each side

> continued

Table 17.7 > *continued*

DAY B: PRESSING, PULLING, TRAPS (continued)

Strength zone	Exercise name	Page number	Workout 1: reload (sets × reps or time)	Workouts 2 and 5 (sets × reps or time)	Workouts 3 and 6 (sets × reps or time)	Workouts 4 and 7 (sets × reps or time)
Traps: scapular elevation	4b. Dumbbell one-arm leaning shrug	90	2 × 10-12 each side	2 × 20-25 each side	3 × 12-15 each side	4 × 8-10 each side

DAY C: QUAD AND CALF FOCUS FOR THE LOWER BODY AND CORE

Strength zone	Exercise name	Page number	Workout 1: reload (sets × reps or time)	Workouts 2 and 5 (sets × reps or time)	Workouts 3 and 6 (sets × reps or time)	Workouts 4 and 7 (sets × reps or time)
*Quads and glutes: knee bending for the lengthened to midrange	1a. Trap bar squat	136	2 × 8-10	3 × 12-15	4 × 5-8	2 × 20-25
Core: linear	1b. Core exercise indicated	198	Reverse crunch 2 × 8-10	Reverse crunch 3 × 10-15	Incline bench reverse crunch 4 × 6-8	Stability ball knee tuck 2 × 20-30
Quads: knee extension for the shortened to midrange	2a. Reverse sled drag	148	2 × 40 yards (36 m)	2 × 100 yards (91 m)	3 × 60-70 yards (55-64 m)	4 × 40 yards (36 m)
Calves: straight knee	2b. Dumbbell one-leg leaning calf raise	180	2 × 12-15 each side	2 × 25-30 each side	3 × 12-15 each side	4 × 8-10 each side
Hips: abduction	3a. Band lateral hip shuffle	170	2 × 10 each side	4 × 15 each side	2 × 30-35 each side	3 × 20-25 each side
Core: lateral	3b. Cable one-arm side bend	204	2 × 10 each side	4 × 8-10 each side	2 × 20 each side	3 × 15 each side
Core: rotational	4a. Cable three-point low-to-high chop	212	2 × 6 in each position, each side	2 × 15 in each position, each side	3 × 10-12 in each position, each side	4 × 6-8 in each position, each side
Calves: bent knee	4b. Machine seated calf raise	185	2 × 15	2 × 25-30	3 × 12-15	4 × 6-8

DAY D: BICEPS, TRICEPS, SHOULDERS

Strength zone	Exercise name	Page number	Workout 1: reload (sets × reps or time)	Workouts 2 and 5 (sets × reps or time)	Workouts 3 and 6 (sets × reps or time)	Workouts 4 and 7 (sets × reps or time)
Middle delts: shortened to midrange	1a. Kettlebell shoulder-to-shoulder press	73	2 × 5-6 each side	3 × 10-12 each side	4 × 6-8 each side	2 × 16-20 each side
Biceps: lengthened to midrange	1b. EZ-Bar preacher curl	100	2 × 10-12	3 × 12-15	4 × 6-8	2 × 20-25

DAY D: BICEPS, TRICEPS, SHOULDERS (continued)

Strength zone	Exercise name	Page number	Workout 1: reload (sets × reps or time)	Workouts 2 and 5 (sets × reps or time)	Workouts 3 and 6 (sets × reps or time)	Workouts 4 and 7 (sets × reps or time)
Triceps: lengthened to midrange	2a. Kettlebell behind-the-head triceps extension	109	2 × 10-12	2 × 20-25	3 × 12-15	4 × 6-8
Middle delts: lengthened to midrange	2b. Dumbbell side-lying side shoulder raise	76	2 × 10-12 each side	2 × 20-25 each side	3 × 12-15 each side	4 × 6-8 each side
Biceps: shortened to midrange	3a. Cable EZ-bar biceps curl	105	2 × 10-12	4 × 6-8	2 × 20-25	3 × 12-15
Rear delts: lengthened to midrange	3b. Cable one-arm rear-delt fly	82	2 × 10-12 each side	4 × 6-8 each side	2 × 20-25 each side	3 × 12-15 each side
Triceps: shortened to midrange	4a. Cable rope triceps extension	114	2 × 10-12	4 × 6-8	2 × 20-25	3 × 12-15
Rear delts: shortened to midrange	4b. Cable rope face pull	79	2 × 10-12	4 × 6-8	2 × 20-25	3 × 12-15

Rest 30 seconds between exercises and 1 to 2 minutes between paired sets or tri-sets.

*As mentioned in chapter 11, due to their multijoint nature, all exercises such as squats, Romanian deadlifts, lunges, step-ups and many variations of those exercises provided in chapters 9 and 10 also load your glutes when they're closer to a lengthened (stretched) range.

TABLE 17.8   Program 3, Four-Day Split

DAY A: GLUTE AND HAMSTRING FOCUS FOR LOWER BODY AND CORE

Strength zone	Exercise name	Page number	Workout 1: reload (sets × reps or time)	Workouts 2 and 5 (sets × reps or time)	Workouts 3 and 6 (sets × reps or time)	Workouts 4 and 7 (sets × reps or time)
*Glutes and hamstrings: hip hinging for the lengthened to midrange	1a. Angled-barbell leaning Romanian deadlift	124	2 × 10-12	4 × 6-8	2 × 17-20	3 × 10-15
Core: linear	1b. Stability ball arc	193	2 × 8-10 each side	4 × 6-8 each side	2 × 14-15 each side	3 × 10-12 each side
Hamstrings: knee flexion for the shortened to midrange	2a. Hamstring exercise indicated	128	Stability ball leg curl 2 × 10-15	Stability ball one-leg curl 3 × 12-20 each side	Nordic hamstring curl 4 × 4-8	Stability ball leg curl 2 × 25-30
Core: lateral	2b. Stability ball side crunch	205	2 × 10 each side	3 × 12-15 each side	4 × 6-10 each side	2 × 20-30 each side
Glutes: hip extension for the shortened to midrange	3a. Weight plate one-leg hip lift	166	2 × 10-12 each side	2 × 25-30 each side	3 × 12-15 each side	4 × 8-10 each side

> continued

Table 17.8   *> continued*

DAY A: GLUTE AND HAMSTRING FOCUS FOR LOWER BODY AND CORE *(continued)*						
Strength zone	**Exercise name**	**Page number**	**Workout 1: reload (sets × reps or time)**	**Workouts 2 and 5 (sets × reps or time)**	**Workouts 3 and 6 (sets × reps or time)**	**Workouts 4 and 7 (sets × reps or time)**
Hips: adduction	3b. NT Loop quadruped hip adduction	176	2 × 10-12 each side	2 × 20-25 each side	3 × 12-15 each side	4 × 8-10 each side
Core: rotational	4. Cable three-point horizontal chop	209	2 × 6-8 in each position, each side	2 × 12-15 in each position, each side	3 × 10 in each position, each side	4 × 6-8 in each position, each side

DAY B: PRESSING, PULLING, TRAPS						
Strength zone	**Exercise name**	**Page number**	**Workout 1: reload (sets × reps or time)**	**Workouts 2 and 5 (sets × reps or time)**	**Workouts 3 and 6 (sets × reps or time)**	**Workouts 4 and 7 (sets × reps or time)**
Chest: horizontal or decline pressing for the lengthened to midrange	1a. Dumbbell bench press	26	2 × 10-12	4 × 5-8	2 × 20-25	3 × 10-15
Lats: horizontal pulling for the shortened to midrange	1b. Dumbbell one-arm bench row	61	2 × 10-12 each side	4 × 6-8 each side	2 × 20-25 each side	3 × 10-12 each side
Chest: incline pressing for the lengthened to midrange	2a. Angled-barbell shoulder-to-shoulder press	35	2 × 20 total	3 × 24-30 total	4 × 12-16 total	2 × 40 total
Lats: vertical or diagonal pulling with arms outside for the lengthened to midrange	2b. Cable fighters lat pull-down	51	2 × 10-12 each side	3 × 12-15 each side	4 × 8-10 each side	2 × 20-25 each side
Chest: horizontal or diagonal shoulder adduction for the shortened to midrange	3a. Machine pec fly	43	2 × 10-12	2 × 20-25	3 × 12-15	4 × 8-10
Traps: scapular retraction	3b. Dumbbell bent-over horizontal shrug	91	2 × 10-12	2 × 25	3 × 15	4 × 10
Lats: vertical or diagonal pulling with arms inside for the lengthened to midrange	4a. Cable straight-arm compound pull-down	57	2 × 10-12	2 × 20-25	3 × 12-15	4 × 8-10
Traps: scapular elevation	4b. Cable wide-grip angled upright row	88	2 × 10-12	2 × 30	3 × 15-20	4 × 10-12

DAY C: QUAD AND CALF FOCUS FOR LOWER BODY AND CORE

Strength zone	Exercise name	Page number	Workout 1: reload (sets × reps or time)	Workouts 2 and 5 (sets × reps or time)	Workouts 3 and 6 (sets × reps or time)	Workouts 4 and 7 (sets × reps or time)
*Quads and glutes: knee bending for the lengthened to midrange	1a. Dumbbell step-up	139	2 × 8-10 each side	3 × 12-15 each side	4 × 5-8 each side	2 × 20 each side
Core: lateral	1b. Off-bench lateral hold	203	2 × 12-15 sec each side	3 × 25-30 sec each side	4 × 15-20 sec each side	2 × 35-40 sec each side
Quads: knee extension for the shortened to midrange	2a. Machine unilateral leg extension	148	2 × 10-12 each side	2 × 20-25 each side	3 × 12-15 each side	4 × 6-8 each side
Core: rotational	2b. Dumbbell plank row	207	2 × 8 each side	2 × 12-15 each side	3 × 8-10 each side	4 × 6-8 each side
Hips: abduction	3a. Machine seated hip abduction	169	2 × 10-12	2 × 20-25	3 × 10-15	4 × 6-8
Calves: bent knee	3b. Dumbbell half-kneeling calf raise	183	2 × 10-12 each side	2 × 25-30 each side	3 × 15-20 each side	4 × 8-12 each side
Calves: straight knee	4a. Machine ankles-together calf raise	182	2 × 15	4 × 8-10	2 × 25-30	3 × 12-15
Core: linear	4b. Band leg lowering	192	2 × 20-30 sec	4 × 30 sec	2 × 50 sec	3 × 40 sec

DAY D: BICEPS, TRICEPS, SHOULDERS

Strength zone	Exercise name	Page number	Workout 1: reload (sets × reps or time)	Workouts 2 and 5 (sets × reps or time)	Workouts 3 and 6 (sets × reps or time)	Workouts 4 and 7 (sets × reps or time)
Middle delts: shortened to midrange	1a. Machine overhead press	75	2 × 10-12	4 × 6-8	2 × 20-25	3 × 10-15
Biceps: shortened to midrange	1b. EZ-bar biceps curl	102	2 × 10-12	4 × 6-8	2 × 20-25	3 × 10-15
Triceps: lengthened to midrange	2a. Cable rope overhead triceps extension	108	2 × 10-12	2 × 20-25	3 × 12-15	4 × 6-8
Middle delts: lengthened to midrange	2b. NT Loop side shoulder raise	77	2 × 10-12 each side	2 × 20-25 each side	3 × 12-15 each side	4 × 6-8 each side
Biceps: lengthened to midrange	3a. Cable one-arm face-away biceps curl	99	2 × 10-12 each side	4 × 6-8 each side	2 × 20 each side	3 × 12-15 each side
Rear delts: lengthened to midrange	3b. Low-cable rear-delt fly	82	2 × 10-12 each side	4 × 6-8 each side	2 × 20-25 each side	3 × 12-15 each side

> *continued*

Table 17.8   > *continued*

DAY D: BICEPS, TRICEPS, SHOULDERS *(continued)*

Strength zone	Exercise name	Page number	Workout 1: reload (sets × reps or time)	Workouts 2 and 5 (sets × reps or time)	Workouts 3 and 6 (sets × reps or time)	Workouts 4 and 7 (sets × reps or time)
Triceps: shortened to midrange	4a. Suspension trainer skull crusher	114	2 × 10-12	4 × 8-10	2 × 20-25	3 × 15
Rear delts: shortened to midrange	4b. Suspension trainer wide-grip row	80	2 × 10-12	4 × 8-10	2 × 20-25	3 × 15

Rest 30 seconds between exercises and 1 to 2 minutes between paired sets or tri-sets.

*As mentioned in chapter 11, due to their multijoint nature, all exercises such as squats, Romanian deadlifts, lunges, step-ups and many variations of those exercises provided in chapters 9 and 10 also load your glutes when they're closer to a lengthened (stretched) range.

TABLE 17.9   Program 4, Four-Day Split

DAY A: GLUTE AND HAMSTRING FOCUS FOR LOWER BODY AND CORE

Strength zone	Exercise name	Page number	Workout 1: reload (sets × reps or time)	Workouts 2 and 5 (sets × reps or time)	Workouts 3 and 6 (sets × reps or time)	Workouts 4 and 7 (sets × reps or time)
*Glutes and hamstrings: hip hinging for the lengthened to midrange	1a. Dumbbell one-leg one-arm Romanian deadlift	123	2 × 10-12 each side	4 × 6-8 each side	2 × 20 each side	3 × 12-15 each side
Core: linear	1b. Suspension trainer arm fallout	195	2 × 8-10	4 × 6-8	2 × 20	3 × 12-15
Hamstrings: knee flexion for the shortened to midrange	2a. Machine seated one-leg curl	126	2 × 8-10 each side	3 × 10-15 each side	4 × 6-8 each side	2 × 20-25 each side
Core: rotational	2b. Cross-body plank	208	2 × 15 sec	4 × 20 sec	2 × 40 sec	3 × 30 sec
Glutes: hip extension for the shortened to midrange	3a. NT Loop glute walk	168	2 × 30 sec	2 × 50 sec	3 × 40 sec	4 × 30 sec
Hips: adduction	3b. Hip adduction exercise indicated	173	Side-lying hip adduction 2 × 8 each side	Side-lying hip adduction 2 × 20-25 each side	Side-lying hip adduction leg scissors 3 × 12-15 each side	Bent-knee Copenhagen hip adduction 4 × 8-10
Core: lateral	4. Dumbbell unilateral farmers walk	201	2 × 30 sec each side	2 × 50-60 sec each side	3 × 40 sec each side	4 × 20-30 sec each side

DAY B: PRESSING, PULLING, TRAPS

Strength zone	Exercise name	Page number	Workout 1: reload (sets × reps or time)	Workouts 2 and 5 (sets × reps or time)	Workouts 3 and 6 (sets × reps or time)	Workouts 4 and 7 (sets × reps or time)
Lats: horizontal pulling for the shortened to midrange	1a. Machine row	64	2 × 10-12	4 × 5-8	2 × 20-25	3 × 10-15
Traps: scapular retraction	1b. Machine row horizontal shrug	94	2 × 10-12	4 × 5-8	2 × 20-25	3 × 10-15
Chest: horizontal or decline pressing for the lengthened to midrange	1c. Push-up exercise indicated	30	Push-up 2 × 12-15	Lock-off push-up 4 × 6-8 each side	Push-up 2 × max reps	Box crossover push-up 3 × max reps
Lats: vertical or diagonal pulling with arms outside for the lengthened to midrange	2a. Cable one-arm half-kneeling lat pull-down	50	2 × 10-12 each side	3 × 10-15 each side	4 × 6-8 each side	2 × 20 each side
Chest: horizontal or diagonal shoulder adduction for the shortened to midrange	2b. Cable one-arm diagonal pec fly	39	2 × 10-12 each side	3 × 10-15 each side	4 × 6-8 each side	2 × 20 each side
Lats: vertical or diagonal pulling with arms inside for the lengthened to midrange	3a. Underhand-grip lat pull-down	55	2 × 10-12	2 × 20-25	3 × 12-15	4 × 8-10
Traps: scapular elevation	3b. Dumbbell one-arm leaning shrug	90	2 × 10-12 each side	2 × 20-25 each side	3 × 12-15 each side	4 × 8-10 each side
Chest: incline pressing for the lengthened to midrange	4. Machine incline chest press	37	2 × 10-12	2 × 20-25	3 × 12-15	4 × 8-10

DAY C: QUAD AND CALF FOCUS FOR LOWER BODY AND CORE

Strength zone	Exercise name	Page number	Workout 1: reload (sets × reps or time)	Workouts 2 and 5 (sets × reps or time)	Workouts 3 and 6 (sets × reps or time)	Workouts 4 and 7 (sets × reps or time)
*Quads and glutes: knee bending for the lengthened to midrange	1a. Dumbbell reverse lunge with NT Loop knee resistance	140	2 × 8-10 each side	3 × 12-15 each side	4 × 6-8 each side	2 × 20 each side
Core: rotational	1b. Cable one-arm press	213	2 × 8-10 each side	3 × 15 each side	4 × 8-10 each side	2 × 20-25 each side

> continued

Table 17.9 > *continued*

DAY C: QUAD AND CALF FOCUS FOR LOWER BODY AND CORE *(continued)*

Strength zone	Exercise name	Page number	Workout 1: reload (sets × reps or time)	Workouts 2 and 5 (sets × reps or time)	Workouts 3 and 6 (sets × reps or time)	Workouts 4 and 7 (sets × reps or time)
Calves: bent knee	2a. Machine seated calf raise	185	2 × 10-12	2 × 25-30	3 × 15-20	4 × 8-12
Core: lateral	2b. Weight plate around the world	206	2 × 6 each side	2 × 12 each side	3 × 8 each side	4 × 6 each side
Hips: abduction	3a. Machine seated hip abduction	169	2 × 10-12	2 × 25	3 × 12-15	4 × 8-10
Calves: straight knee	3b. Dumbbell one-leg leaning calf raise	180	2 × 10-12 each side	2 × 25-30 each side	3 × 12-15 each side	4 × 8-12 each side
Quads: knee extension for the shortened to midrange	4a. Unilateral reverse sled drag	149	2 × 30 yards (27 m) each leg	4 × 20-30 yards (18-27 m) each leg	2 × 80 yards (73 m) each leg	3 × 50-60 yards (46-55 m) each leg
Core: linear	4b. Core exercise indicated	192	Stability ball rollout 2 × 10-12	Ab wheel rollout 4 × 5-6	Stability ball rollout 2 × 20	Arm walkout 3 × 8

DAY D: BICEPS, TRICEPS, SHOULDERS

Strength zone	Exercise name	Page number	Workout 1: reload (sets × reps or time)	Workouts 2 and 5 (sets × reps or time)	Workouts 3 and 6 (sets × reps or time)	Workouts 4 and 7 (sets × reps or time)
Triceps: lengthened to midrange	1a. Dumbbell one-arm behind-the-head triceps extension	110	2 × 10-12 each side	4 × 8-10 each side	2 × 20-25 each side	3 × 12-15 each side
Rear delts: shortened to midrange	1b. Dumbbell rear-delt fly	78	2 × 10-12	4 × 6-8	2 × 20-25	3 × 12-15 each side
Biceps: lengthened to midrange	2a. EZ-bar preacher curl	100	2 × 10-12	4 × 6-8	2 × 20-25	3 × 10-15
Middle delts: lengthened to midrange	2b. NT Loop Mini side shoulder raise	77	2 × 10-12 each side	4 × 6-8 each side	2 × 20-25 each side	3 × 12-15 each side
Middle delts: shortened to midrange	3a. Dumbbell side shoulder raise	72	2 × 10-12	2 × 20-25	3 × 12-15	4 × 6-8
Triceps: shortened to midrange	3b. Cable one-arm triceps kickback	115	2 × 10-12 each side	2 × 20-25 each side	3 × 12-15 each side	4 × 8-10 each side

DAY D: BICEPS, TRICEPS, SHOULDERS *(continued)*

Strength zone	Exercise name	Page number	Workout 1: reload (sets × reps or time)	Workouts 2 and 5 (sets × reps or time)	Workouts 3 and 6 (sets × reps or time)	Workouts 4 and 7 (sets × reps or time)
Biceps: shortened to midrange	4a. Dumbbell concentration biceps curl	103	2 × 10-12 each side	3 × 12-15 each side	4 × 6-8 each side	2 × 20 each side
Rear delts: lengthened to midrange	4b. Dumbbell side-lying rear-delt fly	81	2 × 10-12 each side	3 × 12-15 each side	4 × 6-8 each side	2 × 20-25 each side

Rest 30 seconds between exercises and 1 to 2 minutes between paired sets or tri-sets.

*As mentioned in chapter 11 due to their multijoint nature, all exercises such as squats, Romanian deadlifts, lunges, step-ups and many variations of those exercises provided in chapters 9 and 10 also load your glutes when they're closer to a lengthened (stretched) range.

TABLE 17.10   Program 5, Four-Day Split

DAY A: GLUTE AND HAMSTRING FOCUS FOR LOWER BODY AND CORE

Strength zone	Exercise name	Page number	Workout 1: reload (sets × reps or time)	Workouts 2 and 5 (sets × reps or time)	Workouts 3 and 6 (sets × reps or time)	Workouts 4 and 7 (sets × reps or time)
*Glutes and hamstrings: hip hinging for the lengthened to midrange	1a. Dumbbell lateral Romanian deadlift lunge	122	2 × 10-12 each side	4 × 6-8 each side	2 × 20 each side	3 × 10-15 each side
Core: linear	1b. Core exercise indicated	198	Reverse crunch 2 × 8	Incline bench reverse crunch 4 × 6-8	Reverse crunch 2 × 15-20	Stability ball pike rollout 3 × 8-12
Hamstrings: knee flexion for the shortened to midrange	2a. Hamstring exercise indicated	128	Stability ball leg curl 2 × 10-15	Stability ball one-leg curl 3 × 12-15 each side	Nordic hamstring curl 4 × 5-8	Stability ball leg curl 2 × 25-30
Core: lateral	2b. Cable one-arm side bend	204	2 × 8-10 each side	3 × 12-15 each side	4 × 8-10 each side	2 × 20-25 each side
Glutes: hip extension for the shortened to midrange	3a. 45-degree hip extension	166	2 × 10-12	2 × 20-30	3 × 12-15	4 × 6-10
Hips: adduction	3b. NT Loop quadruped hip adduction	176	2 × 10-12 each side	2 × 20 each side	3 × 12-15 each side	4 × 8-10 each side
Core: rotational	4. Cable three-point horizontal chop	209	2 × 6-8 in each position, each side	2 × 12-15 in each position, each side	3 × 10 in each position, each side	4 × 6-8 in each position, each side

> continued

Table 17.10 > *continued*

DAY B: PRESSING, PULLING, TRAPS

Strength zone	Exercise name	Page number	Workout 1: reload (sets × reps or time)	Workouts 2 and 5 (sets × reps or time)	Workouts 3 and 6 (sets × reps or time)	Workouts 4 and 7 (sets × reps or time)
Lats: vertical or diagonal pulling with arms outside for the lengthened to midrange	1a. Pull-up (assisted if needed with band or machine)	48	2 × 8-10	4 × 5-8	2 × 20-25	3 × 10-12
Traps: scapular elevation	1b. Barbell wide-grip shrug	89	2 × 8-10	4 × 8-10	2 × 20-25	3 × 12-15
Lats: horizontal pulling for the shortened to midrange	2a. Barbell bent-over row	59	2 × 10-12	3 × 10-15	4 × 6-8	2 × 20-25
Chest: incline pressing for the lengthened to midrange	2b. Dumbbell incline bench press	34	2 × 10-12	3 × 10-15	4 × 6-8	2 × 20-25
Lats: vertical or diagonal pulling with arms inside for the lengthened to midrange	3a. Cable one-arm half-kneeling neutral-grip lat pull-down	56	2 × 10-12 each side	2 × 20-25 each side	3 × 12-15 each side	4 × 8-10 each side
Chest: horizontal or diagonal shoulder adduction for the shortened to midrange	3b. Cable one-arm horizontal pec fly	39	2 × 10-12 each side	2 × 20-25 each side	3 × 12-15 each side	4 × 8-10 each side
Chest: horizontal or decline pressing for the lengthened to midrange	4a. Dumbbell decline hip bridge press	27	2 × 10-12	2 × 20-25	3 × 12-15	4 × 6-8
Traps: scapular retraction	4b. Dumbbell bench one-arm horizontal shrug	92	2 × 10-12 each side	2 × 20-25 each side	3 × 12-15 each side	4 × 8-10 each side

DAY C: QUAD AND CALF FOCUS FOR LOWER BODY AND CORE

Strength zone	Exercise name	Page number	Workout 1: reload (sets × reps or time)	Workouts 2 and 5 (sets × reps or time)	Workouts 3 and 6 (sets × reps or time)	Workouts 4 and 7 (sets × reps or time)
*Quads and glutes: knee bending for the lengthened to midrange	1a. Barbell squat	134	2 × 8-10	3 × 10-15	4 × 6-8	2 × 20-25
Core: linear	1b. Core exercise indicated	192	Stability ball rollout 2 × 8-10	Ab wheel rollout 3 × 12-15	Arm walkout 4 × 5-8	Stability ball rollout 2 × 20-25

DAY C: QUAD AND CALF FOCUS FOR LOWER BODY AND CORE *(continued)*

Strength zone	Exercise name	Page number	Workout 1: reload (sets × reps or time)	Workouts 2 and 5 (sets × reps or time)	Workouts 3 and 6 (sets × reps or time)	Workouts 4 and 7 (sets × reps or time)
Quads: knee extension for the shortened to midrange	2a. NT Loop inverted leg extension exercise indicated	151	NT Loop inverted leg extension 2 × 10-12	NT Loop inverted leg extension 2 × 20-25	NT Loop inverted leg extension 3 × 12-15	NT Loop feet-elevated inverted leg extension 4 × 6-10
Core: rotational	2b. Cable same-side one-arm press	214	2 × 10-12 each side	2 × 20-25 each side	3 × 12-15 each side	4 × 8-10 each side
Calves: straight knee	3a. Dumbbell foot-elevated calf raise	181	2 × 12-15 each side	2 × 25-30 each side	3 × 15 each side	4 × 8-12 each side
Hips: abduction	3b. Hip abduction exercise indicated	171	Weight plate side-lying hip abduction 2 × 10-12 each side	Weight plate side-lying hip abduction 2 × 20-30 each side	Dynamic bent-knee side elbow plank with hip abduction 3 × 12-15 each side	Dynamic side elbow plank with hip abduction 4 × 6-10 each side
Calves: bent knee	4a. Dumbbell one-leg seated calf raise	184	2 × 10-12 each side	2 × 25-30 each side	3 × 15 each side	4 × 8-12 each side
Core: lateral	4b. Off-bench lateral hold	203	2 × 10-15 sec each side	2 × 30 sec each side	3 × 20 sec each side	4 × 10-15 sec each side

DAY D: BICEPS, TRICEPS, SHOULDERS

Strength zone	Exercise name	Page number	Workout 1: reload (sets × reps or time)	Workouts 2 and 5 (sets × reps or time)	Workouts 3 and 6 (sets × reps or time)	Workouts 4 and 7 (sets × reps or time)
Biceps: lengthened to midrange	1a. Dumbbell incline bench one-arm preacher curl	101	2 × 10-12 each side	4 × 8-10 each side	2 × 20-25 each side	3 × 12-15 each side
Middle and rear delts: shortened to midrange	1b. Dumbbell incline bench 45-degree row	70	2 × 10-12	4 × 8-10	2 × 20-25	3 × 12-15
Triceps: shortened to midrange	2a. Machine triceps extension	117	2 × 10-12	2 × 20-25	3 × 12-15	4 × 8-10
Rear delts: lengthened to midrange	2b. NT Loop Mini rear-delt fly	84	2 × 10-12 each side	2 × 20-25 each side	3 × 12-15 each side	4 × 8-10 each side
Middle delts: lengthened to midrange	3a. NT Loop side shoulder raise	77	2 × 10-12 each side	4 × 6-10 each side	2 × 20-25 each side	3 × 12-15 each side

> continued

Table 17.10   > *continued*

DAY D: BICEPS, TRICEPS, SHOULDERS *(continued)*

Strength zone	Exercise name	Page number	Workout 1: reload (sets × reps or time)	Workouts 2 and 5 (sets × reps or time)	Workouts 3 and 6 (sets × reps or time)	Workouts 4 and 7 (sets × reps or time)
Triceps: lengthened to midrange	3b. NT Loop overhead triceps press	111	2 × 10-12	4 × 6-8	2 × 20-25	3 × 12-15
Biceps: shortened to midrange	4. Dumbbell incline bench biceps curl	104	2 × 10-12	4 × 6-8	2 × 20-25	3 × 12-15

Rest 30 seconds between exercises and 1 to 2 minutes between paired sets or tri-sets.

*As mentioned in chapter 11, due to their multijoint nature, all exercises such as squats, Romanian deadlifts, lunges, step-ups and many variations of those exercises provided in chapters 9 and 10 also load your glutes when they're closer to a lengthened (stretched) range.

CHAPTER 18

The Most Effective Muscle-Building Strategies

Now that you're armed with a battery of exercises to build strength through the true full range of motion for every major muscle group and workout programs for your experience level and training schedule, what's next? What you need to know are the practical guidelines for reaching your muscle-building goals that will always work and never go out of date. Science-backed, gym-proven strategies for how to gain muscle. This chapter covers it all.

Proven Muscle-Building Training Principles

Over the years I've come to recognize and rely on a handful of basic, proven principles that allow everyone to maintain long-term, sustainable results. Stick to these and forget the fads.

The Best Rep Ranges

Mechanical tension drives muscle growth. Research shows that lifting a lighter load to failure produces gains in muscle size similar to those produced by lifting a heavy load to failure (1). The scientific evidence on rep ranges tells us that there's no magical range for maximizing muscle size. You can use both heavy, low-rep (1-5) sets along with medium-load, high-rep (15-20+) sets if you'd like. But many people focused on building muscle are usually not interested in using weights so heavy that they can only do five or fewer reps with it. And that's fine. Doing some sets in the six to eight rep range serves as a nice middle ground.

The amount of weight you're using also determines the quality of reps you're doing. If the load is too heavy, you may not be able to do good-quality reps. That said, at any given time at any big-box gym, you'll see at least one guy doing biceps curls or shoulder raises, and he'll have to thrust his lower back into it each time he brings the weight up. It's easy to make this mistake. After all, you're in the gym to lift weights, and everyone knows heavy loads are an effective stimulus for muscle growth, right? Well, sort of.

Training to maximize muscle isn't about becoming a weightlifter as many seem to think. It's about using weights as a tool to increase your muscle size and strength. Simply moving as much weight as you can is a less effective and a risky approach. Here's what happens when you use weights that are too heavy:

- You reduce the time under (mechanical) tension because you're forced to use momentum to cheat.
- You're unable to lower the weight slowly and with control, further reducing your time under (mechanical) tension.
- You use more muscles, which reduces the accumulated pump (metabolic stress) in muscles you're trying to target.

Training to maximize muscle isn't just about moving the weight from one point to another as you would when powerlifting or Olympic weightlifting. It's about controlling the weight through the entire range of motion. The point of emphasis on each rep is to avoid swinging the weight up or cheating by using other parts of your body to move the load.

The Best Tempo

Perform the concentric (lifting) portion of each rep at a normal tempo and maintain control during the lowering portion for about three seconds on each rep. When you're trying to maximize gains, controlling the weight and minimizing momentum also applies to the eccentric (lowering) portion of each rep. People who cheat the weight up normally also let the weight come crashing back down. When getting the most gains from each rep are the focus, maintaining deliberate control is paramount.

Letting the weight swing down without control may be even more ineffective than you think. Evidence demonstrates that a slower (four-second) eccentric action during biceps curls produces more arm growth than a one-second eccentric action (2). This makes perfect sense. Lowering slowly creates more mechanical tension on the working muscles than a shorter eccentric portion does.

And because cheating creates an overload of mechanical tension only in a small range of the motion, it's more likely that you'll use a weight that's too heavy for you, making the muscles deal with forces that exceed the structural integrity of your tendons and ligaments. Injuring yourself isn't conducive to building muscle. If you want to maximize your size gains, maximize your time under tension by using strict form and a controlled eccentric portion lasting about three to five seconds, with three seconds being a sweet spot that doesn't take too long on each rep.

The Best Weight

The amount of weight you use on each set is determined by the number of reps you're doing relative to your strength level. Choose a load that leaves you unable to perform any more reps than indicated on your workout program, but without cheating by using additional jerking, twitching, or momentum. If your program calls for three sets of 8 to 12 reps, grab a weight that allows you to complete at least 8 reps using proper form, but not so light that you can do more than 12 reps before reaching technical failure.

Also, if you're using the same weight for each set, you may be able to do 12 reps on the first set, 11 on the next set, and 10 on the third set because of accumulated fatigue. Or you can reduce the weight you're using with each consecutive set to achieve the higher end of the given rep range on each consecutive set. Both methods are effective, but using the same weight on each set often makes the most logistical sense, especially when training in a busy gym.

The Best Number of Sets

I remember listening to a two-hour debate from a couple of science-based coaches who both specialize in hypertrophy (i.e., muscle growth) training. Their entire debate concluded with the agreement that 12 to 20 total sets per muscle per week is a good rule of thumb for hypertrophy—an idea that's been around for years.

That said, if you're looking to bring up certain lagging muscle groups, the first thing you need to do is count the total number of sets you're doing each week for those muscles to see whether you're getting at least 12 sets per week on each area. If you're already hitting that minimum, then it's time to add a few more total sets per week to those muscle groups. You can apply this to any of the workout plans for strength zone training in this book by simply adding a few extra sets of the exercises that hit the muscle groups you want to develop most.

The Best Training Splits

The best type of training split is determined by how many days per week you're training. It all comes down to getting in enough training volume of each muscle group throughout the week. If you're training two or three times per week, total-body workouts are best. If you're training four times per week, an upper-body, lower-body split is the best. If you're training five or six times per week, a body-part split is best in order to allow sufficient recovery of each muscle group between workouts. You can use either a three-day-on and one-day-off rotation, or use a four-day-on, one-day-off rotation.

Regardless of which setup you use, you have flexibility. You can always throw in a few extra sets for a muscle group that is not the focus of a particular day's workout if you want to spark more growth.

The Best Rest Periods

A review of the research found that resting three to five minutes between sets produced the greatest increases in strength by allowing your body the optimal amount of time to recover. Higher levels of muscular power were demonstrated over multiple sets with three to five minutes of rest than with one minute of rest between sets (3). Resting longer than three to five minutes doesn't further increase performance. Plus, you have only so much time to work out anyway.

Speaking of maximizing your workout time, the workout plans in this book use a lot of paired sets, such as pairing a chest exercise with a back exercise, a lower-body exercise with an ab exercise, and an arm exercise with a shoulder exercise. What's a paired set? You might guess supersets, but there is a difference. Whereas there is no rest between exercises within a superset, you rest strategically between exercises when doing a paired set.

Don't get me wrong. There's nothing at all wrong with straight sets. You can use them effectively to get seriously big and strong if you have the time. But paired-set training may be more effective than traditional set training at enabling you to handle maximum volume in your workout. In fact, researchers who compared paired-set versus traditional-set protocols suggested that anyone who wants to maximize workout efficiency and minimize time should try paired sets (4).

The Best Training Equipment for Size and Strength

Some lifters and trainers center their programs on certain pieces of equipment, like the barbell or kettlebell. Many of these people also like to demonize other types of equipment, like machines.

The reality is, no single piece of equipment is best for all jobs. From barbells to machines, dumbbells to kettlebells, and bands to medicine balls, each has a unique use that other implements can't match. I'd like to thank Coach Vince McConnell for his contributions to this section. Let's review.

Plate-Loaded Machines

Unique use: More tension on specific muscles. Heavy, stable loading.

Free weights excel by forcing you to use your stabilizing muscles. Plate-loaded machines excel by providing you more stability, which allows you to work certain areas of your body harder. Free weights fall short when it comes to keeping consistent tension on the muscles throughout the range of motion. That's the area where selectorized machines, discussed next, excel.

Selectorized Machines

Unique use: Tension through more of the range of motion, especially with movement patterns that have a curve to them, such as leg extension, leg curl, and pullover.

Selectorized machines use a cam system, in which a bean-shaped mechanism on the machine rotates as you do each rep. The cam offers consistent resistance throughout the range of motion. This also gives you much more time under tension because your muscles don't get the same chance to rest at the bottom or top position of the range like they do when using free weights.

Selectorized machines also offer the same stability benefits as plate-loaded machines. This is why there's no reason to avoid machines. In fact, for strength and muscle, machines should be used in conjunction with free weights.

Barbell

Unique use: Lifting heavy loads for max strength training—absolute loading.

The barbell allows you to work against the highest amount of overall load of any piece of common gym equipment in the free weight category.

Trap Bar

Unique use: Lifting heavy while saving your lower back.

The trap bar is also best suited for lifting big loads. However, its unique benefit over the barbell is that it allows you to get closer to the weight. This is why many people find the trap bar deadlift to be better for their lower back than the barbell

That said, paired sets allow you to rest longer between sets of the same muscle group while maximizing your overall training time by doing a set targeting a different muscle group. And when training for muscle gains, getting ample rest between sets hitting the same muscle group is important for getting the most out of each set.

Proven Muscle-Building Nutrition Principles

In the world of nutrition, new diet trends emerge, gain popularity, and then fall out of fashion. When a new diet trend comes along, the mainstream jumps on deadlift. Beyond competitive powerlifting, there's no need to use a barbell for the deadlift, and the trap bar is a smarter option for most people.

Dumbbells

Unique use: Unilateral lifts for the upper body. Bilateral lifts with emphasis on each side of the body working with a higher degree of independence. Heavy lifting with less restriction relative to your grip and path of movement.

While you can't load to the same total capacity as you can with a bar, dumbbells are more versatile than the barbell and most lifters find them easier on their joints. The path of motion is freer, so lifters can more easily adjust an exercise to accommodate a problem they might be dealing with.

Kettlebells

Unique use: Exercises that originate from traditional kettlebell lifting: swings, Turkish get-ups, snatches, windmills, goblet squats, and bottoms-up variations.

A lot of dumbbell exercises can be performed with a kettlebell. Because of the kettlebell's unique structure (handle relative to center of mass), they're great for grip work, and they can be used for unique shoulder exercises like the shoulder-to-shoulder press.

The best use for kettlebells isn't exercises for gaining strength and size, but rather for explosive lifts like swings, cleans, and snatches. You have to control the kettlebell to either catch it softly as it flips over or decelerate it on the back end of each rep.

Adjustable Cable Column

Unique use: Creating horizontal and diagonal lines of force. User-friendly angles. Various grip options (handle, bar, or rope).

All free weight and body weight exercises are loaded by gravity, which is a vertical line of force. But with cables, you're able to create a horizontal and diagonal line of force to work against, so workouts can be more comprehensive. Cables help you create a more balanced workout by allowing you to load planes of motion that gravity doesn't load through free weight exercises.

Resistance Bands

Unique use: Their portability.

Resistance bands can be a valid stand-alone tool when you can't make it to the gym. And when you're in the gym, bands can be used in place of an adjustable cable column. You can build muscle with bands when you know how to use them in a way that maximizes their benefits.

it, becomes bored, and then moves on to the next big thing. The pattern keeps repeating, and even trainers and coaches can fall into the trend trap.

We need to avoid getting caught up in these nutrition trends. Have you fallen for any of them? We need to focus instead on the basic principles that always work and will never go out of style. To do that, let's look back at the lessons we've learned so far.

I'd like to thank Dani Shugart for her contributions to this section.

Avoid the Diet Trend Traps

Diet trends fall in and out of favor like clothing styles. And it's often thought that every new wave is better than the previous one. However, history proves otherwise.

Every era has its fans and its great-looking celebrities. They're on board with the hot diet methods of their respective time. So you can't look at whatever methods athletes and celebrities are using as the "secret" to their success. Because in a different era they'd be doing something else. In 1972 the Atkins diet was created, and variations have made a comeback every decade since. (Believe it or not, before it became a hit among the masses, the extremely low-carb diet was first administered by a doctor named William Banting in the 1800s.)

In the 1960s Weight Watchers was founded, and its weight loss diet became popular, but it wasn't the only popular diet plan. If you are a member of the baby boomer generation, you might've tried the SlimFast diet, the grapefruit diet, or the sleeping beauty diet, which had people taking sedatives and sacking out in place of eating food.

In the 1980s and 1990s there was Jenny Craig, the cabbage soup diet, and general eating styles (like the Ornish diet) that encouraged cutting back on fat. Vegetarian diets rose in popularity too. In the mid-1990s the Zone Diet made its debut as one of the first plans to require dieters to consider specific percentages of macronutrients (carbohydrate, protein, fat). It led the way to diets low in sugar and processed carbohydrate, like the South Beach diet.

Then in the 2000s, with the help of the Internet, all sorts of diets emerged: Mediterranean, paleo, gluten free, Whole30, vegan, intermittent fasting, and alkaline. And once again, we saw a very-low-carb diet, but this time it was called keto (something bodybuilders learned about from Dan Duchaine's Body Opus plan back in 1996).

In every diet trend there's always a specific enemy. In many diets, it's not a type of nutrient (e.g., fat, carbohydrate) that's the enemy, but a specific type of food. Many of these diets take foods that a small portion of the population are allergic to, like gluten or dairy, and advise everyone to avoid them as well, which is like saying that because some people are allergic to dogs, no one should get a dog. Other diets demand that you eliminate a whole host of common foods they claim are the cause of sickness and disease. To confuse matters, these diets often make mutually incompatible claims as to which foods cause disease and which prevents disease. The same foods on the no-no list in one diet might be the magic bullet cure-all in another diet. If this alone isn't enough to highlight why these diets are based more on great marketing than on good science, keep in mind that every few years there seems to be a new perfect diet that claims to be better than the last.

The International Society of Sports Nutrition (ISSN) has provided a list of conclusions and recommendations in their position paper on diets and body composition. Here are a few of major takeaways (5):

• There are many diet types and eating styles. The various diet archetypes are wide ranging in total energy and macronutrient distribution. Each type carries varying degrees of supporting data and unfounded claims.

• A wide range of dietary approaches (from low fat to low carb and ketogenic and all points in between) can be similarly effective for improving body composition, and this allows flexibility with program design. To date, no controlled, inpatient isocaloric (calories matched) diet comparison, where protein is matched between groups, has reported a clinically meaningful fat-loss or thermic (metabolic) advantage to the lower-carbohydrate or ketogenic diet.

• Common threads run through the diets in terms of the mechanism of action for weight loss and weight gain, but there are also potentially unique means by which certain diets achieve their intended objectives—factors that facilitate greater satiety, ease of compliance, and support of training demands.

• Diets focused primarily on fat loss—and weight loss beyond initial reductions in body water—operate under the fundamental mechanism of a sustained caloric deficit. This net hypocaloric (reduced calorie) balance can either be imposed daily or over the course of the week.

• The collective body of research about intermittent caloric restriction (intermittent fasting) demonstrates no significant advantage over daily caloric restriction for improving body composition.

• Increasing dietary protein to levels significantly beyond current recommendations for athletic populations may improve body composition. The ISSN's original 2007 position on protein intake (1.4-2.0 grams per kilogram of body weight) has gained further support from subsequent investigations arriving at similar requirements in athletic populations. Higher protein intakes (of 2.3-3.1 gram per kilogram of body weight) may be required to maximize muscle retention in lean, resistance-trained subjects in hypocaloric conditions. Emerging research on very high protein intakes (greater than 3 grams per kilogram of body weight) has demonstrated that the known thermic, satiating, and lean-mass-preserving effects of dietary protein might be amplified in resistance training subjects. (Divide your body weight in pounds by 2.2 to figure out your weight in kilograms.)

• Most existing research showing adaptive thermogenesis (a slowing of metabolism) has involved diets that combine aggressive caloric restriction with low protein intakes and an absence of resistance training, essentially creating a perfect storm for slowing metabolism. Research that has mindfully included resistance training and adequate protein has circumvented the problem of adaptive thermogenesis and muscle loss, despite very low-calorie intakes.

• The long-term success of a diet depends on how well it is followed.

As you can see, the relationship between how many calories you consume per day and the number you expend per day is the single most important factor when it comes to determining whether you lose fat.

Does Muscle Growth Require More Calories?

Everyone talks about needing a calorie deficit for fat loss, but is a calorie surplus needed to build muscle? Not necessarily. This is because stored fat is stored energy. And that energy is available for the body to use as fuel for the muscle-building process.

That said, several studies show that you can simultaneously build muscle and lose fat. Research has demonstrated this in a variety of populations:

• Overweight, sedentary adult males (6)
• Older men and women (7)
• Physically active healthy men (8)
• Young women (9)

But hold on. Get this part straight: Your body can't turn fat into muscle or vice versa. Fat is fat; muscle is muscle. If you're overweight, your body can use your stored energy (fat) to fuel the muscle-building process when the calories needed to build muscle aren't coming from additional food intake.

Fat Loss and Calories: Quantity Versus Quality

Any time someone says that the relationship between how many calories you consume per day and the number you burn per day is the single most important factor when it comes to determining whether you lose fat, someone else tries to refute it by bringing up the fact that the quality of the calories you eat matters. They present it as an either-or proposition.

Research into the potential advantages of diets emphasizing protein, fat, or carbohydrate has found that reduced-calorie diets result in clinically meaningful fat loss regardless of which macronutrients they emphasize. While the research doesn't discount that some calories are more nutrient dense than others, it demonstrates that you can be well nourished and also overfed. Food quality and food quantity are important factors that should be considered together. As important as it is to eat high-quality, nutrient-dense foods for general health, you can still gain fat from eating healthfully if you eat too many calories relative to what you're expending.

The Lesson

Above all, the most important factor in losing fat and improving health is adherence. So what *is* the best diet? It's the one you'll stick with over the long term because multiple dietary approaches will result in fat loss if you're in a calorie deficit and protein intake is sufficient. Whether you're in a calorie deficit or not, make sure it contains enough protein. That's the main piece of diet advice to follow if you're trying to build muscle. The rule of thumb is at least one gram of protein per pound (.45 kg) of body weight.

The fact is, when you strip away the big claims, in all the popular diets, people eat more lower-calorie, nutrient-dense foods while consuming fewer higher-calorie, nutrient-poor foods. The reason people swear by just about every type of diet isn't because of a special eating formula, but because the diet got them to eat more nutritious foods on a regular basis than they were before. And, by focusing on the quality of the foods they eat, they're more likely to end up taking in fewer calories without actually counting them.

You can commit to a diet and remain skeptical of its seemingly miraculous claims. You can test things out and avoid being taken in by marketing hype. And if you do enough research, you'll probably start to see that the reason why most diets work is because they get people to eat meals that are made up of mostly high-quality meats, eggs, fish (or protein substitutes, for vegetarians and vegans), fruits, and vegetables. And these diets control calories by limiting the intake of refined foods, simple sugars, hydrogenated oil, and alcohol.

You most likely already knew these things, but the goal of marketing is to make you think you need something more—like a special diet formula or magic bullet supplement. This explains why just about every person or athlete I've ever trained who has a great physique has told me about the countless times they are asked "what do you eat?" and "what supplements do you take?" as if they know secrets about nutrition that aren't readily available, secrets that explain the reason they look so good.

I've jokingly recommended they give these people what they want by telling them something crazy like, "I eat reticulated python meat for muscle and put powdered bumblebee urine on my thighs and belly before I work out to accelerate fat loss in those areas." Of course, this is pure nonsense, but it does demonstrate how we often think we need to use exotic nutrition practices and make the process of improving our health and fitness way more complicated and unrealistic than it needs to be. Sometimes everyone just needs to be reminded to keep it simple.

REFERENCES

Chapter 1

1. Ebersole KT, Housh TJ, Johnson GO, Perry SR, Bull AJ, Cramer JT. Mechanomyographic and electromyographic responses to unilateral isometric training. *J Strength Cond Res*. 2002 May;16(2):192-201.

2. Folland JP, Hawker K, Leach B, Little T, Jones DA. Strength training: isometric training at a range of joint angles versus dynamic training. *J Sports Sci*. 2005 Aug;23(8):817-24.

3. Kitai TA, Sale DG. Specificity of joint angle in isometric training. *Eur J Appl Physiol Occup Physiol*. 1989;58(7):744-8.

4. Brughelli M, Cronin J. Altering the length-tension relationship with eccentric exercise: implications for performance and injury. *Sports Med*. 2007;37(9):807-26.

5. Butterfield TA. Eccentric exercise in vivo: strain-induced muscle damage and adaptation in a stable system. *Exerc Sport Sci Rev*. 2010 Apr;38(2):51-60.

Chapter 3

1. Saeterbakken AH, Mo DA, Scott S, Andersen V. The effects of bench press variations in competitive athletes on muscle activity and performance. *J Hum Kinet*. 2017 Jun 22;57:61-71. doi:10.1515/hukin-2017-0047.

2. Trebs AA, Brandenburg JP, Pitney WA. An electromyography analysis of 3 muscles surrounding the shoulder joint during the performance of a chest press exercise at several positions. *J Strength Cond Res*. 2010 Jul;24(7):1925-30.

3. Barnett C, Kippers V, Turner P. Effects of variations of the bench press exercise on the EMG activity of five shoulder muscles. *J Strength Cond Res*. 1995 Nov;9(4):222-7. doi:10.1519/00124278-199511000-00003.

Chapter 4

1. Paton ME, Brown JM. Functional differentiation within latissimus dorsi. *Electromyogr Clin Neurophysiol*. 1995 Aug-Sep;35(5):301-9.

2. Park SY, Yoo WG. Differential activation of parts of the latissimus dorsi with various isometric shoulder exercises. *J Electromyogr Kinesiol*. 2014 Apr;24(2):253-7.

3. Signorile JF, Zink AJ, Szwed SP. A comparative electromyographical investigation of muscle utilization patterns using various hand positions during the lat pull-down. *J Strength Cond Res*. 2002 Nov;16(4):539-46.

4. Andersen V, Fimland MS, Wiik E, Skoglund A, Saeterbakken AH. Effects of grip width on muscle strength and activation in the lat pull-down. *J Strength Cond Res*. 2014 Apr;28(4):1135-42.

Chapter 5

1. Barnett C, Kippers V, Turner P. Effects of variations of the bench press exercise on the EMG activity of five shoulder muscles. *J Strength Cond Res*, 1995 Nov;9(4):222-7.

2. Sweeney, SP. Electromyographic analysis of the deltoid muscle during various shoulder exercises. University of Wisconsin-La Crosse Master's Thesis: 2014-05. Published online: https://minds.wisconsin.edu/bitstream/handle/1793/70129/SweeneySamanthaThesis.pdf?sequence=1&isAllowed=y

3. Johnston TB. (1937). The movements of the shoulder-joint a plea for the use of the 'plane of the scapula' as the plane of reference for movements occurring at the humero-scapular joint. *BJS*, 1937 Oct;25(98), 252-60.

4. Greenfield B. Special considerations in shoulder exercises: plane of the scapula. In Andrews, JR, Wilk KE, editors. The athlete's shoulder. New York: Churchill Livingstone, New York; 1994. pp. 513-22.

Chapter 6

1. Bressel ME, Bressel E, Heise GD. Lower trapezius activity during supported and unsupported scapular retraction exercise. *Phys Ther Sport.* 2001 Nov; 2(4):178-85.

2. De Mey K, Danneels L, Cagnie B, Van den Bosch L, Flier J, Cools AM. Kinetic chain influences on upper and lower trapezius muscle activation during eight variations of a scapular retraction exercise in overhead athletes. *J Sci Med Sport.* 2013 Jan;16(1):65-70.

3. Pizzari T, Wickham J, Balster S, Ganderton C and Watson L. Modifying a shrug exercise can facilitate the upward rotator muscles of the scapula. Clin Biomech 29 : 201-205, 2014.

4. Handa T, Kato H, Hasegawa S, Okada J, Kato, K. Comparative electromyographical investigation of the biceps brachii, latissimus dorsi, and trapezius muscles during five pull exercises. *Japanese J Phys Fit Sports Med.* 2005;54(2):159-68.

5. Schoenfeld B, Kolber MJ, Haimes JE. The upright row: implications for preventing subacromial impingement. *Strength Cond J.* 2011 Oct;33(5):25-8.

6. McAllister MJ, Schilling BK, Hammond KG, Weiss LW, Farney T. Effect of grip width on electromyographic activity during the upright row. *J Strength Cond Res.* 2013 Jan;27(1):181-7.

Chapter 7

1. Jarrett C, Weir D, Stuffmann E, Jain S, Miller MC, Schmidt C. (2011). Anatomic and biomechanical analysis of the short and long head components of the distal biceps tendon. *Journal of shoulder and elbow surgery* / American Shoulder and Elbow Surgeons ... [et al.]. 21. 942-8. 10.1016/j.jse.2011.04.030.

Chapter 9

1. Arnason A, Andersen TE, Holme I, Engebretsen L, Bahr R. Prevention of hamstring strains in elite soccer: an intervention study. *Scand J Med Sci Sports.* 2008 Feb;18(1):40-8.

2. Petersen J, Thorborg K, Nielsen MB, Budtz-Jørgensen E, Hölmich P. Preventive effect of eccentric training on acute hamstring injuries in men's soccer: a cluster-randomized controlled trial. *Am J Sports Med.* 2011 Nov;39(11):2296-303.

3. van der Horst N, Smits DW, Petersen J, Goedhart EA, Backx FJ. The preventive effect of the Nordic hamstring exercise on hamstring injuries in amateur soccer players: a randomized controlled trial. *Am J Sports Med.* 2015 Jun;43(6):1316-23.

4. Askling C, Karlsson J, Thorstensson A. Hamstring injury occurrence in elite soccer players after preseason strength training with eccentric overload. *Scand J Med Sci Sports.* 2003 Aug;13(4):244-50.

5. Schoenfeld BJ, Contreras B, Tiryaki-Sonmez G, Wilson JM, Kolber MJ, Peterson MD. Regional differences in muscle activation during hamstrings exercise. *J Strength Cond Res.* 2015 Jan;29(1):159-64.

Chapter 10

1. Ebben WP, Feldmann CR, Dayne A, Mitsche D, Alexander P, Knetzger KJ. Muscle activation during lower body resistance training. *Int J of Sports Med.* 2009 Jan;30(1):1-8.

2. Ema R, Wakahara T, Miyamoto N, Kanehisa H, Kawakami Y. Inhomogeneous architectural changes of the quadriceps femoris induced by resistance training. *Eur J Appl Physiol.* 2013 Nov;113(11):26912-703.

3. Beardsley C. Can you "just squat" for maximal leg development? Retrieved 2018 from www.strengthandconditioningresearch.com.

4. Treubig D. Why you should be using knee extensions after ACL reconstruction. Modern Manual Therapy Blog. 2016 Aug. Available from: www.themanualtherapist.com/2016/08/why-you-should-be-using-knee-extensions.html.

5. Askling C, Karlsson J, Thorstensson, A. Hamstring injury occurrence in elite soccer players after preseason strength training with eccentric overload. *Scand J Med Sci Sports.* 2003 Aug;13(4):244-50.

6. Tumminello N, Vigotsky A. Are the seated leg extension, leg curl, and adduction machine exercises non-functional or risky? *NSCA Personal Training Quarterly.* 2017 June;4(4):50-3.

7. Zalawadia DA, Ruparelia DS, Shah DS, Parekh DD, Patel DS, Rathod DSP, Patel DSV. Study of femoral neck anteversion of adult dry femora in Gujarat region: study of femoral neck anteversion. *Natl J Integr Res Med.* 2010 July-Sept;1(3):7-11.

8. Kingsley PC, Olsmtead KL. A study to determine the angle of anteversion of the neck of femur. *J Bone Joint Surg Am*. 1948 Jul;30A(3):745-51.

9. D'Lima DD, Urquhart AG, Buehler KO, Walker RH, Colwell CW Jr. The effect of the orientation of the acetabular and femoral components on the range of motion of the hip at different head-neck ratios. *J Bone Joint Surg Am*. 2000 Mar;82(3):315-21.

10. Yi C, Ma C, Wang Q, Zhang G, Cao Y. Acetabular configuration and its impact on cup coverage of a subtype of Crowe type 4 DDH with bi-pseudoacetabulum. *Hip Int*. 2013 Mar-Apr;23(2):135-42. doi: 10.5301/hipint.5000015. Epub 2013 Apr 4.

11. Calatayud J, Martin F, Gargallo P, García-Redondo J, Colado JC, Marín PJ. The validity and reliability of a new instrumented device for measuring ankle dorsiflexion range of motion. *Int J Sports Phys Ther*. 2015 Apr;10(2):197-202.

12. Malliaras P, Cook JL, Kent P. Reduced ankle dorsiflexion range may increase the risk of patellar tendon injury among volleyball players. *J Sci Med Sport*. 2006 Aug;9(4):304-9.

13. Dill KE, Begalle RL, Frank BS, Zinder SM, Padua DA. Altered knee and ankle kinematics during squatting in those with limited weight-bearing-lunge ankle-dorsiflexion range of motion. *J Athl Train*, 2014 Nov-Dec;49(6):723–32.

Chapter 11

1. Farrokhi S, Pollard CD, Souza RB, Chen YJ, Reischl S, Powers CM. Trunk position influences the kinematics, kinetics, and muscle activity of the lead lower extremity during the forward lunge exercise. *J Orthop Sports Phys Ther*. 2008 Jul;38(7):403-9.

2. Schütz P, List R, Zemp R, Schellenberg F, Taylor WR, Lorenzetti S. Joint angles of the ankle, knee, and hip and loading conditions during split squats. *J Appl Biomech*. 2014 Jun;30(3):373-80.

3. Tyler TF, Nicholas SJ, Campbell RJ, McHugh MP. The association of hip strength and flexibility with the incidence of adductor muscle strains in professional ice hockey players. *Am J Sports Med*. 2001 Mar-Apr;29(2):124-8.

4. Whittaker JL, Small C, Maffey L, Emery, CA. Risk factors for groin injury in sport: an updated systematic review. *Br J Sports Med*. 2015 Jun;49(12):803-9.

5. Clark DR, Lambert MI, Hunter AM. Muscle activation in the loaded free barbell squat: a brief review. *J Strength Cond Res* 2012 Apr;26(4):1169-78.

6. Dwyer MK, Boudreau SN, Mattacola CG, Uhl TL, Lattermann C. Comparison of lower extremity kinematics and hip muscle activation during rehabilitation tasks between sexes. *J Athl Train*, 2010 Mar-Apr;45(2):181-90.

7. Graves JE, Pollock ML, Jones AE, Colvin AB, Leggett SH. Specificity of limited range of motion variable resistance training. *Med Sci Sports Exerc*. 1989 Feb;21(1):84-9.

8. McMahon GE, Morse CI, Burden A, Winwood K, Onambele GL. Impact of range of motion during ecologically valid resistance training protocols on muscle size, subcutaneous fat, and strength. *J Strength Cond Res*. 2014 Jan;28(1):245-55.

9. Tumminello N, Vigotsky A. Are the seated leg extension, leg curl, and adduction machine exercises non-functional or risky? *NSCA Personal Training Quarterly*. 2017 Jun;4(4):50-3.

10. Farrokhi S, Pollard CD, Souza RB, Chen YJ, Reischl S, Powers CM. Trunk position influences the kinematics, kinetics, and muscle activity of the lead lower extremity during the forward lunge exercise. *J Orthop Sports Phys Ther*. 2008 Jul;38(7):403-9.

11. Schütz P, List R, Zemp R, Schellenberg F, Taylor WR, Lorenzetti S. Joint angles of the ankle, knee, and hip and loading conditions during split squats. *J Appl Biomech*. 2014 Jun;30(3):373-80.

12. WB, Hreljac A, Fleisig GS, Wilk KE, Moorman CT 3rd, Imamura R, Andrews JR. Patellofemoral joint force and stress between a short- and long-step forward lunge. *J Orthop Sports Phys Ther*. 2008 Nov;38(11):681-90. doi: 10.2519/jospt.2008.2694.

13. Stastny P, Lehnert M, Zaatar AM, Svoboda Z, Xaverova Z. Does the dumbbell-carrying position change the muscle activity in split squats and walking lunges? *J Strength Cond Res*. 2015 Nov;29(11):3177-87.

Chapter 12

1. Möck S, Hartmann R, Wirth K, Rosenkranz G, Mickel C. Correlation of dynamic strength in the standing calf raise with sprinting performance in consecutive sections up to 30 meters. *Res Sports Med*. 2018 Oct-Dec;26(4):474-81.

2. Hébert-Losier K, Schneiders AG, García JA, Sullivan SJ, Simoneau GG. Influence of knee flexion angle and age on triceps surae muscle activity during heel raises. *J Strength Cond Res.* 2012 Nov;26(11):3124-33.

3. Tamaki H, Kitada K, Akamine T, Sakou T, Kurata H. (1996). Electromyogram patterns during plantarflexions at various angular velocities and knee angles in human triceps surae muscles. *Eur J Appl Physiol Occup Physiol.* 1996;75(1):1-6.

4. Price TB, Kamen G, Damon BM, Knight CA, Applegate B, Gore JC, Signorile JF. Comparison of MRI with EMG to study muscle activity associated with dynamic plantar flexion. *Magn Reson Imaging.* 2003 Oct;21(8):853-61.

5. Signorile JE, Applegate B, Ducque M, Cole N, Zink, A. Selective recruitment of the triceps surae muscles with changes in knee angle. *J Strength Cond Res.* 2002 Aug;16(3):433-39.

Chapter 13

1. McGill S, Schoenfeld B. Choosing exercises – "the crunch." *Personal Training Quarterly.* 2017 Apr;4(2):20-2.

2. Shinkle J, Nesser TW, Demchak TJ, McMannus DM. Effect of core strength on the measure of power in the extremities. *J Strength Cond Res.* 2012 Feb;26(2):373-80.

3. Schoenfeld BJ, Morey J. Abdominal crunches are/are not a safe and effective exercise. *Strength Cond J.* 2016 Dec;38(6):61-4.

4. Brughelli M, Cronin J. Altering the length-tension relationship with eccentric exercise. *Sports Med.* 2007;37(9):807-26.

5. Butterfield TA. Eccentric exercise in vivo: strain-induced muscle damage and adaptation in a stable system. *Exerc Sport Sci Rev.* 2010 Apr;38(2):51-60.

Chapter 14

1. Cheung K, Hume P, Maxwell L. Delayed onset muscle soreness: treatment strategies and performance factors. *Sports Med.* 2003 Oct;33(2):145-64.

Chapters 15, 16, and 17

1. Rhea MR, Ball SD, Phillips WT, Burkett LN. A comparison of linear and daily undulating periodized programs with equated volume and intensity for strength. *J Strength Cond Res.* 2002 May;16(2):250-5.

2. Prestes J, Frollini AB, de Lima C, Donatto FF, Foschini D, de Cássia Marqueti R, Figueira A Jr, Fleck SJ. Comparison between linear and daily undulating periodized resistance training to increase strength. *J Strength Cond Res.* 2009 Dec;23(9):2437-42.

3. Miranda F, Simão R, Rhea M, Bunker D, Prestes J, Leite RD, Miranda H, de Salles BF, Novaes J. Effects of linear vs. daily undulatory periodized resistance training on maximal and sub-maximal strength gains. *J Strength Cond Res.* 2011 Jul;25(7):1824-30.

4. Simão R, Spineti J, de Salles BF, Matta T, Fernandes L, Fleck SJ, Rhea MR, Strom-Olsen HE. Comparison between nonlinear and linear periodized resistance training: hypertrophic and strength effects. *J Strength Cond Res.* 2012 May;26(5):1389-95.

Chapter 18

1. Mitchell CJ, Churchward-Venne TA, West DW, Burd NA, Breen L, Baker SK, Phillips SM. Resistance exercise load does not determine training-mediated hypertrophic gains in young men. *J Appl Physiol (1985).* 2012 Jul;113(1):71-7.

2. Pereira PEA, Motoyama YL, Esteves GJ, Quinelato WC, Botte L, Tanaka KH, Azevedo P. Resistance training with slow speed of movement is better for hypertrophy and muscle strength gains than fast speed of movement. *Int. J. Appl. Exerc. Physiol.* 2016 Jul;5(2):37-43, 2016.

3. de Salles BF, Simão R, Miranda F, Novaes Jda S, Lemos A, Willardson JM. Rest interval between sets in strength training. *Sports Med.* 2009;39(9):765-77.

4. Robbins DW, Young WB, Behm DG. The effect of an upper-body agonist-antagonist resistance training protocol on volume load and efficiency. *J Strength Cond Res.* 2010 Oct;24(10):2632-40.

5. Aragon AA, Schoenfeld BJ, Wildman R, Kleiner S, VanDusseldorp T, Taylor L, Earnest CP, Arciero PJ, Wilborn C, Kalman DS, Stout JR, Willoughby DS, Campbell B, Arent SM, Ban-

nock L, Smith-Ryan AE, Antonio J. International society of sports nutrition position stand: diets and body composition. *J Int Soc Sports Nutr*. 2017 Jun 14;14:16.

6. Wallace MB, Mills BD, Browning CL. Effects of cross-training on markers of insulin resistance/hyperinsulinemia. *Med Sci Sports Exerc*. 1997 Sep;29(9):1170-5.

7. Iglay HB, Thyfault JP, Apolzan JW, Campbell WW. Resistance training and dietary protein: effects on glucose tolerance and contents of skeletal muscle insulin signaling proteins in older persons. *Am J Clin Nutr*. 2007 Apr;85(4):1005-13.

8. Dolezal BA, Potteiger JA. Concurrent resistance and endurance training influence basal metabolic rate in nondieting individuals. J Appl Physiol (1985). 1998 Aug;85(2):695-700.

9. Josse AR, Tang JE, Tarnopolsky MA, Phillips SM. Body composition and strength changes in women with milk and resistance exercise. *Med Sci Sports Exerc*. 2010 Jun;42(6):1122-30.

ABOUT THE AUTHOR

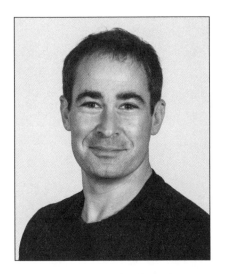

Nick Tumminello is an internationally recognized fitness professional with over 20 years of industry experience. He is the inventor of the NT Loop (NTLoop.com), which is a world-class resistance band.

With over 20 years of hands-on experience, Nick has trained thousands of clients, including professional NFL players, figure and bodybuilding athletes, and plenty of ordinary people. Still coaching clients today, Nick understands the challenges that everyday athletes and active adults face.

Tumminello has been a fitness professional since 1998 and co-owned a private training center in Baltimore, Maryland, from 2001 to 2011. He has worked with a variety of exercise enthusiasts of all ages and fitness levels, including physique and performance athletes from the amateur level to the professional ranks. From 2002 to 2011, Tumminello was the strength and conditioning coach for the Ground Control MMA team. He has been a consultant and expert for clothing and equipment companies such as Sorinex, Dynamax, Hylete, Reebok, and Power Systems.

Nick has authored three best-selling books: *Strength Training for Fat Loss*, *Building Muscle and Performance*, and *Your Workout PERFECTED*. He has been featured in two exercise books on the *New York Times* best seller list, on the home page of Yahoo! and YouTube, and in the *ACE Personal Trainer Manual*. In 2015 Tumminello was inducted into the Personal Trainer Hall of Fame. Nick was the 2016 NSCA Personal Trainer of the Year, and he is the editor in chief of the National Strength and Conditioning Association's *Personal Training Quarterly* journal.

From massive industry conferences to private team development events, Nick has racked up hundreds of speaking engagements all over the world. He is passionate about bringing the best fitness and performance information to trainers, athletes, and active adults in the most practical way possible.

When the best coaches and organizations in the fitness industry want proven, research-backed information, Nick is their trusted resource.

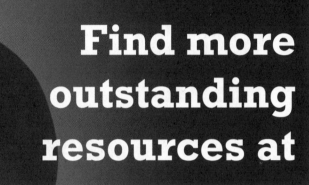
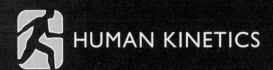

You read the book—now complete the companion CE exam to earn continuing education credit!

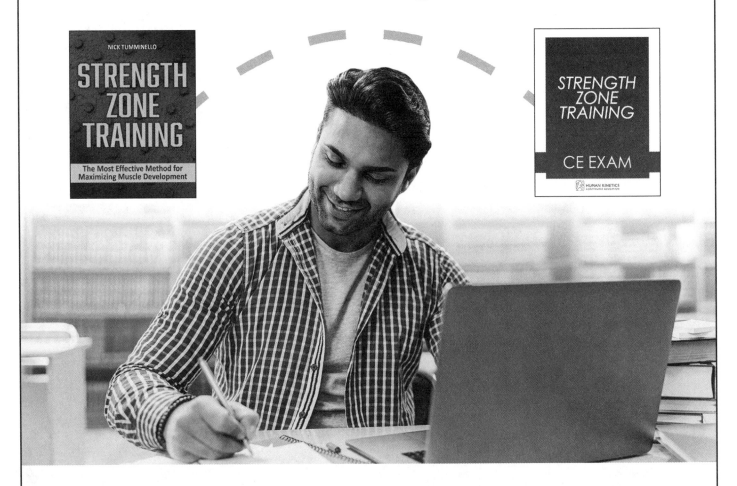

Find and purchase the companion CE exam here:
US.HumanKinetics.com/collections/CE-Exam
Canada.HumanKinetics.com/collections/CE-Exam

50% off the companion CE exam with this code

SZT2023

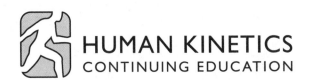

HUMAN KINETICS
CONTINUING EDUCATION

...idual looking to start an exercise program or improve ... ...arpen your tools of program design, Strength Zone Tr... ...—especially full range of motion training—make it a g...

Dan Dalrymple, CSCS, RSCC*E, MSCC
Two-Time NFL Strength and Conditioning Coach of the ...

"Effort gets results. Smart effort gets maximum results. Coach Nick's strategies in Strength Zone Training *eliminate wasted effort and amplify results. That means faster progress, better performance, and the ability to keep it all going."*

Chris Shugart
Chief Content Officer at T-Nation.com

"Nick Tumminello is one of the best at using the science of exercise to develop practical training approaches. He has an astute ability to take complex topics and make them understandable for the masses."

Brad Schoenfeld, PhD
Author of *Science and Development of Muscle Hypertrophy*

STRENGTH ZONE TRAINING

Don't waste your time doing workouts that leave large gaps in your strength or load you up with unnecessary, redundant exercises. Take a strategic approach to your workouts by using a proven system that focuses on training through each joint's true full range of motion.

In *Strength Zone Training*, world-renowned personal trainer Nick Tumminello, who has become known as the trainer of trainers, shows you the following:

- **How to build strength through the true full range of motion**
- **The redundant exercises you just don't need to do**
- **The exercises to maximize upper body and lower body strength that are missing from your workout**
- **The angles most people don't do exercises for but should**
- **The best exercises to include in your program to train each muscle group**
- **A better strategy to follow when choosing your exercises**
- **Beginner and advanced workout plans for any schedule**

You'll find exercises addressing every area of the body, with details on how to perform the exercise as well as coaching tips. Select exercises are depicted with a hybrid of photo and art highlighting the various movement zones. In addition to the exercises, you'll find four chapters of fully comprehensive workout plans so you can choose one that is right for you, regardless of your training level or weekly schedule.

Strength Zone Training is the blueprint for building muscle with a purpose. Choose your exercises and get ready to dominate!

CE EXAM AVAILABLE

Human Kinetics

ISBN 978-1-7182-1147-6

52795

9 781718 211476

US $27.95